Group Therapy for Complex Trauma

I0093610

Group Therapy for Complex Trauma provides a roadmap for profession-als trying to address the many issues that arise in group treatment. It's an excellent training resource for mental health professionals working in insti-tutions that provide higher levels of acute care, including inpatient, partial hospitalization, and/or intensive outpatient programs, as well as those run-ning groups in traditional outpatient settings.

Chapters pull the most recent theory and practice into one concise resource, addressing not only how to treat complex trauma but also why doing so matters. They also provide guidance for troubleshooting situations that often arise when conducting groups with a population that is often highly dysregulated.

The second section includes exercises, and handouts that can be repro-duced and shared with participants, enabling them to follow along during the group session and to complete exercises and review material in their own time.

Judith A. Margolin, PsyD, is a certified advanced schema therapist, vis-iting faculty at Rutgers University, and supervising psychologist at Penn Medicine Princeton Health. She specializes in the treatment of trauma and dissociation.

Group Therapy for Complex Trauma

A Schema-Informed Approach

Judith A. Margolin

Routledge
Taylor & Francis Group

NEW YORK AND LONDON

Designed cover image: Getty Images

First published 2026
by Routledge
605 Third Avenue, New York, NY 10158

and by Routledge
4 Park Square, Milton Park, Abingdon, Oxon, OX14 4RN

Routledge is an imprint of the Taylor & Francis Group, an informa business

ISBN: 9781032568065 (hbk)
ISBN: 9781032568058 (pbk)
ISBN: 9781003462958 (ebk)

DOI: 10.4324/9781003462958

Typeset in Optima
by codeMantra

This book is dedicated to my husband, Moshe, whose infinite patience and wisdom supported the completion of this project.

And to all those on their healing journey from complex trauma. May you find strength, hope, and resilience within these pages.

Contents

Foreword   *xi*
Acknowledgments   *xiii*
About the Author   *xv*
List of Handouts   *xvi*
List of Exercises   *xvii*
List of Figures   *xviii*

PART 1
Foundations: Theoretical Underpinnings and
Treatment Considerations   1

Chapter 1   Introduction   3

Chapter 2   Early Childhood Trauma and Complex
             Post-Traumatic Stress Disorder   8

Chapter 3   Schema Therapy and Early Childhood Trauma   27

Chapter 4   Building Safety in the Group   43

Chapter 5   Therapeutic Challenges and the Role of Leadership   52

Chapter 6   Trauma, Mindfulness, and the Healthy Adult   72

Chapter 7   Trauma, Substance Use Disorders, Eating
             Disorders, and Behavioral Addictions   82

Chapter 8   Theoretical Underpinnings and Treatment
             Considerations: A Summary   91

PART 2
Session Protocols 101

Chapter 9   Group Structure and Framework   103

Session 1   Beginning the Group   109

Session 2   Schema Therapy   125

Session 3   Post-Traumatic Stress Disorder and
               Complex Post-Traumatic Stress Disorder   141

Session 4   The Window of Tolerance   152

Session 5   Emotion Regulation   165

Session 6   The Neurobiology of Trauma   178

Session 7   Trauma and the Body   190

Session 8   Traumatic Memory   202

Session 9   Intrusive Symptoms of PTSD: Flashbacks,
               Nightmares, and Intrusive Memories   212

Session 10   Trauma and Dissociation   224

Session 11   Trauma and Attachment   244

Session 12   The Trauma Triangle   255

Session 13   Shame and the Inner Critic   268

Session 14   Self-Compassion   282

Session 15   Developing Healthy Relationships   291

Sessions 16–17   Making Sense of It All:
               Recovery, Reconnection, and Integration   300

PART 3
A Roadmap for Recovery from Complex Trauma 311

Chapter 10   Recovering from Complex Trauma   313

Index   319

Foreword

Dr. Judith Margolin once again offers an invaluable resource with *Group Therapy for Complex Trauma: A Schema-Informed Approach*. Building on the foundations of her groundbreaking work, *Breaking the Silence* (1999), this book incorporates the latest advancements in understanding complex trauma, attachment, and neurobiology. Dr. Margolin seamlessly integrates contemporary research and diverse psychological approaches into a structured trauma-informed and schema-based group therapy format.

What truly distinguishes this book on groups for complex trauma is its schema-informed perspective. This approach goes beyond symptom relief and management to address unconscious, implicit, and deeply held distorted belief systems—maladaptive schemas—that arise from traumatic experiences and unmet childhood needs. By identifying and challenging these distorted schemas (e.g., I am unlovable and I am damaged), survivors gain a deeper appreciation of trauma's impact. Interventions are designed to encourage participants to cultivate a more accurate and affirming self-view, emphasizing not what is wrong with you but how you learned to cope. Central to this process is fostering a strong "adult healthy self." With the development and reinforcement of self-compassion, empathy, and acceptance, the "adult healthy self" is empowered to support and help other internal parts, like the vulnerable child or punitive inner critic (labeled as modes in schema therapy).

A detailed 20-session program with clearly defined goals, themes, and experiential exercises is outlined. Although not designed this way, each session could stand on its own, making this book a critical resource for group therapists and a valuable tool for individual clinicians. Concepts such as the window of tolerance, dissociation, and emotion regulation strategies can be easily adapted for one-on-one work, broadening the book's relevance across therapeutic modalities.

The group content relies on psychoeducation, skill-building (e.g., mindfulness and grounding techniques), experiential exercises, and group dynamics to address the lasting impact trauma leaves behind. Margolin characterizes this legacy as a "failure of integration" which results from "dysregulation, disruption, distortion, disorientation, disconnection, and defensiveness" (six D's). Alongside practical session plans, Margolin thoughtfully highlights factors critical to group success such as transference, leadership skills, and managing group conflict.

With a strong focus on safety, connection, and creating a supportive group space, survivors can explore their experiences and overcome feelings of shame, isolation, and loneliness. Packed with practical tools, session outlines, thoughtful guidance, and rich insights, *Group Therapy for Complex Trauma* is an essential guide for clinicians committed to fostering meaningful growth and healing for trauma survivors.

Marsha Heiman, PhD
Private Practice, Metuchen, NJ Author of *Learning to Live in Harmony*: *A Primer for Trauma Survivors and Those Who Dissociate*

Acknowledgments

First and foremost, I extend my deepest gratitude to my clients, survivors of complex trauma, who bravely shared their stories and experiences. I have learned so much from you all. Your resilience and courage have been the driving force behind this work.

I am indebted to the mental health professionals and trauma specialists who lent their expertise and added depth and nuance to this work, in particular, my colleagues at Princeton House Behavioral Health, Princeton, NJ, Kate Diviao, Katie Scozzari, Lisa Canzano, Jocelyn Elderton, Sarah Carstens, and Kat Masterson for the collaborative spirit and thought-provoking discussions that jump-started and enriched this work immeasurably. I am especially grateful to Ishwari Store, my dear friend and colleague, who enriched this work with insightful reading framed by her understanding of the needs of this population. Her keen eye and astute feedback helped refine and elevate this manuscript.

To my mentors and advisors, Wendy Behary, David Edwards, and Joan Farrell, your guidance, expertise, constructive criticism, and support throughout this journey have been invaluable. Your insights have shaped and enriched this book and my understanding of Schema Therapy's approach to trauma and healing. I am also grateful for the support and encouragement offered by my friends and colleagues, Laura Skivone, Karen Cohen, and Nancy Talbot, as well as my community of Schema Therapists, especially Robin Spiro, John Gaswieski, Theresa Reitz, Elizabeth Lacy, Marsha Blank, Megan Fry, and Catherine Wood.

My heartfelt appreciation goes to my dear friends Harold Heft and Fran Mascia Lees for reading and editing early drafts, providing emotional support, and being a sounding board throughout this process.

To my beloved family, particularly my spouse, Moshe Margolin, thank you for your patience and understanding during the long hours and emotional challenges of writing about such a sensitive topic. This book could never have been written without your unwavering support and editorial comments. Thank you to my children and grandchildren, Ayelet, Gidon,

Noa, Mickey, Andrea, Shaun, Ethan, Jake, Romi, and Arya, for always being there even when this endeavor pulled me out of your orbit.

Lastly, I want to express my gratitude to all the researchers, clinicians, and advocates who have paved the way in the field of complex trauma. Your groundbreaking work has laid the foundation for this exploration.

Judith Margolin
March 1, 2025

About the Author

Judith A. Margolin, PsyD, is a certified advanced schema therapist, supervisor of schema therapy, and visiting faculty in the Graduate School of Applied and Professional Psychology at Rutgers University in New Jersey. She is a clinical supervisor and member of the medical staff at Penn Medicine Princeton Health and was a supervising psychologist and clinical director of the Women's Trauma program at Princeton House Behavioral Health. She has presented nationally and internationally on complex trauma, dissociative identity disorder, and schema therapy. Dr. Margolin is also the author of one of the earliest books on group therapy for sexual abuse, *Breaking the Silence: Group Therapy for Childhood Sexual Abuse—A Practitioner's Manual* (1999).

Handouts

1.1 Sample Group Guidelines 116
1.2 Sample Group Format 120
1.3 Identifying Needs 122
2.1 Walking Through My Modes 138
3.1 Understanding PTSD and Complex Trauma 148
4.1 Managing Your Window of Tolerance and Level of Arousal 157
4.2 Strategies to Help Identify and Monitor the State of Arousal 159
5.1 Understanding Emotions 169
5.2 Developing your Healthy Adult Mode 172
5.3 Emotion Regulation Strategies 174
6.1 Understanding Your Brain's Response to Trauma 187
7.1 How Can I Learn to Live in My Body? 198
8.1 Trauma Memory Questionnaire 207
9.1 Take Charge of Your Triggers 218
9.2 Managing Intrusive Symptoms 220
10.1 Your Dissociative Experience 234
10.2 Structural Dissociation, Action Tendencies and Modes 236
10.3 Recognizing the Presence of the Action Heroes and Modes 238
10.4 Structural Dissociation Model 240
11.1 Attachment Styles 248
11.2 Exploring Relationship Challenges 251
12.1 Breaking the Cycle 262
12.2 Strengthening the Healthy Adult Mode: Supporting Your
Vulnerable Child Mode 263
13.1 Talking about Shame and Guilt 275
14.1 Quieting the Voice of the Inner Critic 285
15.1 Trauma and Relationships 295
16.1 Your Healing Journey: Recovery, Reconnection and
Integration 305

Exercises

2.1   Introducing Imagery: The Ice Cream Shoppe   135

2.2   Modes on the Bus Exercise   136

3.1   Safe Place Imagery   149

3.2   The Safety Bubble Exercise   150

4.1   Breath Awareness   162

4.2   Mountain Meditation   163

5.1   Emotion Labeling and Breath Awareness   171

7.1   Felt Sense Focusing   197

8.1   Exploring a Raisin Mindfully   209

8.2   Stretching   210

9.1   Sensory Awareness   222

11.1   Secure Base Visualization   253

12.1   Role Awareness Meditation   265

12.2   Strengthening the Healthy Adult Mode   266

13.1   Challenging the Inner Critic's Messages   277

13.2   Compassionate Chair Work with the Critic Mode   278

15.1   Establishing Connections   297

15.2   Passing Claps   298

16.1   Future-Oriented Imagery   307

16.2   The Stone Ceremony   308

Figures

4.1 The Window of Tolerance and Zones of Arousal 154
6.1 The Triune Brain, Nervous System Integration, and
Information Processing 181
6.2 Brain Structures and Pathways Involved in Threat Detection 183
6.3 The Polyvagal Ladder: Basic Psychological States and
Schema Modes 184
10.1 The Structural Dissociation Model 229
12.1 The Trauma Triangle 259
12.2 The Roles of the Trauma Triangle 261
13.1 Shame vs. Guilt 271
14.1 The Three Functions of Emotion: Drive, Protection, and
Soothing 285

Part 1

Foundations

Theoretical Underpinnings and Treatment Considerations

Chapter 1

Introduction

Over the past four decades, much has been learned about early childhood trauma and the treatment of its symptoms. Definitions of trauma have expanded to include a range of experiences that overwhelm the individual's capacity to cope. These are as nuanced as the treatment approaches therapists use to help their patients heal from the effects of their early traumatic experiences. Combining individual and group therapy and utilizing a well-stocked toolbox stands out for its effectiveness as a trauma-focused approach that best serves the patient's needs.

The aftermath of early childhood trauma is characterized by a failure of integration of core functions that results from a combination of the six D's—dysregulation, disruption, distortion, disorientation, disconnection, and defensiveness. This impaired integration impacts the individual's sense of who they are, their place in the world, and how they relate to others after what happened. Operating from a place of dysregulation, disruption, disconnection, disorientation, distortion, and defensiveness affects the brain, the body, relationships, and identity. For instance, the ability to manage the onslaught of *disorienting* and *dysregulating* emotions and physical sensations can interfere with and *disrupt* daily functioning. What one knows and believes about oneself becomes *distorted* and contributes to *disconnection* and *distancing* from others. Survival *defenses* are activated to protect the person when the world seems so threatening.

Chronic threat disrupts the brain's "steady state" or homeostasis, as normal functions fail to return to baseline when survival tendencies (fight/flight/freeze/submit/attach) remain activated. The body "keeps score" as physical health is compromised and the ability to self-regulate goes awry. Anger, agitation, anxiety, sleep difficulties or numbing, dissociation, and shutdown interfere with the ability to live in the present. Suicidal or homicidal ideation, self-harm, substance abuse, and eating disorders threaten the person's safety in their attempt to cope and find short-term relief.

DOI: 10.4324/9781003462958-2

Early childhood trauma disturbs attachment in primary relationships when those who were supposed to protect may have been the source of the danger. Basic needs for safety, security, nurturance, guidance, love, and affection often go unmet. Personal narratives about self and others are colored by shame, guilt, defectiveness, and self-blame. They become shaped by the secrecy and isolation that shroud early trauma.

Ongoing danger and threat interfere with coregulation and social engagement opportunities, which are foundational to developing essential self-regulatory capacities. Anxiety, fear of rejection or abandonment, avoidance, disconnection, and isolation come to characterize the individual's modes of relating. Trust is shattered and the roles of victim, perpetrator, and rescuer become embedded in these interactions.

Treatment options vary, and the importance of defining the most appropriate course of therapy that best fits each patient must be addressed. The patient's needs are best served when armed with a well-stocked toolbox that incorporates group treatment, informed by Schema Therapy (ST), as an adjunct to individual therapy for Complex Trauma.

There are many ways to present the amount and variety of information discussed in this book. The author's most significant challenge is determining the most effective way of doing this. My first book, *Breaking the Silence: Group Therapy for Childhood Sexual Abuse: A Practitioner's Manual* (Margolin, 1999), evolved from my work as a Rutgers University graduate student and clinic coordinator. At that time, we repeatedly listened as our clients broke the silence and secrecy surrounding their past. They spoke of the isolation, shame, and loneliness stemming from traumatic experiences. They asked that we develop a group where they could begin to share these experiences with others who had also been abused.

At that time, knowledge about and research into the lasting impact of early childhood trauma was in its infancy. Even less was known or written about group treatment for survivors of abuse. My colleagues and I combed the literature as we compiled a time-limited psychoeducational program that also offered a forum to explore and confront the sequelae of the early trauma. The amount of research into childhood trauma and its manifestations in adults has grown exponentially each year since then. Today, we stand armed with a rich body of knowledge and treatment approaches that further enhance recovery and healing from early childhood trauma.

After leaving my position as the Director of a partial hospitalization/intensive outpatient Women's Trauma Program in 2007, I serendipitously embarked on a new phase in my professional development after attending a workshop on ST. ST is an integrative approach that combines elements of cognitive-behavioral, psychodynamic, and gestalt therapies to address maladaptive schemas, or deeply ingrained patterns of thoughts, feelings, and behaviors. The concepts of unmet needs and the development of maladaptive schema and dysfunctional modes helped shed light on the behaviors displayed by many of the women who passed through the Women's Trauma Program. The dysregulation, disconnection, and disruption in their lives that were reflected in their negative beliefs about themselves and in their rapid shifts into different self-states ranging from spacing out and numbness to intense anxiety or lashing out in anger made sense when seen from this perspective. ST offers a nonpathologizing way to understand and address these phenomena.

Group therapy offers an ideal environment to explore the impact of trauma on the brain, body, relationships, and the self. ST provides a valuable lens to understand how self-defeating patterns of feelings, thoughts, and behaviors can develop out of adversity. Combining both can be a powerful tool to support individuals as they recover from the debilitating impact of early childhood abuse. This book provides a group therapy model that combines all we have learned about trauma in the past 30 years with a conceptualization based on ST principles and the six D's. It addresses what the therapist needs to know to support the group in understanding the impact of early childhood trauma (dysregulation, disruption, distortion, disorientation, disconnection, and defensiveness) and the development of maladaptive schema and ways of coping.

This book provides a roadmap for professionals who wish to use the group format to help individuals struggling to make sense of their early traumatic experiences. It is structured to guide the reader through the fundamental issues of group treatment for complex trauma, offering a comprehensive resource for conducting trauma-focused groups in various settings. The content is designed to engage you in healing and recovery, addressing specific challenges that arise for therapists and their clients.

Part I provides the empirical foundation for Schema-informed group treatment of Complex Trauma. Research supporting this approach is presented. Chapter 2 addresses the impact of early childhood trauma and the diagnosis of Complex Post-Traumatic Stress Disorder (CPTSD). Chapter 3 introduces ST and examines its application in the treatment of early childhood trauma. Chapter 4 discusses the fundamental role of building safety in trauma-informed group therapy. Chapter 5 explores the complex leadership role and therapeutic challenges when facilitating trauma-informed therapy groups. Chapter 6 discusses the complementary roles of Mindfulness and the Healthy Adult mode in supporting trauma recovery, fostering emotional regulation, self-compassion, and adaptive functioning. The complex interrelationship between trauma and comorbid issues of addictions and eating disorders are discussed in Chapter 7, even though no one session is dedicated to these topics. Chapter 8 summarizes the theoretical underpinnings and treatment considerations highlighted in Part I.

Part 2 provides specific protocols for each theme-based session. Current theory and practice guidelines are presented to support practitioners in delivering these services and understanding the relevance of each topic to trauma-informed care. Mindfulness, grounding, and experiential exercises are included throughout the book to help participants practice skills and apply the material to their own experiences. Chapter 9 outlines the group's structure and framework for this group therapy program for complex trauma.

Session 1 begins the process of group formation and the development of safety and group cohesion. Introductions, a review of the group's structure and content, group and individual goals, expectations, and concerns, are discussed in the first session. Mindfulness and grounding are introduced early in the program to help participants better regulate their emotions. Core needs and their relationship to the development of self-defeating patterns are illustrated by the story of Ella and the Thunderstorm and the analogy of the Dandelion and the Orchid.

Session 2 addresses the core elements of ST, Group ST, and their interface with trauma-focused treatment. Session 3 examines the complex nature and profound impact of trauma, distinguishing between Post-Traumatic Stress Disorder and CPTSD. Special attention is given to the systemic effects of trauma on an individual's sense of self, ability to regulate emotions, and capacity to maintain relationships. Sessions 4 and 5 explore the critical role of emotion regulation in trauma recovery. The concept of the Window of Tolerance, the theoretical framework of optimal arousal zones, hyperarousal and hypoarousal, and the interconnection between maladaptive schema activation, mode flipping, and arousal states are introduced, emphasizing the narrowing of one's capacity for emotional regulation after trauma. Sessions 6, 7, and 8 survey the impact of traumatic stress on the nervous system, the body, and memory. These sessions assess the neurobiological effects of early childhood trauma on brain structure and function, nervous system regulation and information processing, the connection between trauma and its physical manifestations in the body, and how traumatic memories are encoded, stored, and retrieved differently from regular memories. Direct manifestations of traumatic memory and trauma-related emotional dysregulation are presented in the Session 9 discussion of intrusive memories, flashbacks, and nightmares. Session 10 considers the complex relationship between childhood trauma and dissociation as a defensive survival strategy. It presents the Structural Dissociation model and ST explanations of how traumatic experiences lead to the fragmentation of personality and the development of distinct coping modes.

Trauma's impact on relationships is introduced in Sessions 11 and 12. These sessions observe the interplay between attachment and emotional regulation, exploring how trauma impacts attachment styles, roles (the Trauma Triangle), and dysfunctional relational patterns. Sessions 13 and

14 discuss the development of shame and guilt, the functions of the inner critic, and the antidotes of mindfulness and self-compassion. Three unstructured sessions are included in the program to allow completion of previous core topics or flexibility to dive deeper into issues relevant to the particular group. These open sessions can be used at any time during the group at the leaders' discretion.

The final sessions move the group towards the third phase of trauma recovery. Session 15 addresses the development of healthy relationships. Sessions 16 and 17 speak to trauma recovery, reconnection, integration, and post-traumatic growth and are dedicated to saying goodbye as the group ends. The transition from fragmentation to coherence is highlighted through the participants' healing journey in the group. Central to the discussion are the concepts of Post Traumatic Growth and the recursive spiral of trauma recovery. The group concludes with a Stone Ceremony celebrating each member's progress and achievements.

Part 3, Chapter 10 summarizes *Group Therapy for Complex Trauma: A Schema-Informed Approach*, recapping this comprehensive framework that bridges psychoeducation, experiential learning, and schema-informed interventions to provide a structured, compassionate roadmap for reclaiming agency and rebuilding a life fractured by trauma.

Reference

Margolin, J.A (1999). *Breaking the Silence: Group Therapy for Childhood Sexual Abuse: A Practitioner's Manual*. New York: Haworth Press.

Chapter 2

Early Childhood Trauma and Complex Post-Traumatic Stress Disorder

Early childhood trauma may be one of the most damaging experiences endured by today's youth. Secrecy, social isolation, and a lack of control have long characterized the experience of early childhood trauma. Assumptions about safety, trust, and invulnerability to harm may have been shattered, developmental tasks compromised, and primary relationships disrupted. As survivors came forward to disclose their experiences, we learned more about the impact of these early adverse events.

What permits one child to emerge seemingly unscathed while another may be severely incapacitated? How does the meaning of the event influence survival? How are these wounds carried forth into adulthood, and what treatments are effective in helping these individuals move beyond the adverse effects of their early experiences? How can one grow and thrive in the aftermath of these profound disruptions? (Margolin, 1999) Over the years, research in areas such as traumatic stress, neurobiology, attachment, and the mind-body connection, for example, burgeoned and has begun to answer some of these early questions.

Trauma is considered something so painful and shocking that it overwhelms an individual's ability to cope. The brain's ability to self-organize, regulate emotions, and integrate these unfathomable experiences becomes compromised, resulting in the intrusive reexperiencing of the trauma, avoidance of reminders of the past, heightened arousal, and negative alterations in the way they feel and think about themselves and the world. Mental, emotional, and physical health are compromised as these beliefs about self, others, and the world are compromised.

Early Childhood Trauma [Complex Post-Traumatic Stress Disorder (CPTSD)] can develop in response to prolonged, repeated, and often inescapable exposure to traumatic events, particularly those of an interpersonal nature (Herman, 1992; Courtois & Ford, 2012; WHO ICD-11, 2022).

DOI: 10.4324/9781003462958-3

Unlike single-incident trauma, sometimes associated with classic PTSD, complex trauma typically involves chronic abuse, neglect, or other adverse experiences beginning in childhood. Complex trauma encompasses the terror and helplessness similar to all psychological trauma, in addition to a shattering of the survivor's experience due to the fundamental betrayal of core protective relationships over a prolonged period (Herman, 1992; Freyd, 1994; van der Kolk et al., 1996; Courtois & Ford, 2012).

The impact of complex trauma is almost always more extensive and debilitating than single-incident PTSD, affecting a person's sense of self, relationships, and ability to regulate emotions. In addition to the core symptoms of PTSD (intrusion, avoidance, heightened arousal, and negative alterations in cognitions and mood), the consequences of childhood-onset interpersonal trauma and relational injury can lead to an altered sense of reality about the self, others, and the world, relational disruptions and potential revictimization, difficulties regulating emotions and impairments in physical health (Burback et al., 2024).

"Trauma survivors have symptoms instead of memories" (Fisher, 2022). Mood changes, negative affect and beliefs, feelings of shame, guilt, helplessness, hopelessness, worthlessness, dissociation, self-harm, chronic suicidal ideation, and health problems linked to the body's stress response are all potential manifestations of these traumatic experiences. Disrupted sleep, disordered eating, and substance use often accompany early childhood trauma.

Survivors interpret the abuse through their system of meaning embedded in their early maladaptive schemas. The relationship between life experiences, systems of meaning, and associated emotions helps determine the individual's unique experience of the traumatic event, affecting later psychological and relational functioning (McCann et al., 1988 in Margolin, 1999). Understanding these relationships allows treatment to be molded to meet the individual's needs.

Treatment of Complex Trauma

Herman (1992) suggested that recovery evolves in stages, beginning with developing a solid therapeutic alliance and establishing safety and stability in the individual's life. This then allows the individual to begin the tasks of remembering, reconstructing, and mourning the past. Finally, integrating the traumatic past allows the individual to reconnect with everyday life meaningfully. The treatment sequencing and strategy choice within each phase are essential considerations (Courtois, 1991).

This journey begins with the decision to heal and a commitment to treatment. It progresses through the realization that this happened, it happened to me, and it is not happening now and involves resolving responsibility, self-blame, shame, and guilt, identifying and managing emotions, restructuring maladaptive beliefs, mourning losses, increasing self-acceptance and self-compassion, and re-establishing healthy relationships. Treatment explores the impact of the past on current functioning and proceeds as a recursive spiral that moves back and forth as clients advance and relapse through the various healing tasks (Bass & Davis, 1988; Kepner, 1995).

New and effective interventions have been developed to address CPTSD, drawing from different theoretical orientations for individual and group treatments. Cognitive-behavioral theory underlies many trauma-focused therapies like Trauma-Focused Cognitive Behavior Therapy (TFCBT), Cognitive Processing Therapy (CPT), or Prolonged Exposure (PE) (Chard, 2005;Resick, 2008; Ehlers et al., 2013; Foa et al., 2007). TFCBT focuses on the re-evaluation of cognitive patterns and assumptions to help the person reconceptualize their understanding of traumatic experiences, their understanding of themselves, and their ability to cope. Exposure to the trauma narrative and triggers helps reduce avoidance and maladaptive associations with the trauma. CPT helps individuals process traumatic experiences by addressing and modifying unhelpful thoughts and beliefs associated with the trauma to create a new appreciation of the traumatic event. PE employs a gradual exposure approach to trauma-related memories, feelings, and situations, teaching individuals that trauma-related stimuli are not dangerous and do not need to be avoided.

Eye Movement Desensitization and Reprocessing (EMDR; Shapiro, 2017) is a structured therapy that emphasizes the modification of dysfunctional thoughts and behaviors with a reduction in the vividness and emotional impact of trauma memories. Patients focus on the trauma memory while experiencing bilateral stimulation, typically through eye movements. Schema Therapy (ST, Young et al., 2003; Younan et al., 2018; Huntjens et al., 2019; Lee & de Haan, 2020) is an integrative therapy that focuses on the development of maladaptive schema and dysfunctional coping as consequences of unmet needs during childhood and adolescence. Blending traditional cognitive behavioral treatment with experiential and interpersonal elements, it uses the therapeutic relationship as an essential vehicle to bring about the healing of maladaptive schemas emerging from early trauma.

Psychodynamic approaches, such as Brief Eclectic Psychotherapy for PTSD (Sachsse et al., 2008; Gersons et al., 2020), emphasize shame, guilt, and the relationship between the patient and therapist to modify thoughts and feelings that are the result of a traumatic event. Narrative Exposure Therapy (NET, Schauer et al., 2011) integrates both traumatic and non-traumatic experiences and cognitive, affective, and sensory memories of a patient's trauma to create a coherent narrative of the patient's life. Somatic therapies such as Somatosensory Psychotherapy (Ogden & Fisher,

2015) and Somatic Experiencing (Levine, 1999) emphasize the connection between mind and body with the belief that trauma is stored not only in the mind but also in the body. These therapies focus on addressing the physical manifestations of trauma. Self-compassion and mindfulness-based interventions (Neff, 2015; Gilbert, 2023) are promising adjuncts to traditional treatments for childhood trauma, offering therapeutic benefits by targeting symptoms of avoidance and negative cognitions, including self-blame, shame, and guilt, by increasing present-moment awareness, acceptance, and emotional regulation.

Overall, trauma-focused therapies are strongly recommended for the treatment of Complex Trauma (APA, 2024). Approaches that directly focus on the details of the trauma assist the patient in processing the cognitions, emotions, somatic reactions, and memories associated with the trauma. It is believed that once these are processed sufficiently to arrive at a point of resolution, completion, or a change of perspective, trauma symptoms should decline or remit. Incorporating non-trauma-focused treatment elements such as mindfulness or self-compassion training also enhances the treatment of Complex Trauma. As a trauma-informed therapist, it is vital to have a deep toolbox with a wide range of both trauma-focused and resilience-fostering interventions.

Treatment Approaches

Primary, processing-focused, and secondary, resourcing-focused approaches have been suggested as two very different approaches to trauma treatment (Ogden & Minton, 2000; Solomon & Heide, 2005; Ford, 2018, as cited in Tempone-Wiltshire, J., 2024). Processing-focused models specifically focus on processing the cognitive, affective, and sensory aspects of the traumatic experience. Resourcing-focused models emphasize emotion regulation and skill building (Tempone-Wiltshire, 2024). A phased approach to trauma treatment has been recommended for complex trauma populations, especially for those with dissociation, comorbidities, or active suicidal ideation (Herman, 1992). This approach incorporates the resourcing-focused model followed by the processing-focused model.

A phased-based approach to trauma therapy involves distinct stages: stabilization, trauma processing, and integration. In this sequential trauma treatment model, the treatment alliance, affect regulation, education, safety, and skill-building are developed during the early stages of treatment before undertaking trauma-focused memory processing (Stage I safety and stabilization phase). Stage II begins when the client has enough stability, affect modulation, and coping skills to process traumatic material with less post-traumatic impairment (Stage II remembrance and mourning phase). The final stage focuses on present-day life issues and relationships and developing a life less affected by trauma and its consequences (Stage III integration and reconnection phase) (Herman, 1992; Courtois, 2004).

Proponents of the stage-based approach suggest that trauma processing should not be introduced until both external and internal resources have been identified and are in place and that premature exposure to emotionally charged traumatic memories may lead to symptom exacerbation and increased risk (Wolfsdorf & Zlotnick, 2001; Brand et al., 2014; Van Minnen et al., 2015; de Jongh et al., 2016). Trauma-focused interventions are considered too destabilizing for chronically low-functioning patients, including those with severe attachment problems, minimal ego strength and coping capacity, ongoing enmeshment with perpetrators, severe personality pathology, significant medical problems, and ongoing substance abuse and dependency (Cloitre et al., 2012). In this model, trauma-focused exposure and processing are started once the individual has developed sufficient resources (ego strength, commitment to treatment, social support, and economic resources) to effectively manage current life stress and control fears and bodily reactions to those fears. The stabilization phase is considered essential to teach these patients more effective skills to regulate affect, manage interpersonal relationships, and overcome trauma-based ways of responding, including dissociation.

Some argue that the phased approach may not be necessary for all individuals and that a more flexible, individualized approach could be more effective. The phased approach has faced criticism for potentially prolonging treatment, restricting access to or delaying trauma processing (de Jongh et al., 2016). It is also suggested that delaying a focus on the trauma may demoralize patients by communicating the message that they are unable to manage the processing of traumatic material (de Jongh et al., 2016; Angelakis et al., 2020). A meta-analysis of group treatments for adults with symptoms associated with CPTSD found that trauma memory processing interventions for PTSD, depression, and psychological distress were superior to or as effective as usual care and psychoeducational interventions (Ehring et al., 2014; Mahoney et al., 2019). Whether or not a phase-based conceptualization of treatment for complex trauma prevents some clients from recovering as quickly as they could, the intensification of treatment in trauma-focused protocols has been shown to facilitate faster improvement in adaptive functioning (Huntjens et al., 2019). The diversity in clinical presentation in this population necessitates the development of individualized case conceptualizations for each client. These will guide clinical decision-making in determining the focus of treatment and the speed with which to move forward and will have implications when considering adjunctive interventions.

Despite these controversies, the phased-based approach remains a cornerstone in trauma therapy, providing a structured framework for treatment.

Having the opportunity to process trauma-based memories safely is vital when survivors also have sufficient resources to manage any emotional dysregulation that might arise. While often insufficient in themselves for the treatment of trauma, resourcing approaches are essential supplements in effective trauma treatment (Tempone-Wiltshire, 2024) and can be beneficial in managing symptoms. Psychoeducation and skill-building resources offered as part of a phased approach teach the survivor to manage the symptoms of general distress and PTSD, including dissociation. Dialectical Behavior Therapy (DBT), Interpersonal Therapy, Mindfulness, and Self Compassion Therapy are effective in the management of PTSD symptoms, emotion regulation, self-judgment, negative attributions, and, to a lesser extent, depression (Talbot et al., 1998; Follette et al., 2015; Bohus et al., 2020; Taylor et al., 2020; Toshishige et al., 2022). The timing, nature, and intensity of trauma processing interventions must match individual treatment needs and capabilities and still be sufficient to ensure substantial progress is achieved and maintained (Griffin et al., 2023).

Group Treatment

Group therapy offers opportunities for new interpersonal learning, sharing everyday experiences, and developing a cohesive community to provide a context for the central mechanism for change. Successful groups create a curative environment that fosters healing, personal growth, and transformation through shared experiences and group support (Yalom & Leszcz, 2020). Groups leverage nonspecific therapy factors such as collective experiences and shared understanding of group members to foster healing, resilience, and personal growth. The group imparts information, instills hope, reduces isolation, and demonstrates the universality of experiences. The sharing of knowledge and insight helps others address past childhood injuries. At the same time, skill development, modeling, imitation, and interpersonal learning about relationships and intimacy allow for a "corrective experience" and the development of healthier relational patterns. "Group therapy directly and experientially addresses interpersonal and relational difficulties … it provides the opportunity to join others with similar histories to gain perspective on the past and its impact on the present" (Courtois & Ford, 2012, pp. 190–191).

Group therapy fosters optimism as members witness positive changes in others and a sense of belonging and acceptance as they realize they are not alone in their struggles. Contributing positively to others is empowering and enhances the member's sense of self-worth and confidence. The opportunity to observe others in the group disrupts old dysfunctional patterns. It allows room for new behaviors to develop as the group members begin to confront, accept, and find new meaning in the realities of life.

Group Therapy for Complex Trauma

Group Therapy for Complex Trauma is a specialized approach that is beneficial for individuals with complex trauma histories who have experienced profound and often multidimensional traumatic events (Ford et al., 2009; Mendelsohn et al., 2011). Different models have been suggested for group treatment with this population, ranging from long-term, open-ended groups that focus on in-depth examination of the core issues and processing of trauma memories to short-term time-limited groups that provide a structured approach integrating educational and trauma-focused interventions.

Trauma-focused group therapy more directly focuses on the desensitization of traumatic memories while addressing the consequences, symptoms, and current life problems engendered by the traumatic experience. It provides the ideal forum to address the impact of early trauma on present-day experiences by providing education about complex trauma as well as "opportunities to be seen, heard and supported, to gain perspective on the past and its impact on the present within a safe, honest and respectful setting with individuals who share similar experiences and emotions" (Courtois & Ford, 2012, p. 193). These opportunities allow the individual to learn to regulate emotions and interact within relationships through modeling by the group leaders and members.

Experiencing trauma can lead to feelings of shame and the desire to hide and isolate rather than engage and bond with others (Hofmann et al., 2003; Charuvastra & Cloitre, 2008). A lack of social interaction and support may increase the severity of PTSD symptoms and impair a person's ability to regulate their distress (Price et al., 2018). Group-based treatments offer social support for individuals who may be isolated because of their trauma. The group can help mitigate the effects of trauma and reduce PTSD symptoms by providing a forum for people to be in contact with others "like them" (i.e., others who have also experienced a similar trauma) and fostering acceptance, perceived efficacy, support, and solidarity (Cruwys & Gunaseelan, 2015; Muldoon et al., 2019). The goal is to provide a safe, supportive environment where participants can make meaning of their trauma, reduce shame-related cognitions, develop effective coping strategies, and build a sense of community (Courtois & Ford, 2010; Schwartze et al., 2019; Griffin et al., 2023).

The benefit of group therapy became clear after witnessing a Stone Ceremony, a special ceremony marking the end of the group, or, in open-ended groups, when an individual completes their participation. During the Stone Ceremony, the member chooses a stone inscribed with one word that captures their journey (e.g., strength, resilience, hope, trust, etc.). The stone is then passed around to the other members as they witness the growth, progress, and small victories of the person leaving the group. Earlier feelings of shame or defectiveness visibly diminish as the person receives their peers' caring and compassion.

When comparing individual and group treatments for complex trauma, both formats have shown efficacy in reducing symptoms. Individual therapy provides significant symptom reduction and can be a crucible in which the individual safely and securely explores the impact of the trauma while learning new ways to manage its sequelae. Individual therapy is an essential component of trauma-focused treatment, but it does not address all the dimensions necessary for healing. Healthy development requires more than dyadic therapy for experiences encompassing broader "family" dynamics. When applied to treatment for Complex Trauma, group ST is an approach that promotes healing as the group "family" supports the treatment of the complex nature of trauma-related issues. It mirrors family of origin dynamics as a "microcosm of the outside of therapy" world (Farrell, 2012).

The Group Therapy for Complex Trauma literature highlights its potential effectiveness and feasibility. The group offers unique benefits which can be particularly valuable for individuals with complex trauma. It can counteract the sense of betrayal, feelings of powerlessness and stigmatization, and traumatic sexualization, and also address experiences of guilt, shame, and isolation (Finkelhor & Browne, 1985; Carver et al., 1989; Stalker & Fry, 1999; Price et al., 2001; Callahan et al., 2004). It is difficult to resolve issues of secrecy, shame, and stigma in individual treatment alone, and dependency may be reinforced in individual therapy (Herman & Schatzow, 1984; Margolin, 1999). "Group therapy combats the social isolation, allows connection with sources of resilience and self-esteem, and rebuilds relationship capacities" (Mendelsohn et al., 2011, p. 1).

Griffin et al. (2023) argue that the group-based nature of the treatment is most beneficial and may offer advantages over individual-level treatments. They emphasize the beneficial effect of being a member of a group on psychological health as the group provides social and psychological resources to cope with the effects of adverse life events (Jones et al., 2012; Walsh et al., 2015; Haslam et al., 2018; Kearns et al., 2018; Muldoon et al., 2019). Group membership has been associated with lower risk of depression (Sani et al., 2012; Cruwys et al., 2013; Seymour-Smith et al., 2017), greater well-being (Iyer et al., 2009; Sani et al., 2015), lower PTSD symptoms (Muldoon & Downes, 2007; Jones et al., 2012) and increasing a sense of belonging and social support (Haslam et al., 2005; Haslam et al., 2016; Walter et al., 2016; Avanzi et al., 2018). A systematic review and meta-analysis found sufficient evidence to recommend trauma-focused group therapy as an addition to individual trauma-focused interventions (Griffin, et al., 2023). Research studies indicate that group therapy can effectively reduce PTSD symptoms compared to control conditions. However, as a stand-alone treatment, it was either less or equally efficacious compared to individual or combined treatments (Ehring et al., 2014). In a randomized clinical trial of 495 adult participants with BPD in five countries, combined individual and group ST was significantly more effective than optimal treatment as usual and predominantly group ST in reducing the severity of Borderline Personality Disorder, a disorder sharing many commonalities with those of Complex PTSD. These findings add to the evidence for the effectiveness of ST and indicate that the combination of individual and group ST is the more effective ST format. Group therapy for CPTSD can be viewed as an essential complement to the intensive, individual exploration of the trauma (Arntz, 2022).

Both trauma memory processing and psychoeducational approaches are valuable interventions, though the specific benefits may differ based on the type of trauma and individual needs (Griffin et al., 2023). It is important to remember that several factors can influence the success and effectiveness of the group. The nature of the trauma, the composition of the group (particularly gender composition), the identification and degree of fit with other members, the similarity of the shared experience, the social support offered, the association of shame and stigma, and facilitator characteristics are important moderators of treatment outcome and play crucial roles in the success of therapy (Barrera et al., 2013; Sloan et al., 2013; Schwartze et al., 2019).

Models of Group Therapy for Complex Trauma

Skills Training in Affective and Interpersonal Regulation plus Modified Prolonged Exposure (STAIR/MPE) is an example of a Phase I group targeting PTSD symptoms, emotion-regulation deficits and interpersonal difficulties. It is an evidence-based, 2-phase cognitive behavioral treatment designed to address the substantial clinical concern that treatment focusing on the emotional processing of traumatic memories increases the risk of early dropout and symptom exacerbation in those with limited emotion-regulation skills (Cloitre et al., 2002; Levitt & Cloitre, 2005). Seeking Safety (Najavits, 2002) is also a Phase I treatment designed for clients with both PTSD and substance abuse. This model is a structured topic and skill-focused approach that does not address trauma memories and can be offered in individual and group formats. The Trauma Adaptive Recovery Group Education And Therapy (TARGET, Ford & Russo, 2006) relates the symptoms of PTSD and affect dysregulation to survival from trauma. It, too, can be delivered individually or in groups to enhance affect regulation. The Trauma Information Group (TIG, Herman & Kallivayalil, 2019) is an example of a Phase I group that focuses on safety, stability, and self-care. The didactic and time-limited format helps the client better understand trauma, develop effective means of coping with their distress, and increase self-compassion while decreasing shame, stigma, and isolation. The TIG also provides a platform for group members to share their experiences and learn from each other's coping strategies, fostering a sense of community and mutual support.

Phase II groups move beyond the primary educational and stabilization focus with increased attention paid to processing the trauma and making meaning of its impact. Many of these group models continue to incorporate psychoeducation and skill development into their trauma-focused approach, organizing around specific themes that apply to the group members' relationships and their lives and teaching skills necessary for effective functioning (Courtois & Ford, 2008; Lubin & Johnson, 2008; Mendelsohn et al., 2011).

Margolin (1999) provided an early example of a "hybrid" group for adults who experienced childhood sexual abuse. Comprised of both psychoeducational and process-oriented components, the structured approach was directed toward understanding the effects of early abuse on the individual's current functioning through the limited sharing of personal stories, skill development, and the exploration of the sequelae, meaning, and impact of those early experiences. The Trauma Centered Group Psychotherapy (Lubin & Johnson, 2008) is a program that combines education and processing. It is a semi-structured, time-limited, theme-organized model emphasizing women's empowerment, trauma education, and skill development. Early trauma disclosure within a safe environment is encouraged to reduce anticipatory anxiety, overcome avoidance strategies, and enhance group cohesion. The Trauma Recovery Group (Mendelsohn et al., 2011) is a Phase II time-limited group treatment focused on the processing and integration of traumatic memories. Members work toward individualized goals using the relational context of the group.

Inpatient Group ST for Complex Trauma (Younan et al., 2018) is a four-week in-patient group program for adults with complex trauma in a psychiatric hospital setting. This program demonstrated positive effects on psychiatric symptoms and maladaptive schemas following participation in the group ST program (Younan et al., 2018). S.A.F.E.T.Y. is a trauma program for high-risk, emotionally dysregulated women utilizing DBT and trauma-focused treatment in a short-term acute care setting (partial hospitalization/intensive outpatient). Significant reductions in emotion dysregulation and increased stabilization of impulsivity and high-risk behaviors were demonstrated upon completion of routine treatment (Margolin & Krejci, unpublished report, 2020). Examinations of other inpatient and day treatment programs found significant improvements in dissociation, stress reactions, and defense mechanisms, reductions of PTSD symptoms, and improvements in self-esteem, interpersonal problems, and general psychopathology (Boos et al.,1999; Jepsen et al., 2014; Philipps et al., 2019). These findings support the feasibility of trauma-focused group therapy at higher levels of care as well as in traditional outpatient settings.

Limitations of Group Therapy for Complex Trauma

While group therapy offers several advantages, it also has limitations for treating complex trauma. One significant limitation is the potential for re-traumatization, as revisiting trauma memories in a group and hearing others' traumatic experiences may increase the intensity of emotions in some participants. Even though exposure is considered a key component in the treatment of PTSD, it can be potentially harmful when it causes intense and uncontrollable emotional dysregulation, including uncontrolled dissociation (Briere & Runtz, 1988; Courtois & Ford, 2012). It has also been suggested that if participants draw comparisons between the individual's experience of trauma and that of others, it may cause them to delegitimize their own experience (Beck & Coffey, 2005). However, it's important to note that group therapy, when conducted with care and under the guidance of a skilled facilitator, can provide a sense of community and validation, potentially leading to positive outcomes. Additionally, group settings may not provide the level of individual attention and support needed for those with severe symptoms or comorbid conditions. Group therapy may be contraindicated for those with active risk behaviors, including suicidal or homicidal behaviors and active substance abuse, the inability to regulate emotions, control impulsive tendencies or interpersonal aggression, psychosis, or paranoid, schizophrenic, or other personality disorders that would interfere with successful participation in the group (Courtois & Ford, 2012). High drop-out rates are also a concern in some group therapy programs. Difficulty regulating emotions, increased aggression, impulsivity, and the inability to tolerate the intense affect triggered in the group may be contributing factors causing premature dropout.

As previously mentioned, the effectiveness of group therapy and treatment outcomes can vary based on group dynamics and the facilitator's skill. The success of group therapy depends on managing group dynamics, ensuring a safe environment for all participants, group composition, facilitator skills, and the specific therapeutic model used (Shea et al., 2009; Sloan et al., 2013; Younan et al., 2018). However, it is important to highlight that these challenges can be effectively addressed when the group leader is trained in trauma-informed care. A skilled leader can support dysregulated members by intervening appropriately when signs of emotional dysregulation and re-traumatization are recognized and can model an atmosphere of mutual respect and validation in a non-competitive space. This underscores the significant impact that the group leader's skills and training can have on the success of group therapy.

Summary

Both individual and group therapies have their merits. Each is effective in reducing symptoms of complex trauma, such as PTSD and emotional distress.

The choice between them should be guided by the specific needs and preferences of the patient, the nature of their trauma, and the resources available. Combining both approaches may enhance treatment outcomes and offer the most comprehensive benefits for long-term recovery in complex trauma patients. There is consensus that the most effective treatment of CPTSD adopts a trauma-informed approach that emphasizes safety and stabilization along with paced, titrated exposure to trauma-related content. The group fosters healing by sharing experiences in a setting with transparent, predictable, and consistent guidelines, norms, and boundaries. Peer support and validation promote trust and cohesion in the group and provide a model for successful interpersonal relationships. Recovery involves learning skills to manage emotions and identify potential triggers and red flags for re-traumatization.

As a complement to individual therapy, the group is similarly directed toward increasing self-reflective capabilities, regulating emotions and arousal within the Window of Tolerance, developing healthy interpersonal relationships, and developing a straightforward, coherent narrative of the self, past and present. Examining and analyzing one's experiences, thoughts, feelings, and actions without judgment, identifying core values and unmet needs while making intentional changes to align actions with personal values and goals is enhanced within a group. Survival action tendencies and coping responses (fight/flight/freeze/submit/attach), maladaptive schemas, and behavior patterns that interfere with healthy functioning and healthy relationships can be addressed as they play out in the group. Having one's experiences mirrored by the group aids in recognizing, acknowledging, and accepting the impact of the past trauma on one's present-day self and relationships. The group provides another forum to facilitate the development of a coherent narrative. "This happened, and it happened to me, but it is not happening now" accepts that the past happened, that it is not happening now, and that it no longer defines current experiences.

References

American Psychological Association (APA) (2024). Guidelines for working with adults with complex trauma histories. Retrieved from [https://www.apa.org/practice/guidelines/adults-complex-trauma-histories.pdf] Washington, DC: American Psychological Association.

Angelakis, I., Austin, J. L., & Gooding, P. (2020). Association of childhood maltreatment with suicide behaviors among young people: a systematic review and meta-analysis. *JAMA Netw Open*, 3(8): E2012563. https://doi.org/10.1001/Jamanetworkopen.2020.12563

Arntz, A., Jacob, G. A., Lee, C. W., Brand-de Wilde, O. M., Fassbinder, E., Harper, R. P., Lavender, A., Lockwood, G., Malogiannis, I. A., Ruths, F. A., Schweiger, U., Shaw, I. A., Zarbock, G., & Farrell, J. M. (2022). Effectiveness of predominantly group schema therapy and combined individual and group schema therapy for borderline personality disorder: a randomized clinical trial. *JAMA Psychiatry*, 79(4), 287–299. https://doi.org/10.1001/jamapsychiatry.2022.0010

Avanzi, L., Fraccaroli, F., Castelli, L., Marcionetti, J., Crescentini, A., Balducci, C., & van Dick, R.et al. (2018). How to mobilize social support against workload and burnout: the role of organizational identification. *Teaching and Teacher Education*, 69, 154–167 https://doi.org/10.1016/J.Tate.2017.10.001

Barrera, T. L., Mott, J. M., Hofstein, R. F., & Teng, E. J. (2013). A meta-analytic review of exposure in group cognitive behavioral therapy for posttraumatic stress disorder. *Clinical Psychology Review*, 33, 24–32.

Bass, E., & Davis, L. (1988). *The Courage to Heal: A Guide For Women Survivors of Child Sexual Abuse*. New York: Perennial Library/Harper & Row Publishers.

Beck, J. G. & Coffey, S. F. (2005). Group cognitive behavioral treatment for PTSD: treatment of motor vehicle accident survivors. *Cognitive and Behavioral Practice*, 12(3), 267–277. https://doi.org/10.1016/S1077-7229(05)80049-5

Bohus, M., Kleindienst, N., Hahn, C., Müller-Engelmann, M., Ludäscher, P., Steil, R., Fydrich, T., Kuehner, C., Resick, P. A., Stiglmayr, C., Schmahl, C., & Priebe, K. (2020). Dialectical behavior therapy for posttraumatic stress disorder (DBT-PTSD) compared with cognitive processing therapy (CPT) in complex presentations of PTSD in women survivors of childhood abuse: a randomized clinical trial. *JAMA Psychiatry*, 77(12), 1235–1245. https://doi.org/10.1001/Jamapsychiatry.2020.2148

Boos, A., Scheifling-Hirschbil, I., & Rüddel, H. (1999). Evaluation of an inpatient therapy group, 'recovery from trauma' within the psychosomatic treatment and rehabilitation of patients with chronic PTSD. *Verhaltenstherapie*, 9(4), 200–210. https://doi.org/10.1159/000030701

Brand, B. L., Loewenstein, R. J., & Spiegel, D. (2014). Dispelling myths about dissociative identity disorder treatment: an empirically based approach. *Psychiatry*, 77(2), 169–89. https://doi.org/10.1521/Psyc.2014.77.2.169

Briere, J., & Runtz, M. (1988). Symptomatology associated with childhood sexual victimization in a non-clinical adult sample. *Child Abuse and Neglect*, 12, 51–59.

Burback, L., Brémault-Phillips, S., Nijdam, M. J., McFarlane, A., & Vermetten, E. (2024). Treatment of posttraumatic stress disorder: a state-of-the-art review. *Current Neuropharmacology*, 22(4), 557–635. https://doi.org/10.2174/15701 59X21666230428091433

Carver, C. M., Stalker, C., Stewart, E., & Abraham, B. (1989). The impact of group therapy for adult survivors of childhood sexual abuse. *The Canadian Journal of Psychiatry / La Revue Canadienne De Psychiatrie*, 34(8), 753–758.

Chard, K. M. (2005). An evaluation of cognitive processing therapy for the treatment of posttraumatic stress disorder related to childhood sexual abuse. *Journal of Consulting and Clinical Psychology*, 73, 965–971. https://psycnet.apa.org/doi/10.1037/0022-006X.73.5.965

Charuvastra, A., & Cloitre, M. (2008). Social bonds and posttraumatic stress disorder. Annual *Review of Psychology*, 59, 301–328. https://doi.org/10.1146/Annurev.Psych.58.110405.085650

Cloitre, M., Courtois, C. A., Ford, J. D., Green, B. L., Alexander, P., Briere, J., Herman, J. L., Lanius, R., Stolbach, B. C., Spinazzola, J., Van der Kolk, B. A., & Van der Hart, O. (2012).

The ISTSS Expert Consensus Treatment Guidelines for Complex PTSD in Adults. https://www.istss.org/ISTSS_Main/media/Documents/ISTSS-Expert-ConcesnsusGuidelines-for-Complex-PTSD-Updated-060315.pdf

Cloitre, M., Koenen, K. C., Cohen, L. R., & Han, H. (2002). Skills training in affective and interpersonal regulation followed by exposure: a phase-based treatment for PTSD related to childhood abuse. *Journal of Consulting and Clinical Psychology*, 70(5), 1067.

Cognitive Processing Therapy (CPT) | Lifepsychologyclinic. https://www.lifepsychologyclinic.com/cognitive-processing-therapy-cpt

Courtois C. A. (1991). Theory, sequencing, and strategy in treating adult survivors. *New Directions for Mental Health Services*, 51, 47–60. https://doi.org/10.1002/Yd.23319915106

Courtois, C. A. (2004). Complex trauma, complex reactions. *Psychotherapy: Theory, Research, Practice, Training*, 41 (4), 412–425.

C.A. Courtois & J.D. Ford (Eds.) (2010). Treating Complex Traumatic Stress Disorders: An Evidence-Based Guide. New York: The Guilford Press.

Courtois, C.A. & Ford, J.D. (2012). *Treatment of Complex Trauma: A Sequenced, Relationship-Based Approach.* New York: The Guilford Press.

Cruwys, T., Dingle, G. A., Haslam, C., Haslam, S. A., Jetten, J., & Morton, T. A. (2013). Social group memberships protect against future depression, alleviate depression symptoms, and prevent depression relapse. *Social Science & Medicine*, 98, 179–186.

Cruwys, T., & Gunaseelan, S. (2015). "Depression is who i am": mental illness identity, stigma and wellbeing. *Journal of Affective Disorders*, 189, 36–42. https://doi.org/10.1016/J.Jad.2015.09.012

De Jongh, A., Resick, P. A., Zoellner, L. A., Van Minnen, A., Lee, C. W., Monson, C. M., Foa, E. B., Wheeler, K., Broeke, E. T., Feeny, N., Rauch, S. A., Chard, K. M., Mueser, K. T., Sloan, D. M., Van Der Gaag, M., Rothbaum, B. O., Neuner, F., De Roos, C., Hehenkamp, L. M., Rosner, R., & Bicanic I. A. (2016). Critical analysis of the current treatment guidelines for complex PTSD in adults. *Depress Anxiety*, 33(5), 359–369. https://doi.org/10.1002/Da.22469

Ehring, T., Welboren, R., Morina, N., Wicherts, J. M., Freitag, J. & Emmelkamp, P. M. G. (2014). Meta-analysis of psychological treatments for posttraumatic stress disorder in adult survivors of childhood abuse. *Clinical Psychology Review*, 34(8), 645–657.

Ehlers, A., Grey, N., Wild, J., Stott, R., Liness, S., Deale, A., Handley, R., Albert, I., Cullen, D., Hackmann, A., Manley, J., McManus, F., Brady, F., Salkovskis, P., & Clark, D. M. (2013). Implementation of cognitive therapy for PTSD in routine clinical care: effectiveness and moderators of outcome in a consecutive sample. *Behavior Research and Therapy*, 51(11), 742–752.

Farrell, J.M (2012). Introduction to Group Schema Therapy. In Vreeswijk, M., Broersen, J. & Nadort, M. (Eds.) *The Wiley-Blackwell handbook of schema therapy, theory, research, and practice.* Oxford, UK: Wiley-Blackwell, 337–339.

Finkelhor, D. & Browne, A. (1985). The traumatic impact of child sexual abuse: a conceptualization. *American Journal of Orthopsychiatry*, 55(4), 530–541, https://doi.org/10.1111/J.1939-0025.1985.Tb02703.X

Fisher, J. (2022). *The Living Legacy of Trauma Flip Chart: A Psychoeducational In-Session Tool for Clients and Therapists.* Eau Claire, WI: Pesi Publishing.

Foa, E. B., Hembree, E. A., & Rothbaum, B. O. (2007). *Prolonged Exposure Therapy for PTSD: Emotional Processing of Traumatic Experiences: Therapist Guide.* New York: Oxford University Press.

Follette, V.M., Briere, J., Rozelle, D., Hopper, J.W., & Rome, D. I. (2015). Mindfulness-Oriented Interventions for Trauma: Integrating Contemplative Practices. United Kingdom: Guilford Publications.

Ford, J. D., & Russo, E. (2006). Trauma-focused, present-centered, emotional self-regulation approach to integrated treatment for posttraumatic stress and addiction: trauma adaptive recovery group education and therapy (target). *American Journal of Psychotherapy*, 60(4), 335–355.

Ford, J. D., Fallot, R. D., & Harris, M. (2009). Group therapy. In C. A. Courtois & J. D. Ford (Eds.), *Treating Complex Traumatic Stress Disorders: An Evidence-Based Guide.* New York: Guilford Press, 415–440.

Ford, J.D. (2018) Trauma Memory Processing in Posttraumatic Stress Disorder Psychotherapy: A Unifying Framework. *Journal of Traumatic Stress*, 31(6), 791–945.

Freyd, J. J. (1994). Betrayal trauma: traumatic amnesia as an adaptive response to childhood abuse. *Ethics & Behavior*, 4(4), 307–329.

Gersons, B. P. R., Nijdam, M. J., Smid, G. E., & Meewisse, M.-L. (2020). Brief eclectic psychotherapy for PTSD. In L. F. Bufka, C. V. Wright, & R. W. Halfond (Eds.), *Casebook to the APA Clinical Practice Guideline for the Treatment of PTSD.* Washington, DC: American Psychological Association, 139–161.

Gilbert, P. (2023). Self-compassion: an evolutionary, biopsychosocial, and social mentality approach. In A. Finlay-Jones, K. Bluth, & K. Neff (Eds.), *Handbook of Self-Compassion.* Switzerland: Springer Nature Switzerland AG, 53–69.

Griffin, S. M., Lebedová, A., Ahern, E., McMahon, G., Bradshaw, D., & Muldoon, O. T. (2023). Group-based interventions for posttraumatic stress disorder: a systematic review and meta-analysis of the role of trauma type. *Campbell Systematic Reviews*, 19(2), E1328. https://doi.org/10.1002/Cl2.1328

Haslam, S. A., O'Brien, A., Jetten, J., Vormedal, K., & Penna, S. (2005). Taking the strain: social identity, social support, and the experience of stress. *British Journal of Social Psychology*, 44(3), 355–370. https://doi.org/10.1348/014466605X37468

Haslam, C., Cruwys, T., Milne, M., Kan, C. -H., & Haslam, S. A. (2016). Group ties protect cognitive health by promoting social identification and social support. *Journal of Aging and Health*, 28(2), 244–266. https://doi.org/10.1177/0898264315589578

Haslam, C., Jetten, J., Cruwys, T., Dingle, G., & Haslam, S.A. (2018). *The New Psychology of Health: Unlocking the Social Cure (1st ed.).* Routledge. https://doi.org/10.4324/9781315648569

Herman, J., & Schatzow, E. (1984). Time-limited group therapy for women with a history of incest. *International Journal of Group Psychotherapy*, 34(4), 605–616.

Herman, J. L. (1992). Complex PTSD: a syndrome in survivors of prolonged and repeated trauma. *Journal of Traumatic Stress*, 5, 377–391.

Herman, J. L., & Kallivayalil, D. (2019). *Group Trauma Treatment in Early Recovery: Promoting Safety and Self-Care* (1st ed.). New York: Guilford Press.

Hofmann, S. G., Litz, B. T., & Weathers, F. W. (2003). Social anxiety, depression, and PTSD in Vietnam veterans. *Journal of Anxiety Disorders*, 17(5), 573–582.

Huntjens, R. J. C., Rijkeboer, M. M., & Arntz, A. (2019). Schema therapy for dissociative identity disorder (did): rationale and study protocol. *European Journal of Psychotraumatology*, 10(1):1571377. https://doi.org/10.1080/20008198.2019.1571377

Iyer, A., Jetten, J., Tsivrikos, D., Postmes, T., & Haslam, S. A. (2009). The more (and the more compatible), the merrier: multiple group memberships and identity compatibility as predictors of adjustment after life transitions. *British Journal of Social Psychology*, 48(4), 707–733. https://doi.org/10.1348/014466608X397628

Jepsen, E. K. K., Langeland, W., Sexton, H., & Heir, T. (2014). Inpatient treatment for early sexually abused adults: a naturalistic 12-month follow-up study. *Psychological Trauma: Theory, Research, Practice, and Policy* 6(2), 142–51. https://doi.org/10.1037/A0031646

Jones, J. M., Williams, W. H., Jetten, J., Haslam, S. A., Harris, A., & Gleibs, I. H. (2012). The role of psychological symptoms and social group memberships in the development of post-traumatic stress after traumatic injury. *British Journal of Health Psychology*, 17(4), 798–811.

Kearns, M., Muldoon, O. T., Msetfi, R. M., & Surgenor, P. W. G. (2018). Identification reduces the stigma of mental ill-health: a community-based study. *American Journal of Community Psychology*, 61(1–2), 229–239. https://doi.org/10.1002/Ajcp.12220

Kepner, J. I. (1995). *Healing Tasks: Psychotherapy with Adult Survivors of Childhood Abuse*. San Francisco, CA, Jossey-Bass Publishers.

Lee, C. W., & De Haan, K. B. (2020). Working with trauma memories and complex post-traumatic stress disorder. In G. Heath, & H. Startup (Eds.), *Creative Methods in Schema Therapy: Advances and Innovation in Clinical Practice*. Routledge/Taylor & Francis Group, 124–137.

Levine, P. A. (1999). *Healing Trauma: Restoring the Wisdom of Your Body*. Louisville, CO: Sounds True, Inc.

Levitt, J. T., & Cloître, M. (2005). A clinician's guide to STAIR/MPE: treatment for PTSD related to childhood abuse. *Cognitive and Behavioral Practice*, *12*, 40–52. https://doi.org/10.1016/S1077-7229(05)80038-0

Lubin, H. & Johnson, D. R. (2008). *Trauma-Centered Group Psychotherapy for Women*. New York: Guilford Publications, Inc.

Mahoney, A., Karatzias, T., & Hutton, P. (2019). A systematic review and meta-analysis of group treatments for adults with symptoms associated with complex post-traumatic stress disorder. *Journal of affective disorders*, *243*, 305–321. https://doi.org/10.1016/j.jad.2018.09.059

Margolin, J. (1999). *Breaking the Silence: Group Therapy for Childhood Sexual Abuse*. New York: The Haworth Maltreatment and Trauma Press.

Margolin, J. & Krejci, J. (2020). Utilizing dialectical behavior therapy and trauma informed care to enhance emotion regulation and symptom stabilization in an acute partial hospital/intensive outpatient treatment setting. Unpublished Report.

McCann, I. L., Sakheim, D. K., & Abrahamson, D. J. (1988). Trauma and victimization: a model of psychological adaptation. *The Counseling Psychologist*, 16(4), 531–594.

Mendelsohn, M., Herman, J. L., Schatzow, E., Kallivayalil, D., Coco, M., & Levitan, J. (2011). *The Trauma Recovery Group: A Guide for Practitioners*. New York: Guilford Publications.

Muldoon, O. T., & Downes, C. (2007). Social identification and post-traumatic stress symptoms in post-conflict northern Ireland. *British Journal of Psychiatry*, 191(2), 146–149. https://doi.org/10.1192/Bjp.Bp.106.022038

Muldoon, O. T., Haslam, S. A., Haslam, C., Cruwys, T., Kearns, M., & Jetten, J. (2019). The social psychology of responses to trauma: social identity pathways associated with divergent traumatic responses. *European Review of Social Psychology*, 30(1), 311–348. https://doi.org/10.1080/10463283.2020.1711628

Najavits, L. M. (2002). *Seeking Safety: A Treatment Manual for PTSD and Substance Abuse*. New York: Guilford Press.

Neff, K. (2015). *Self-Compassion: The Proven Power of Being Kind to Yourself*. New York: William Morrow.

Ogden, P., & Fisher, J. (2015). *Sensorimotor Psychotherapy: Interventions For Trauma and Attachment (Norton Series on Interpersonal Neurobiology)*. New York: W. W. Norton & Company.

Ogden, P., & Minton, K. (2000). Sensorimotor Psychotherapy: One Method for Processing Traumatic Memory. Traumatology, 6(3), 149–173.Philipps, A., Silbermann, A., Morawa, E., Stemmler, M., & Erim, Y. (2019). Effectiveness of a multimodal, day clinic group-based treatment program for trauma-related disorders: differential therapy outcome for complex PTSD vs. Non-complex trauma-related disorders. *Frontiers in Psychiatry*, 10:800. https://doi.org/10.3389/Fpsyt.2019.00800

Price, M., Lancaster, C. L., Gros, D. F., Legrand, A. C., Van Stolk-Cooke, K., & Acierno, R. (2018). An examination of social support and PTSD treatment response during prolonged exposure. *Psychiatry*, 81(3), 258–270. https://doi.org/10.1080/00332747.2017.1402569

Price, J. L., Hilsenroth, M. J., Petretic-Jackson, P. A., & Bonge, D. (2001). A review of individual psychotherapy outcomes for adult survivors of childhood sexual abuse. *Clinical Psychology Review*, 21(7), 1095–1121. https://doi.org/10.1016/S0272-7358(00)00086-6

Resick, P. A., Galovski, T. E., Uhlmansiek, M. O. B., Scher, C. D., Clum, G. A., Young-Xu, Y. (2008). A randomized clinical trial to dismantle components of cognitive processing therapy for posttraumatic stress disorder in female victims of interpersonal violence. *Journal of Consulting and Clinical Psychology*, 76, 243–258.

Sachsse, U., Vogel, C., & Leichsenring, F. (2006). Results of psychodynamically oriented trauma-focused inpatient treatment for women with complex posttraumatic stress disorder (PTSD) and borderline personality disorder (BPD). *Bull Menninger Clinic*, 70 (2), 125–44. https://doi.org/10.1521/Bumc.2006.70.2.125

Sani, F., Herrera, M., Wakefield, J. R., Boroch, O., & Gulyas, C. (2012). Comparing social contact and group identification as predictors of mental health. *The British journal of social psychology*, 51(4), 781–790. https://doi.org/10.1111/j.2044-8309.2012.02101.x

Sani, F., Madhok, V., Norbury, M., Dugard, P., & Wakefield, J. R. H. (2015). Greater number of group identifications is associated with lower odds of being depressed: evidence from a Scottish community sample. *Social Psychiatry and Psychiatric Epidemiology*, 50 (9), 1389–1397. https://doi.org/10.1007/S00127-015-1076-4

Schauer, M., Neuner, F., & Elbert, T. (2011). *Narrative Exposure Therapy: A Short-Term Treatment for Traumatic Stress Disorders* (2nd ed.). Cambridge, MA: Hogrefe Publishing.

Schwartze, D., Barkowski, S., Strauss, B., Knaevelsrud, C., & Rosendahl, J. (2019). Efficacy of group psychotherapy for posttraumatic stress disorder: systematic review and meta-analysis of randomized controlled trials. *Psychotherapy Research*, 29(4), 415–431. https://doi.org/10.1080/10503307.2017.1405168

Seymour-Smith, M., Cruwys, T., Haslam, S. A., & Brodribb, W. (2017). Loss of group memberships predicts depression in postpartum mothers. *Social Psychiatry and Psychiatric Epidemiology*, 52(2), 201–210. https://doi.org/10.1007/S00127-016-1315-3

Shapiro, F. (2017). *Eye Movement Desensitization and Reprocessing (EMDR) Therapy: Basic Principles, Protocols, and Procedures*. New York: Guilford Publications.

Shea, M. T., Devitt-Murphy, M., Ready, D. J., & Schnurr, P. P. (2009). Group therapy. In E. B. Foa, T. M. Keane, M. J. Friedman, & J. A. Cohen (Eds.) *Effective Treatments for PTSD: Practice Guidelines from the International Society for Traumatic Stress Studies*. New York: Guilford Publications.

Sloan DM, Feinstein BA, Gallagher MW, Beck JG, Keane TM. (2013). Efficacy of group treatment for posttraumatic stress disorder symptoms: a meta-analysis. *Psychological Trauma: Theory, Research, Practice, and Policy*, 5(2), 176–83. https://doi.org/10.1037/A0026291

Solomon, E. P., & Heide, K. M. (2005). The biology of trauma: implications for treatment. *Journal of Interpersonal Violence*, 20(1), 51–60.

Stalker, C. A. & Fry, R. (1999). A comparison of short-term group and individual therapy for sexually abused women. *The Canadian Journal of Psychiatry*, 44, 168–174.

Talbot, N. L., Houghtalen, R., Cyrulik, S., Betz, A., Barkun, M., Duberstein, P., & Wynne, L. C. (1998). Women's safety in recovery: group therapy for patients with a history of childhood sexual abuse. *Psychiatric Services*, 49 (2), 213–217.

Taylor, J., Mclean, L., Korner, A., Stratton, E. & Glozier, N. (2020). Mindfulness and yoga for psychological trauma: systematic review and meta-analysis. *Journal of Trauma & Dissociation*, 21(5), 536–573. https://doi.org/10.1080/15299732.2020.1760167

Tempone-Wiltshire, J. (2024). The role of mindfulness and embodiment in group-based trauma treatment. *Psychotherapy and Counselling Journal of Australia*, 12(1), 1–27. https://doi.org/10.59158/001c.94979

Toshishige, Y., Kondo, M., & Akechi, T., (2022). Interpersonal psychotherapy for complex posttraumatic stress disorder related to childhood physical and emotional abuse with great severity of depression: a case report. *Asia-Pacific Psychiatry*, 14(3), e12504. https://doi.org/10.1111/Appy.12504

Van Der Kolk, B. A., Van Der Hart, O., & Marmar, C. R. (1996). Dissociation and information processing in posttraumatic stress disorder. In B. A. Van Der Kolk, A. C. McFarlane, & L. Weisaeth (Eds.), *Traumatic Stress: The Effects of Overwhelming Experience on Mind, Body, and Society*. New York: Guilford Press, 303–327.

van Minnen, A., Zoellner, L. A., & Harned, M. S. (2015). Changes in comorbid conditions after prolonged exposure for PTSD: a literature review. *Current Psychiatry Reports*, 17(3), 549. https://doi.org/10.1007/S11920-015-0549-1

Walter, Z. C., Jetten, J., Dingle, G. A., Parsell, C., & Johnstone, M. (2016). Two pathways through adversity: predicting well-being and housing outcomes among homeless service users. *British Journal of Social Psychology*, 55(2), 357–374. https://doi.org/10.1111/Bjso.12127

Walsh, R. S., Muldoon, O. T., Gallagher, S., & Fortune, D. G. (2015). Affiliative and "self-as-doer" identities: relationships between social identity, social support, and emotional status amongst survivors of acquired brain injury (ABI). *Neuropsychological Rehabilitation*, 25(4), 555–573. https://doi.org/10.1080/09602011.2014.993658

Wolfsdorf, B. A., & Zlotnick, C. (2001). Affect management in group therapy for women with posttraumatic stress disorder and histories of childhood sexual abuse. *Journal of Clinical Psychology*, 57(2), 169–181. https://doi.org/10.1002/1097-4679(200102)57:2<169::AID-JCLP4>3.0.CO;2-0

World Health Organization. (2022). Geneva, Switzerland: *International Statistical Classification of Diseases and Related Health Problems* (11th ed.). Https://Icd.Who.Int/

Yalom, I. D. & Leszcz, M. (2020). *The Theory and Practice of Group Psychotherapy* (6th ed.). New York: Basic Books.

Younan, R., Farrell, J. & May, T. (2018). "Teaching me to parent myself": the feasibility of an in-patient group schema therapy program for complex trauma. *Behavioral and Cognitive Psychotherapy*, 46(4), 463–478.

Young, J. E., Klosko, J. S., & Weishaar, M. E. (2003). *Schema therapy: A practitioner's guide*. New York: Guilford Press.

Chapter 3

Schema Therapy and Early Childhood Trauma

Schema Therapy is a therapeutic approach designed to address deeply ingrained patterns, known as schemas, that often originate from unmet emotional needs in childhood (Young et al., 2003). The integrative and experiential nature of Schema Therapy makes it a fitting model from which to conceptualize the treatment of early childhood trauma. There is a significant overlap between the goals of Schema Therapy and those of trauma-informed care, both of which focus on changing the meaning of past events while strengthening a psychologically healthy, mature, and reflective way of being in the present. Schema Therapy helps people "disengage from unhelpful patterns of relating to past experiences and strive for healthy and well-balanced behavior" (Roediger et al., 2018, p. 2). The childhood origins of these problems are linked to their expression in current behaviors, thoughts, and maladaptive coping strategies that tend to perpetuate entrenched patterns.

The primary objectives of Schema Therapy in addressing childhood trauma involve several key goals. These include identifying and transforming the self-defeating patterns developed in response to unmet emotional needs during childhood (Early Maladaptive Schema, EMS). Therapists play a central and reassuring role in guiding a process designed to fulfill these unmet needs (e.g., safety and secure attachment), enhance emotional regulation, and promote healthier coping mechanisms (Boterhoven de Haan, et al., 2021; Van Dijk, et al., 2023). The modification of the maladaptive schemas and dysfunctional coping modes through techniques such as limited reparenting, empathic confrontation, imagery rescripting, and mode dialogues promotes healing, especially in the context of trauma. Strengthening the Healthy Adult (HA) mode helps moderate the dysfunctional modes and supports behavioral change. The group format offers a supportive environment where participants can collaboratively practice challenging dysfunctional coping while reinforcing the HA mode and promoting personal healing and growth after early childhood trauma.

DOI: 10.4324/9781003462958-4

Schemas

Schemas are enduring, lifelong patterns encompassing memories, body sensations, emotions, and thoughts that form the lens through which we view our world. They develop early in life and guide our understanding of feelings, behaviors, life experiences, and beliefs about self and others. They can result from adverse childhood experiences relating to a *toxic frustration of needs, traumatization, overindulgence or overprotectiveness,* and *overidentification with significant others* (Young et al., 2003; Edwards, 2013). They continue to be elaborated and superimposed on later life experiences, often without conscious awareness of their impact. Schemas are self-perpetuating and resistant to change as they fight for their survival.

Schema formation is significantly influenced by whether or not basic needs (safety, predictability, secure and loving relationships, competence, autonomy, independence, freedom to express emotions openly, clear boundaries, spontaneity, and playfulness) are met. Attachment theory posits that a safe haven (attachment) provides a secure base for venturing into the world (autonomy). Roediger et al. (2018) build on this when they describe these basic needs as two "legs" or poles necessary to maintain balance and flexibility. The attachment leg reflects the "we," the essential need for connection to survive, while the autonomy leg represents the "me," the equally important need for autonomy, self-reliance, and assertiveness.

Core maladaptive schemas develop when primary attachment and autonomy needs are unmet due to adverse experiences, leading to pervasive feelings of disconnection, rejection, helplessness, dependency, and inadequacy. Automatic and unconscious self-destructive beliefs and behavior patterns cause a confusing, emotionally distressing, and imbalanced view of self and others. The child may come to believe she is fundamentally flawed, unlovable, unsafe, and unwanted, that others will intentionally cause harm, that emotional needs will never be met, or that others will leave them (Mistrust/Abuse, Emotional Deprivation, Abandonment/Instability, and Defectiveness/Shame) (Young, 1990; Yalcin et al., 2022). The persistent fear of imminent disaster or harm, the belief that one needs significant help to handle daily responsibilities, and the pervasive feeling of loneliness and alienation can lead to schemas that significantly limit autonomy, independence, and competence. Other-directed schemas (e.g., self-sacrifice, unrelenting standards, or emotional inhibition) may develop as automatic, compensatory coping styles to avoid activating core maladaptive schema. Mistrust/Abuse, Vulnerability to Harm, and Emotional Deprivation schema are especially significant in the development of PTSD (Karatzias et al., 2016).

Young (1990) identified 18 EMS, further elaborated by Yalcin (2022). These include:

1 Abandonment: The expectation that one will lose anyone with whom an emotional attachment is formed, that close relationships will end ("Eventually people I love will leave me").
2 Mistrust: The expectation that others will hurt, abuse, humiliate, cheat, lie, manipulate, or take advantage (I can't let my guard down or trust anyone).
3 Emotional Deprivation: The expectation that others will not adequately meet one's need for healthy emotional support (nurturance, empathy, protection) ("I don't matter, I can't rely on anyone to meet my needs")
4 Defectiveness/Shame: The feeling that one is defective, bad, unwanted, inferior, unloveable ("I'm not good enough", "there is something wrong with me").
5 Social Isolation: Feeling isolated from the rest of the world, different ("I don't belong; I'm different").
6 Failure: The belief that one has or will fail relative to others ("Nothing I do is as good as other people; I won't succeed no matter how hard I try").
7 Dependence: Feels incapable of functioning independently without help from others. ("I am helpless; I can't cope alone").
8 Vulnerability to Harm/Illness: Exaggerated fear that imminent catastrophe will strike and can't be prevented ("I'm not safe; I can't protect myself; I am vulnerable").
9 Enmeshment/Undeveloped self: Excessive emotional involvement and closeness with significant others at the expense of full individuation and normal social development ("I don't know who I am; I can't separate myself from others").
10 Subjugation: Excessive surrendering of control (of needs/emotions) because one feels coerced to avoid anger, retaliation, and abandonment ("I am powerless; If I say what I really feel, I will be punished").
11 Self-Sacrifice: Excessive focus on voluntarily meeting the needs of others in daily situations at the expense of one's gratification—to prevent causing pain, avoid guilt, and maintain connection. ("My own needs aren't important; It is selfish to do things for myself").
12 Emotion Constriction: The excessive inhibition or disconnection of spontaneous emotion, action, or expression due to underlying shame/embarrassment ("Showing emotions means I'm weak/vulnerable; It is foolish to be emotional").
13 Fear of Losing Control: The excessive inhibition or disconnection of spontaneous emotion, action, or expression due to a fear that one would otherwise lose control of their impulses (fear of being overwhelmed, fear of other's responses, fear of harming oneself/others, fear

of overindulging). ("If I show how I feel, it will cause damage; I won't be able to stop; I won't be able to cope").

14 Unrelenting Standards: The belief that one must meet high internalized standards to avoid criticism that results in significant impairment in pleasure, relaxation, self-esteem, and relationships (perfectionism, rigid rules, preoccupation with time/efficiency). ("I have to be perfect; I can't accept 'good enough'").

15 Entitlement-Grandiosity: The belief that one is superior to others, entitled to special rights and privileges, not bound by rules ("I deserve special treatment; I should be able to do whatever I want").

16 Insufficient Self-Control: Pervasive difficulty or refusal to exercise self-control and frustration tolerance to achieve one's goals—"discomfort avoidance." ("I can't control my behavior; I can't tolerate discomfort).

17 Approval-Seeking: Excessive emphasis on gaining approval, recognition, or attention from others or fitting in at the expense of developing a secure sense of self. ("I only have value if others say so; I am only worthwhile if I am getting attention/praise").

18 Negativity/Pessimism: Pervasive focus on the negative aspects of life while minimizing or neglecting the positive aspects ("Bad things always happen to me; If things are good, it is only temporary").

19 Punitiveness (Attacking Self-Internalizing): Self-directed hypercriticalness towards one's mistakes, suffering, imperfection, the belief that one should be punished for failing to meet expectations that leads to self-blame, self-directed anger, and lack of forgiveness. ("I deserve to be punished; I should have known better").

20 Punitiveness (Attacking Others-Externalizing): Hypercriticalness towards others' mistakes, suffering, or imperfections; the belief they should be punished for their indiscretions; preoccupation with concepts of justice. ("There is no excuse for mistakes; It's all their fault").

Schemas are hidden and "sleep" in the background until they "wake up." A situation similar to a defining childhood experience may trigger or activate a schema (Roediger et al., 2018, p. 23) that distorts and disrupts present awareness and experiences. The responses to schema activation include schema surrender (giving in to the schema), schema avoidance (dodging the schema), and schema compensation (fighting the schema). For example, the COVID-19 pandemic may have triggered a schema associated with a lack of safety or vulnerability to harm. One person might avoid public places or wash down all groceries even after the threat has passed. At the same time, another might defy precautions or reject vaccinations as they fight the vulnerability to harm schema. A failing marriage may trigger a schema related to rejection, abandonment, or failure, avoiding further intimate connections or seeking new relationships that perpetuate the schema.

The EMS most often associated with early childhood trauma include abandonment, mistrust/abuse, emotional deprivation, and defectiveness schemas, depending on the nature of the trauma. Repeatedly triggered schemas become rigid, inflexible, and self-defeating reactions embedded in the body, even when they are no longer applicable. This can lead to the reenactment of past traumatic experiences in relationships, the selection of partners that mirror early childhood relationships, and difficulty maintaining healthy boundaries and independent functioning. A person may also struggle to regulate their emotions, experience chronic anxiety and hypervigilance, and have persistent negative expectations about relationships and safety that make it difficult to trust others and form secure attachments.

Schema Modes

When schemas are activated, we can experience sudden, intense floods of feelings, thoughts, and behaviors embodying different internal states. These *schema modes* are the moment-to-moment emotional states that shape how we respond and cope when our "emotional buttons" are pushed. Each mode feels different, with different subjectively experienced qualities (Lazarus & Rafaeli, 2023). Dysfunction occurs when a mode, as "a part of the self," is "cut off from other parts of the self" (Young et al., 2003, p. 40, as cited in Edwards, 2022, p. 2).

Modes show up in the therapy room in a way that represents the broad spectrum of human reactions. A person with an emotional deprivation schema might surrender to the schema, believing the schema to be valid without trying to make things better ("I am unlovable and will never have a loving relationship"), actively avoid situations that trigger painful emotional states ("If I don't get close to anyone I can't be hurt"), or overcompensate by fighting back against the schema ("I can take care of myself. I do not need anyone"). Another person might challenge beliefs resulting from their early experiences as they acknowledge that they *are* worthy of the connection and relationships essential to functioning as a healthy adult.

Difficult life situations trigger reactions comparable to defensive action tendencies. The coping modes help avoid the threat or pain of those experiences through surrender, avoidance, or overcompensating responses that fight against them. For example, if a tiger is in the tree, we may automatically "flip" into a survival mode where we fight back, run away, freeze, reach out to another for rescue, or surrender to the threat. These responses become maladaptive "emotional painkillers" when they result in self-defeating patterns that lead to over or underreactions that hurt us or others in the absence of any threat (Young et al., 2003; Edwards, 2013).

Modes may also reflect a mixture of behaviors or experiences as a collection or sequence rather than one distinct singular state. Simpson (2020) provides an example of a Helpless Surrenderer mode, which encompasses feelings of being dependent, helpless, and needing to be rescued. Depending on context, this mode may manifest with different "flavors" or combinations. It can present as a mixture of surrender or overcompensatory behaviors, aggrieved, passive-aggressive, histrionic (theatrical), sullen ("teenager"), entitled, hopeless, pessimistic, complaining or submissive. A hypervigilant attachment-seeking feature associated with this mode may also be considered a way of coping with abandonment (Edwards, 2022). This example illustrates the complexity inherent in the concept of schema modes.

Over 80 modes have been identified and classified into the four broad categories of *healthy adult, child modes, inner critic (parent) modes, and coping modes (including surrender, detached/avoidant, overcompensator, and ruminative, repetitive, unproductive thinking)*. "The identification and analysis of schema modes is central to Schema Therapy as a basis for case conceptualization and as a guide to practice" (Edwards, 2022, p. 2). Modes may follow each other in *mode sequences* (e.g., a fight with one's partner might activate the vulnerable child (VC) mode and an associated inner critic mode, followed by a switch into a coping mode such as compliant surrender or avoidant protector). *Default modes* are modes that are relatively stable over time. They are often mistaken as a Healthy Adult but may be an overcompensating coping mode. *Blended modes* occur when multiple modes appear simultaneously, often complicating the identification of the person's current mode (e.g., lonely/scared child; helpless surrender/self-pity-victim mode). The reader is referred to Edwards (2022) for an in-depth discussion of schema modes and their importance in case conceptualization.

- *Child modes* are essential survival-based responses that reflect the enduring emotional vulnerability of a young child. The VC mode often carries the emotional weight of past traumas. The VC feels alone, abandoned, unworthy, defective, and unloved because her core emotional needs were not met. The *Angry Child* feels enraged or frustrated, venting the more powerful anger in ways that may hide the underlying vulnerability. The anger or rage may bring attention to the child's unmet need for independence and autonomy ("What about me?"). An *Impulsive or Undisciplined Child* acts in selfish or uncontrolled ways to get her needs met. She may not be able to tolerate a delay of gratification or limit setting and may become easily frustrated. The *Happy Child* (HC) feels loved, safe, and capable. She is playful, joyous, and spontaneous.

- *Dysfunctional Coping Modes* can be viewed as survival defenses that individuals develop to cope with trauma, as a way to protect themselves from the pain of the VC. These include avoidant, overcompensatory, or surrender modes. A person might give in or submit to others as a way to avoid conflict or rejection (Compliant Surrender CS-surrender), avoid painful feelings by shutting down and detaching from emotions (Detached Protector DP-flight/freeze), or engage in activities or substances that soothe or distract (Detached Self-Soother DSS flight/active avoidance), or seek dominance or control as a way to fight against or overcompensate for feelings of vulnerability (Overcompensation-Self-Aggrandizer, Bully/Attack).
- *Inner Critic modes* are internalized critical or demanding voices that often stem from traumatic experiences with caregivers. These internalized messages can be directed toward the self or towards others. The internal voices make unrealistic demands (demanding criticism to be better, try harder, and be perfect) or harsh judgments (the punitive and critical mode that is harsh and unforgiving—you are worthless, unlovable, and a loser).

A Perfectionistic Overcontroller may try to be perfect to avoid underlying vulnerability; a Suspicious Overcontroller may be hypervigilant, rigid, and controlling, or a bully may lash out at others to defend against and hide any weakness. An Avoidant Protector might avoid social interactions to keep others at a distance; an Angry Protector might use anger to drive people away, or a Detached Self-Soother might do or use something to take the pain away, such as using drugs, daydreaming or overfocusing on work. A Compliant Surrenderer might sacrifice their own needs by giving in, pleasing, or appeasing people to gain their approval.

- **The Healthy Adult Mode:** A special word about this mode. It is described as a suite of modes that address the dimensions of healthy functioning by answering the question, "How would a mature, compassionate, and psychologically minded person think, feel, and act in this situation?" (Edwards, 2022). In this mode, a person can step back and reflect on one's experience and that of others (meta-awareness, distancing, diffusion, and detached mindfulness). They can evaluate everyday experiences without denying or avoiding their reality. A Healthy Adult has a clear and consistent sense of their identity concerning personal beliefs, values, and motivations, takes responsibility for their actions, and can be emotionally genuine in relationships with a sense of caring and connection that extends beyond the self.

The Healthy Adult represents an individual's wise, kind, and self-compassionate self, the internal 'good parent' that integrates the functioning of the other modes. It plays a crucial role in healing from trauma. The Healthy Adult (HA) mode offers empathy and emotional support and recognizes and acknowledges feelings compassionately. The HA offers a balanced perspective on challenging situations. It helps to set limits for emotional child modes and moderates dysfunctional critic modes. Somewhat like a 'project manager,' it prioritizes the Vulnerable Child, listens to the Angry Child, directs Maladaptive Coping Modes, challenges and negotiates with the Critic modes, and fosters the spontaneity and happiness of the Happy Child mode. The HA mode adopts a mindful approach to solving problems and making healthier choices when coping with difficult situations.

"Experience shapes what we see and how we see it; a person with a history of abuse and maltreatment looks out at the world mistrustfully and may see a neutral face as threatening" (Edwards, 2014, p. 10). Healing from the effects of early childhood trauma requires understanding the childhood origins of the maladaptive schemas and coping modes that perpetuate the entrenched behavior patterns reflected in their current behaviors and thoughts. Strengthening the HA mode helps transform these dysfunctional strategies into adaptive responses that meet core emotional needs in a healthier, more balanced way.

Schema Healing

Techniques such as limited reparenting, empathic confrontation, imagery rescripting, and mode dialogues serve as the backbone of Schema Therapy, facilitating the modification of maladaptive schemas. Various cognitive, perceptual, and somatic techniques that promote behavioral change are introduced throughout this manual.

- **Limited Reparenting and Empathic Confrontation:** *Limited Reparenting* is a cornerstone of Schema Therapy designed to meet the unmet childhood needs of clients within the bounds of a professional therapeutic relationship. Clients can internalize the "corrective experience" of a caring, nurturing, genuine, and supportive relationship that offsets experiences that were neglectful, unpredictable, or abusive. *Empathic Confrontation* gently challenges the client's self-defeating patterns, maladaptive behaviors, and negative beliefs while validating their origins, fostering self-awareness, and promoting healthier coping strategies. For example, clients might discuss how they tend to isolate themselves for fear of rejection. The therapist, using empathic confrontation, might acknowledge the pain behind this behavior while gently pointing out how it reinforces their abandonment schema and interferes with their need for connection.

- **Experiential Interventions:** Schema Therapy effects behavior change through experiential interventions that activate the emotional intensity necessary for change (imagery rescripting, mode dialogues, and chair work). Emotion-focused and cognitive exercises are core strategies that supplement traditional cognitive behavior techniques. These interventions help rescript the client's painful early experiences and challenge the self-defeating patterns and maladaptive beliefs. The therapy relationship, imagery rescripting, mode dialogues, and chair work activate the emotional memory, promote rapid changes in the brain, and weaken the impact of self-defeating patterns as new information is connected to the activated schema (Roediger et al., 2018).
- **Imagery and Imagery Rescripting** involves revisiting and reimagining past traumatic experiences more positively and adaptively. Imagery creates an "affect bridge" that links schema to their childhood origins. It can be used diagnostically (to identify unmet needs), to build resources (safe place imagery, caring for the VC), and to create a corrective emotional experience that changes the meaning of the early experiences and strengthens the HA mode. Rescripting the narrative provides emotional resolution for past traumas, empowering clients to modify their maladaptive schemas and core negative beliefs and envision a different future.
- **Mode Dialogues** (and Chair Work) help clients understand and interact with different aspects of themselves. Speaking from the chair, representing the voice of different modes and symptoms, or another person increases awareness of different emotional states and coping mechanisms, facilitates internal communication and integration, supports perspective changes, reduces experiential avoidance, and strengthens the HA mode.

The reader is referred to Roediger et al. (2018), Kellogg & Garcia Torres (2021), and van der Winjgaart (2021) for in-depth instructions for all these interventions.

The Goal of Schema Therapy

The primary goal of ST is to strengthen the HA mode so that a person is a "good parent" to themselves. They can then better achieve an emotionally regulated life with fulfilling relationships and personal and professional satisfaction. The Healthy Adult meets the VC's need for care and comfort, and it substitutes maladaptive coping modes with more adaptive responses that reflect their adult experience. The Healthy Adult expresses emotions directly and assertively and makes wise decisions rather than resorting to self-defeating patterns that may have negative consequences. It replaces the messages of the inner critic modes with a self-compassionate voice.

Group Schema Therapy

Group Schema Therapy combines the therapeutic factors of groups described by Yalom (Yalom & Lesczez, 2005) with Schema Therapy's hallmark cognitive, experiential, and behavioral pattern-breaking interventions. It offers advantages that enhance individual ST: mutual support, trust, and a sense of belonging between group members, as well as more opportunities to experiment with expressing emotions and new behaviors. For example, the empathic confrontation offered by group members in response to undesirable behavior might be more effective than confrontation by a therapist alone (Farrell, 2012; Farrell & Shaw, 2012).

Farrell and Shaw (2012) developed a distinctive and comprehensive approach to treatment for Borderline Personality Disorder that differs from other approaches. This Group Schema Therapy approach has been effective in reducing Borderline Personality Disorder (BPD) symptoms, improving quality of life, and with fewer dropouts in both outpatient and inpatient settings. A recent study found that the combination of group and individual ST required one year less treatment than individual ST alone (Arntz et al., 2022). Its effectiveness has also been demonstrated as a short-term treatment for patients not requiring long-term treatment (Broersen & van Vreeswijk, 2012), with those who have mixed personality disorders (Skewes et al., 2015; Nenadić et al., 2017; Dadomoa et al., 2018), severe anxiety (Straarup et al., 2022; Balj et al., 2024), eating disorders (Simpson, 2020) and in a psychodynamic format that integrates knowledge and techniques from ST, psychodynamic and group dynamic therapies (Aalders & Van Dijk, 2012).

Schema Therapy and the Trauma-Focused Group

Schema Therapy offers a promising approach for the group treatment of Complex Trauma. There is a significant overlap between Complex Trauma and BPD, with a majority of BPD clients having a history of trauma (Cloitre et al., 2013). Both groups struggle to regulate emotions, maintain a coherent sense of self, and sustain healthy relationships. These complex reactions to severe stressors are viewed as adaptations to the environment where there is no escape or opportunity to learn standard developmental skills (Courtois & Ford, 2009).

The rapid mode shifts in BPD can be compared to the innate survival actions and dissociated states seen in complex trauma, with modes such as the abandoned child mode reflecting the reexperiencing of traumatic past events (Farrell & Shaw, 2012). Shaw et al. (2014) developed a protocol to treat Dissociative Identity Disorder within a group Schema Therapy format. The initial exploration phase focuses on assessment, connection, safety, and establishing a shared definition of problems. During this phase, the patient receives education on the emotional and developmental needs of children, schemas, modes, dissociation, and PTSD. The Schema Therapy Mode Model is used in the second phase of treatment to increase mode awareness and facilitate change. (It should be noted that there is no published research on this form of group therapy).

Younan et al. (2017) demonstrated a reduction of general symptom severity and maladaptive schema modes in patients participating in a four-week inpatient Group Schema Therapy Program for Complex Trauma, which addressed emotion regulation, the narration of trauma memory, cognitive restructuring, identity, and attachment issues. Patients developed a better understanding of the biopsychosocial impact of their experiences, their dysregulation, and complex reactions. Results suggest implementing a modified GST protocol is also feasible for in-patient psychiatric settings.

Incorporating Schema Therapy principles into Group Therapy for Complex Trauma promotes healing on multiple levels as the group "family" supports the treatment of the multifaceted nature of trauma-related issues. This approach helps remediate the interpersonal effects of the schema-driven and mode behaviors of patients. It can mirror family of origin dynamics and can be viewed as a "microcosm of the "outside of therapy" world" (Farrell & Shaw, 2012). Healthy development requires more than individual therapy in experiences that include "family" dynamics.

The group augments the healing experiences for vulnerable group members as it weaves the curative benefits of groups with the active ingredients of ST (limited reparenting, empathic confrontation, experiential and cognitive change, and behavioral pattern breaking). Core symptoms such as abandonment, emptiness, defectiveness, isolation, mistrust, and a lack of belonging are targeted in an environment that offers mutual support, validation by group members, healing internal models of unsafe attachment, and the opportunity to experiment with emotional expression and new behaviors safely.

The therapist is the stable, consistent, supportive, affirming "good parent" who balances the individual needs of each member with the group's collective needs, just as a parent would manage siblings in a family. The therapist and the group provide a corrective emotional experience by offering compassion, validation, and healthy attachment in meeting needs unmet in childhood. This creates a safe, contained environment where patients can explore and begin to understand the effects of their trauma on their current lives. Limited reparenting from the schema perspective requires the therapist to be actively involved, genuine, and "real" in a way that extends the therapeutic alliance. The therapist actively supports, nurtures, sets limits, and challenges ineffective behaviors as the individual's needs are balanced with the group's cumulative needs. The group becomes a safe and supportive family developed and maintained by the "parent-therapists."

Farrell and Shaw (2012) describe using mode imagery in groups. They first introduce the imagery experience using an image of a child in an ice cream shop. They teach safe place imagery before engaging an image of the VC. The group explores their experiences during the imagery exercises. The therapists and the group may delve further when a member has a particularly intense emotional reaction to the imagery to identify the triggers, activated modes, and underlying unmet needs. The individual focus is brief and is aimed at issues shared by the group as the group is brought into individual work rather than individual therapy with the group as observers.

A genuine, accepting, and validating family and peer group offers "corrective experiences" as it helps meet core emotional needs to heal the sequelae of the early traumatic experiences. Psychoeducation about trauma and unmet needs allows bonding around similarities in early experiences. The group provides the opportunity to practice skills as members observe others with similar experiences, identify their cognitive distortions and impulsive actions, learn to tolerate intense emotions, and recognize how their behavior affects others. For example, the therapist might note that the group has expressed concern about a member's behavior in the group (e.g., the tendency to dominate conversations) and refer back to the group to discuss how this impacts the group dynamics and to explore what needs the member might be trying to meet through this behavior. Group members can better receive and accept feedback and express vulnerability when they see that others are not rejected or abandoned when they express complex emotions. Group members are also encouraged to share their photographs as young children to enhance the connection to their VC mode. Validation and empathy toward the traumatized "child" help members bond with therapists and each other and strengthen the commitment to treatment.

Schema mode change, emotional awareness, and regulation occur as coping modes and defensive actions used to avoid painful emotions are addressed. Empathic confrontation and cognitive restructuring help modify the negative core beliefs and schema-driven thoughts and behaviors. Patients learn to understand their emotional needs, minimize maladaptive coping, and strengthen healthy responses, thereby replacing dysfunctional patterns that cause problems in adult life with new, adaptive ways of meeting their needs (Farrell & Shaw, 2012). Self-defeating modes are challenged within the group as the collective presence becomes the container for the different emotions. The safety of this container facilitates mode healing, particularly in the practice of emotion-focused exercises. The group learns to trust that the "parents" will protect them from threats to their well-being as difficult emotions are expressed within the group.

A significant component of GST involves increasing emotional awareness by helping patients notice pre-crisis distress and better understand their emotional experiences and subsequent behaviors. The group provides an environment where these skills can be practiced in vivo. The group "container" also helps regulate conflict and emotions while allowing room for their safe expression. For example, therapists set clear limits around destructive or abusive behaviors while identifying the underlying unmet needs that activated the expressed anger or critical modes. The client's needs can be acknowledged, understood, and validated when expressed from a non-destructive, non-threatening posture.

Farrell and Shaw (2012) describe a group exercise that confronts the Inner Critic mode, where the group writes the negative messages of the critic on a cloth parent figure. The therapists later remove this effigy to highlight its powerlessness to harm. This can be followed by developing a representation of the "good parent" and good parent messages. While individual members may not be able to confront their internalized messages, they can see that nothing happens to others when they do. The HC mode can also be engaged when playful and fun activities are introduced into the group. For example, the group can laugh together as they mimic one another's "passing" stretching movements during a mindfulness exercise.

Summary

The curative factors of groups are harnessed within the trauma group to enhance interpersonal relationships and social functioning. A deep toolbox of cognitive, emotional, and interpersonal interventions that incorporates a Schema Therapy approach helps the participants recognize and gradually accept their internalized beliefs, messages, and personal vulnerability and distinguish their different "sides" or modes to facilitate a healthy integration of a coherent self. The concepts of maladaptive schemas and coping modes provide an additional lens through which group members better understand their emotional and behavioral responses to triggering situations and intrusive material. Individual self-regulation capacity builds on the co-regulation within the group, as the external sense of safety and cohesion facilitates the development of internal safety. As their HA mode strengthens, members learn to set clear boundaries and engage in healthy relationships. The therapists and group together become a powerful vehicle for change, providing opportunities for connection, validation, and the corrective experiences crucial for complex trauma recovery.

The regulation of autonomic arousal (widening the window of tolerance, the group members' understanding of emotions, and increasing their ability to identify, tolerate, and regulate their emotional experiences) is a core goal of trauma-focused treatment. PTSD symptoms decrease as the group members learn skills to manage triggers, intrusive symptoms, hyperarousal, and dissociation. They can better stay in their window as they develop resources for stabilization and managing dysregulation. Group discussions and experiences aid the member's thoughtful reflection on the impact of their early experiences. The group learns how early traumatic experiences shape the development of schemas and modes. They learn to identify maladaptive schemas and coping modes and understand their emotional and behavioral responses to triggers. Current information about the effects of early traumatic experiences on the nervous system's ability to process information and memories, detect threats, regulate arousal, and promote social engagement enhances the group's understanding of their experiences. Experiential activities such as imagery, chair work, and mode dialogues are incorporated throughout the text to allow participants to access and process the impact of their past trauma.

This book does not attempt to replicate the Group Schema Therapy approach designed by Farrell and Shaw (2012). Instead, the Schema Therapy framework is presented here as a coherent way to integrate the concepts, perspectives, and exercises from the broader literature on complex trauma.

References

Aalders, H. & Van Dijk, J. (2012). Schema therapy in a psychodynamic group. In M. Van Vreeswijk, J. Broersen, & M. Nadort (Eds.), *The Wiley-Blackwell Handbook of Schema Therapy: Theory, Research and Practice* (1st ed.). New York: John Wiley & Sons, Ltd, 383–390.

Arntz, A., Jacob, G. A., Lee, C. W., et al.(2022) Effectiveness of predominantly group schema therapy and combined individual and group schema therapy for borderline personality disorder: a randomized clinical trial. *JAMA Psychiatry*, 79(4), 287–299. https://doi.org/10.1001/jamapsychiatry.2022.0010

Balj´, A. E., Anja Greeven, A., Deen, M. Van Giezen, A. E., Arntz, A., & Spinhoven, P. (2024) Group schema therapy versus group cognitive behavioral therapy for patients with social anxiety disorder and comorbid avoidant personality disorder: a randomized controlled trial. *Journal of Anxiety Disorders*, 104, 102860. https://doi.org/10.1016/j.janxdis.2024.102860

Broersen, J. & van Vreeswijk, M. (2012). Schema therapy in groups: a short-term schema CBT protocol. In M. van Vreeswijk, J. Broersen, & M. Nadort (Eds.), *The Wiley-Blackwell Handbook of Schema Therapy: Theory, Research, and Practice* (1st ed.). New York: John Wiley & Sons, Ltd, 374–381.

Boterhoven de Haan, K. L., Lee, C.W., Correia, H., Menninga, S., Fassbinder, E., Köehne, S., & Arntz, A. (2021). Patient and therapist perspectives on treatment for adults with PTSD from childhood trauma. *Journal of Clinical Medicine*, 10(5), 954. https://doi.org/10.3390/jcm10050954

Cloitre, M., Garvert, D. W., Brewin, C. R., Bryant, R. A., & Maercker, A. (2013). Evidence for proposed ICD-11 PTSD and Complex PTSD: a latent profile analysis. *European Journal of Psychotraumatology*, 4(1), 10.3402/ejpt.v4i0.20706. https://doi.org/10.3402/ejpt.v4i0.20706

Courtois, C. A., & Ford, J. D. (Eds.). (2009). *Treating complex traumatic stress disorders: An evidence-based guide*. New York: The Guilford Press.

Dadomoa, H., Panzeric, M., Caponcelloc, D., Carmelitad, A., & Grecuccie, A., (2018). Schema therapy for emotional dysregulation in personality disorders: a review. *Current Opinion in Psychiatry*, 31, 43–49.

Edwards, D. (2013). *Using Schema and Schema Modes as a Basis for Formulation and Treatment Planning in Schema Therapy*. www.schematherapysouthafrica.Co.Za

Edwards, D. (2014). Schemas in clinical practice: what are they, and how can we change them? *APA: Independent Practitioner: Bulletin of Psychologists in Independent Practice*, 34(1), 10–13.

Edwards, D. J. (2022). Using schema modes for case conceptualization in schema therapy: an applied clinical approach. *Frontiers in Psychology*, *12*, 763670. https://doi.org/10.3389/fpsyg.2021.763670

Farrell, J.M. (2012). Introduction to group schema therapy. In M. Van Vreeswijk, J. Broersen, & M. Nadort (Eds.), *The Wiley-Blackwell Handbook of Schema Therapy: Theory, Research and Practice*. New York: John Wiley & Sons, Ltd, first edition, 337–340.

Farrell, J.M., & Shaw, I.A. (2012). *Group Schema Therapy for Borderline Personality Disorder: A Step-by-Step Treatment Manual with Patient Workbook*. New York: John Wiley & Sons.

Karatzias, T., Jowett, S., Begley, A., & Deas, S. (2016). Early maladaptive schemas in adult survivors of interpersonal trauma: foundations for a cognitive theory of psychopathology. *The European Journal of Psychotraumatology*, 7, 30713. https://doi.org/10.3402/Ejpt.V7.30713

Kellogg, S. & Garcia Torres, A. (2021). Toward a chairwork psychotherapy. *Practice Innovations*, 6(3), 171–180. https://doi.org/10.1037/pri0000149

Lazarus, G. & Rafaeli, E. (2023). Modes: Cohesive personality states and their interrelationships in organizing concepts in psychopathology. *Journal of Psychopathology and Clinical Science*, 132(3), 238–248. https://doi.org/10.1037/abn0000699

Nenadić, I., Lamberth, S., & Reiss, N., (2017). Group schema therapy for personality disorders: a pilot study for implementation in acute psychiatric in-patient settings. *Psychiatry Research* 253, 9–12.

Ozgur, Y., Ida, M., Christopher, L., & Helen, C. (2022). Revisions to the Young Schema Questionnaire using Rasch Analysis: the YSQ-R. *Australian Psychologist*, 57(1), 8–20. https://doi.org/10.1080/00050067.2021.1979885

Roediger, E., Stevens, B. A., & Brockman, R. (2018). *Contextual Schema Therapy: An Integrative Approach to Personality Disorders, Emotional Dysregulation & Interpersonal Functioning*. Oakland, CA: Context Press.

Shaw, I., Farrell, J., Rijkeboer, M. M., Huntjens, R. J. C., & Arntz, A. (2014). *Schema Therapy for Dissociative Identity Disorder: A Treatment Protocol*. Unpublished Manuscript.

Simpson, S. (2020). Manual of group schema therapy for eating disorders, OaklOa. In S. Simpson & E. Smith (Eds.), *Schema Therapy for Eating Disorders: Theory and Practice for Individual and Group Settings*. London: Routledge, 136–184.

Skewes, S. A., Samson, R. A., Simpson, S. G., & van Vreeswijk, M. (2015). Short-term group schema therapy for mixed personality disorders: a pilot study. *Frontiers in Psychology*, 22(5), 1592. https://doi.org/10.3389/Fpsyg.2014.01592

Straarup, N. S., Renneberg, H. B., Farrell, J., & Younan, R. (2022). Group schema therapy for patients with severe anxiety disorders. *Journal of Clinical Psychology*, 78, 1590–1600. https://doi.org/10.1002/Jclp.23351

Van Dijk, S. D., Veenstra, M. S., Van den Brink, R. H., Van Alphen, S. P., & Oude Voshaar, R. C. (2023). A systematic review of the heterogeneity of schema therapy. *Journal of Personality Disorders*, 37(2), 233–262. https://doi.org/10.1521/pedi.2023.37.2.262

van der Winjgaart, R. (2021). *Imagery Rescripting: Theory and Practice*. Glasgow: Pavilion Publishing & Media Ltd.

Yalcin, O., Marais, I., Lee, C. & Correia, H. (2022). Revisions to the young schema questionnaire using Rasch. analysis: the YSQ-R. *Australian Psychologist*, 57(1), 8–20. https://doi.org/10.1080/00050067.2021.1979885

Yalom, I.D. and Leszcz, M. (2005) *The Theory and Practice of Group Psychotherapy*. 5th Edition. New York: Basic Books.

Younan, R., Farrell, J., & May, T. (2017). Teaching me to parent myself: the feasibility of an inpatient group schema therapy program for complex trauma. *Behavioral and Cognitive Psychotherapy*, 46(4), 463–478. https://doi.org/10.1017/S1352465817000698

Young, J. E. (1990). *Cognitive Therapy for Personality Disorders: A Schema-Focused Approach*. Sarasota, FL: Professional Resource Press.

Young, J. E., Klosko, J., & Weishaar, M. E. (2003). *Schema Therapy: A Practitioner's Guide*. New York: Guilford.

Chapter 4

Building Safety in the Group

Building Safety

Providing a safe space to explore the impact of early childhood trauma is the primary organizing principle for a trauma-informed group. Safety, as it is used here, refers not only to the absence of real-world external threats such as life-threatening experiences, domestic violence, ongoing abuse, addictions, or other harmful situations but also to establishing a stable and predictable atmosphere for all participants. Trust, a fundamental requirement for trauma survivors who join the group with some level of guardedness, mistrust, or suspicion, is something that the group leaders play a crucial role in fostering. Physical and emotional vulnerability can be triggered by the uncertainty of the new environment, new people, and new expectations. Boundaries may feel violated by group dynamics that elicit powerlessness, helplessness, fear, shame, inadequacy, isolation, or anger.

The therapist's role is pivotal in managing the group dynamics, pacing the therapy, and being emotionally available to build and maintain safety. This ongoing process requires consistent monitoring and fine-tuning throughout the group therapy. The therapist is the stable, solid, calm, and wise anchor who manages her reactions with minimal activation and keeps the group from spinning out of control. The image of a wise and grounded Buddha anchored in a sea of chaos, turmoil, and the unknown captures the essence of this role, providing a sense of security and stability to the group.

Lisa described a time she noticed a client quietly withdrawing from the group. The client appeared "lost at sea" as she disappeared amid the group. Lisa guessed that the client, new to the group, may have felt overwhelmed and bewildered by the demands and expectations of the group. She noted the client's withdrawal as she gently "reeled" her back in. A subtle acknowledgment of her presence offered her a lifeline to reconnect to the group. Lisa's nonintrusive observations of the client ("I noticed you nodded your head") signaled to the client and the rest of the group that she was seen and conveyed that her reticence was understood and respected. Lisa and

DOI: 10.4324/9781003462958-5

the group were willing to meet the member where she was until she felt
safe enough to engage gradually at her own pace.

At times, though, the group can feel predatory and threatening for both the leader and the members, like a tiger waiting to pounce. It is a struggle to stay fully present when it feels like walking on eggshells. The therapist may feel like a walking target, with the urge to run away rather than stay the course. The group can be derailed by a lack of cooperation, unwillingness to participate, fear and mistrust, sabotage, inflexibility, hypervigilance, and defensiveness. Therapists may fear not being able to manage the intense emotions in the group (Who let me run this group? Did I open a Pandora's Box?). They may become overly cautious to avoid becoming a perpetrator. Members can feel endangered when pushed too fast or too far beyond their limits, when they feel misunderstood or think the therapist has a different agenda. The client may remain on guard against possible dangers and be unable to relax when the leader cannot manage other members' behaviors (e.g., when another member monopolizes the group or is disruptive). Even in the absence of imminent danger, a non-threatening situation may be dysregulating and perceived as threatening to the person with a narrow Window of Tolerance and difficulty regulating emotions. The therapist is faced with fostering an environment free of real-world threats while still challenging the group to tolerate their discomfort as they address traumatic material. Sometimes, this may mean that clients may be pushed to the edge of their Window of Tolerance.

Consistency, predictability, and respect for personal boundaries increase the feeling of safety within the group. Group leaders who demonstrate consistent, reliable behavior and create predictable routines and structure in sessions build safety into the group process. The active management of group dynamics and balanced participation allows the group to develop without rushing through the process. When clear ground rules and boundaries for respectful interaction are established, and boundary violations are immediately enforced, group members learn what to expect and avoid rude surprises. The group is free to assimilate new information and evolve at its own pace, confident that it is in good hands.

The Therapy Relationship

Safety builds on the relationships in the group, developing resources and strengths and providing a context for the client's life that allows them to understand why they feel and act the way they do ("I am not crazy; this is why I feel this way"). Progress occurs when the participants can access feelings that have been suppressed for so long that they fear going near them. Imagine red fireworks embodying the fear, rage, or urges to fight or run held in these emotions, or the image of a pacing tiger in a cage ready to pounce as long-standing emotions wait to be unleashed.

Members can better regulate, speak up, and share the feelings that may be outside their comfort zone when they feel understood and supported by the group.

The importance of the interpersonal elements of the therapeutic relationship in addressing trauma has been consistently supported in therapy outcome literature (Dalenberg, 2004; Courtois & Ford, 2013; Cronin et al., 2014). The therapeutic relationship is considered the most important gauge of successful treatment and healing (Briere & Scott, 2015). The group leader's role is to be a "good parent" to the group "family." It is to offer "limited reparenting" and a "corrective experience" within the therapeutic relationship's safety, stability, and boundaries. Authenticity and genuineness are the cornerstones for treating complex trauma.

"Limited Reparenting" (Schema Therapy, Young et al., 2003) describes the therapist's role in building a healthy "surrogate" family within the group. The group therapist is a stable, consistent, supportive, affirming "good parent" who balances the individual needs of the patient with the collective needs of the group, similar to the way a parent handles siblings in a family (Farrell & Shaw, 2012). The therapist models healthy parenting by fostering a warm, accepting atmosphere that provides emotional safety for the group and increases the sense of connection and belonging. While the therapist provides some reparenting, group members can also offer each other support and validation, creating a "corrective family" experience.

Warmth, genuineness, acceptance, inclusion, and validation of the patients by the therapists and other group members help heal maladaptive schema (Rogers, 1973). Within this "holding environment," group members can better identify, explore, and "empathically confront" self-defeating core themes and coping responses that interfere with meeting needs (Winnicott, 1969). The therapist can validate group members' feelings and experiences related to their trauma, providing the emotional attunement that may have been lacking in childhood. Group discussions and exercises can focus on identifying and addressing unmet childhood needs in age-appropriate ways. These two interventions, *limited reparenting,* and *empathic confrontation* provide the "corrective emotional experience" and the vehicle for change as the client's self-defeating patterns are empathically challenged (Edwards, 2022). In this context, the group provides the crucible in which the battle is fought, and change can occur.

The "limited reparenting" role can be challenging and requires careful group dynamics and boundaries management. The therapist must be mindful not to create dependency or favoritism (sibling rivalry?) and to encourage appropriate peer support while maintaining their role as group leader. Being a "good parent" also requires that therapists recognize their limitations and vulnerabilities and know when the group triggers them.

What is stirred up when working with clients with complex trauma? When triggered, how can the therapist care for the needs of their own "vulnerable child" along with the needs of the group's "vulnerable children"? Awareness and tolerance of the complexity of all reactions teach group members how to understand and tolerate their vulnerability.

Group Cohesion

Cohesion is considered a central and necessary mechanism of change in groups. Group cohesion is the equivalent of the therapeutic alliance in individual therapy. The consistency, attunement, responsiveness, kindness, compassion, warmth, openness, honesty, empathy, predictability, and flexibility provided by the therapist are all vital in promoting cohesion in the group. While the therapeutic alliance focuses on the patient-therapist relationship, group cohesion encompasses the relationships among all group members and the overall sense of group unity. Schore (2019) suggested that the group's attachment bonds, emotional connections, shared experiences, and coregulation represent the implicit "invisible" glue holding them together as they navigate the impact of their traumatic experiences. Group rituals such as the morning mindfulness practice, check-ins, and shared group exercises create a sense of belonging that fosters cohesion, reinforces the collective experience, and counteracts the isolation often experienced by trauma survivors.

Group cohesion creates a network of supportive relationships that enhance the therapeutic environment. The therapist facilitates shared experiences and mutual support within the group as they encourage the members to offer support and feedback to each other rather than relying solely on the therapist. Recognizing shared experiences deepens the group's connection (e.g., "It sounds like both Sarah and John have experienced similar challenges with trusting others after their traumas," "Has anyone else had a similar experience? What helped you cope?").

"The Connecting Web Exercise" (Farrell & Shaw, 2012) is a way to facilitate bonding and cohesion and establish a felt sense of connection to the group. Just as a spider weaves her web, group members develop their web of connection as they toss a ball of yarn around and hold on to a piece each time it comes to them. They become aware of the strength of connection in the group as they tighten the pull on the yarn or the lack of connection when one or two members release the yarn. The yarn can also make a bracelet that reminds the group of their connection. Beads can be added to signify different experiences in the group. In between sessions, each member can visualize their connection to the group as they feel the pull of the string and experience how all are linked together.

Risk Management

Assessing and managing risk and establishing crisis intervention guidelines begin during intake and screening. This involves the initial risk assessment, psychoeducation, a commitment to safety, and sufficient resources to regulate difficult emotions. Addressing the group's potential to elicit overwhelming emotions and identifying, anticipating, and managing triggers can help reduce the intensity of high-risk urges. Developing relationships with the client's treatment team and a cope-ahead plan to manage crises prepares the client to navigate the urges when they arise. Having sufficient skills and resources to manage personal risk and emotional overwhelm is a prerequisite for group participation, particularly in traditional outpatient settings where minimal resources may exist to manage risk. It may be necessary to screen out individuals if they cannot safely engage in the group's discussions.

Building Skills and Resources

Building safety also means helping the client learn skills and strengthen self-regulation and co-regulation resources. Self-regulation is the ability to calm oneself when either hypo or hyper-aroused. Coregulation uses the soothing aspects of relationships as the bridge to soothing oneself. The client learns they can rely on their internal resources and reach out to others for help. Early childhood trauma often creates a state where the individual does not trust their feelings, does not know what they need, and cannot self-soothe. They may not have had someone to comfort them and have learned to avoid reaching out. Schema coping modes may have been resources or strategies outside a person's conscious awareness that helped them survive. They may have become rigid and automatic over time, so increasing awareness of their origin and function is important. How did this mode or survival strategy help the individual get through difficult times? Is it still helpful?

Feeling safe in the group requires safety in one's own body. Increasing awareness of "mode flipping" helps group members recognize their shifts into dysfunctional coping modes as they develop the resources to help them regulate their emotions without becoming overwhelmed. A resource is anything (skills, objects, relationships, and actions) that supports safety, widens the Window of Tolerance (the zone of optimal arousal where emotional processing and learning can occur concurrently), and helps the client feel safer in their body and better in the moment (Siegel, 1999). These resources increase the person's ability to tolerate a broader range of emotions and somatic experiences and maintain a sense of self that is connected and differentiated from others regardless of what is happening around them, helping them feel empowered and capable (Ogden et al., 2006). Top-down resources include education about trauma-related themes, setting boundaries, managing intrusive symptoms, seeking support, or safety planning. Bottom-up approaches focus on physical and somatic capabilities that widen the Window of Tolerance, including breathing, movement, and visualization.

Enhancing mindfulness, self-awareness, and self-control serves the broader goal of increasing the individual's ability to tolerate a wider range of experiences within their Window of Tolerance (Tempone Wiltshire, 2024). Clients learn to identify distressing sensations held in their bodies and the changes that occur when they practice healthy ways to self-regulate. What do they notice in their body? What sensations do they experience as they practice using different exercises? What helps them feel better? (Do more of this) Worse? (Do less of this). They may already use somatic resources that can be noticed and pointed out. Closing their eyes, taking deep breaths, sighing, turning away, curling up, extending the spine, stroking a part of their body, smiling, and laughing are resources they can utilize when they are outside their Window of Tolerance (Startup & Breidis, 2024). Increasing the usefulness of resources takes time and practice. It is necessary to offer a broad menu as some interventions may be more helpful with individual group members than others.

Resources

1 **Pacing** is a strategic resourcing technique that allows the group to navigate the therapeutic process better. The adage "slower is faster, less is more" guides this approach. It may involve taking breaks during intense therapy sessions or gradually increasing exposure to trauma material to have more control when addressing complex issues.
2 **Distancing, Containment, and Diffusion** create a pause and separation that helps minimize the flooding of emotions. These strategies provide separation from intense, distressing, dysregulating emotions until they can be processed safely within the Window of Tolerance. Therapists serve as a stable container when they remain calm in the face of the client's distressing emotions. The therapist can offer different interventions to help clients avoid dysregulating or overwhelming feelings. Suggestions might include visualizing turning down the volume, switching TV channels, viewing the experience as a picture in a picture or on a fuzzy movie screen, using third-person language to describe experiences, advising a friend in the same situation, imagining locking distressing thoughts/feelings inside a secure container such as a bank vault, writing them down on a piece of paper stored in a box, or putting them in a hot air balloon launched into the atmosphere.

Ginny and Jackie were two group members who reacted differently to group interventions. Ginny voiced skepticism of the containment strategy, stating that she did not believe it possible to "put things on a shelf," especially when flooded by emotions and memories. Jackie, however, shared that she felt more in control of her emotions when she imagined sending a hot air balloon filled with her distressing thoughts and emotions up into the hands of Jesus. Ginny was reminded that practicing these strategies in the Window of Tolerance makes them more accessible when feeling overwhelmed.

3 **Titration** is slowly turning up the dial on a complex topic to find the optimal level of intensity to challenge clients while ensuring they do not become overwhelmed. Instead of diving straight into a complicated topic, the therapist carefully increases the intensity of discussion over time to allow group members to process emotions at a manageable pace. The goal is to find the right balance between promoting growth by gently pushing them slightly outside their comfort zone and still maintaining an optimal level of arousal.

4 **Pendulation** is the rhythmic movement between challenging and calming activities, between a state of activation/arousal when triggered by traumatic content and a state of calm/relaxation. Regulating the nervous system within the Window of Tolerance allows more control and choice when processing difficult experiences. Alternating between discussing the trauma and talking about benign topics like the weather or shifting focus between body sensations and the external environment are examples of pendulation.

5 **Grounding and Postural Adjustments** focus on increasing tolerance to feeling more present in the body. Using stress balls, physio balls, weighted blankets, playdough, clay, soft felt strips, cold objects, playful activities, exercise, walking, essential oils, or strong mints are different ways to access all senses when reconnecting with the body. Changing posture or position, stamping feet, or using a foot cushion helps connect with the body and plant firmly on the ground. Standing tall like a mountain imbues strength compared to feelings generated when slumped over with shoulders turned inward. Squatting against a wall helps the client connect with their body and the space around them.

6 **Orienting** is an external focus on the environment that helps clients tolerate the present moment. Have clients turn their heads one way and look around them, taking in all details of what they observe. These slow movements help activate the thinking brain as they scan the environment and help decrease dissociation.

7 **Somatic Resourcing** includes interventions that help upregulate hypoarousal (moving the body, postural changes, and using sound) or downregulate hyperarousal (sighing and breathing) (Startup and Breidis, 2024).

8 Additional strategies to increase the feeling of safety can be incorporated as part of the mindfulness exercise that begins each group or the grounding that ends the group. Interventions include assembling a **safety box** (photos, objects, and memories representing safe relationships), practicing multi-sensory **safe imagery** (imagining a **safe place**, a "safety bubble" that envelops the client and only allows safe things inside; visualizing an image of a caring, comforting, protective circle of supportive, wise "others"). **Transitional objects** such as a yarn bracelet or soft strips of felt linking members to others in the group may allow them to maintain a sense of safety and connection. Native American practices invite individuals to choose a **power animal totem** with qualities they want to emulate or embody. This technique can help generate a positive sense of self and self-confidence when one lacks the knowledge or affective skills necessary to cope with life's challenges (Hickey, 2001). Reading written or listening to audio **flashcards** is another way to bridge the time between sessions. The flashcard can be written or recorded, addressing specific needs or general messages to the whole group, reinforcing their shared experience.

Summary

The group experience provides the opportunity to build on the innate resources clients have used to survive difficult times. Creating a space where judgment or criticism is discouraged and where individuals feel supported and understood models respect for each member's trauma history. Accepting where each person is in their recovery, how they understand their experiences and problems, and when they are comfortable sharing their experiences and feelings is a central tenet of group therapy. Compassion, patience, attention to the needs of all members, and recognition of strengths are the scaffolding for developing resilience, healing, and recovery. Validating individual experiences and choices encourages self-efficacy and promotes agency over dependency within the support offered by the group community. Conversations that progress at a pace comfortable for the group and the individual participants, where they can share without feeling judged, pressured, pressed for details, or rushed through sensitive topics, are empowering and reduce emotional overwhelm. Establishing and maintaining clear group guidelines that ensure confidentiality and respect individual boundaries fosters the safety and predictability underlying the therapeutic environment.

The group is designed to help members recognize how trauma is expressed through their symptoms, how they interact in their relationships (increased impulsivity, anger and rage, and distrust in relationships), and how they feel about themselves (low self-regard, the belief that they are permanently damaged, or will never recover). Members experience how these effects play out in the group as a microcosm of their lives.

Not everyone has the same level of understanding about complex PTSD. Psychoeducation establishes a common playing field by informing and clarifying misunderstandings or misconceptions. Group discussions, the growing awareness of the impact of their trauma, specific topics, or words may trigger distressing memories or reactions among participants. The group benefits when strategies are in place to manage these responses and provide immediate support if needed.

The successful group balances safety, stability, predictability, support, and acceptance by promoting strengths, capabilities, emotional processing, and growth with established boundaries and guidelines.

References

Briere, J., & Scott, C. (2015). Complex trauma in adolescents and adults. *Psychiatric Clinics of North America*, 38(3), 515–527.

Courtois, C. A., & Ford, J. D. (2013). *Treatment of Complex Trauma: A Sequenced, Relationship-Based Approach.* New York: The Guilford Press.Cronin, E., Brand, B. L., & Mattanah, J. F. (2014). The impact of the therapeutic alliance on treatment outcome in patients with dissociative disorders. *European Journal of Psychotraumatology*, 6(5), 10.3402/ejpt.v5.22676. https://doi.org/10.3402/ejpt.v5.22676

Dalenberg, C. J. (2004). Maintaining the safe and effective therapeutic relationship in the context of distrust and anger: countertransference and complex trauma. *Psychotherapy: Theory, Research, Practice, Training*, 41(4), 438–447.

Edwards, D. J. A. (2022). Kelly's circle of safety and healing: an extended schema therapy narrative and interpretative investigation. *Pragmatic Case Studies in Psychotherapy*, 18(3), 210–261.

Farrell, J. M., & Shaw, I. A. (2012). *Group Schema Therapy for Borderline Personality Disorder.* New York: Wiley-Blackwell.

Hickey, D. A. (2001). The power animal technique: internalizing a positive symbol of strength. In H. G. Kaduson & C. E. Schaefer (Eds.), *101 More Favorite Play Therapy Techniques.* Northvale, NJ: Jason Aronson, 451–454.

Ogden, P., Minton, K., & Pain, C. (2006). *Trauma and the Body: A Sensorimotor Approach to Psychotherapy.* New York: W.W. Norton & Company, Inc.

Rogers, C. R. (1973). *Carl Rogers on Encounter Groups* (1st Harrow ed.). New York: Harper & Row.

Schore, A. N. (2019). *Right Brain Psychotherapy.* New York: Norton.

Siegel, D. J. (1999). *The Developing Mind: How Relationships and the Brain Interact to Shape Who We Are.* New York: Guilford Press.

Startup, H., & Breidis, J. (2024). *Schema Therapy: The Lived Experience of Trauma* Webinar.

Tempone Wiltshire, J. (2024). *The Role of Mindfulness and Embodiment in Group-Based Trauma Treatment.* https://core.ac.uk/download/566457379.pdf

Winnicott, D. W. (1969). The Use of an Object in the Context of Moses and Monotheism. *International Journal of Psycho-Analysis*, 50, 711–716.

Young, J. E., Klosko, J. S. & Weishaar, M. E. (2003) Schema Therapy: A Practitioner's Guide. New York: The Guilford Press.

Chapter 5

Therapeutic Challenges and the Role of Leadership

Facilitating trauma-informed groups is both an art and a science. The group leader is responsible for creating and maintaining the group by building a culture that establishes norms for behavior and deters any threats to the group's cohesiveness. The leader enhances individual and group functioning by providing a shared safe space that allows room for vulnerability and strength, reduces isolation, and provides opportunities for new learning and practice to promote self-understanding and healing.

The art of facilitation involves relating in a warm, empathic, attuned manner, with an awareness and sensitivity to individual and cultural differences the members bring into the group. The art entails listening and responding without judgment, reframing misinterpretations, and repairing disconnections and ruptures when they occur. The therapist actively attends to the group process, reflecting, clarifying, and summarizing what is being discussed. Linking the present to the past, promoting member-to-member interactions, and empathically confronting ineffective behaviors are resources used to help the members progress. Being an effective group leader requires a strong core self and understanding one's relational style, personality, needs, schema, and modes when activated in the group.

The science of facilitation entails planning and structuring the process and content of the group from the beginning to establish predictability and consistency. It requires identifying the characteristics and specific needs of the target audience. It calls for a knowledge of the group dynamics and therapeutic factors as they unfold in the group. It requires the ability to direct and guide the group through this process. It calls for an understanding of the primary and fundamental principles of trauma and requires the ability to remain focused on the goals of trauma-informed care.

At different times, the group leader is a teacher, a model, a mediator, an interpreter, a container, and a "good parent" to the group. She attends to

DOI: 10.4324/9781003462958-6

the group's informational and relational needs by relaying new information clearly and understandably. She models effective ways to engage in the group (giving constructive feedback, sharing thoughts and feelings with "I," "me," rather than "we," "us," providing information rather than asking questions, problem-solving, or giving advice). The leader encourages members to participate fully and interact directly with one another.

The leader has to manage attitudes and behaviors that can unsettle the group. Overwhelming emotions can spread like wildfire through the group. Think about the member who erupts with rage and lashes out at the group or another who abruptly leaves the group without notice. Others may try to soothe and reassure the group by making comments that lessen the emotional intensity of what is happening, attempt to control or monopolize, or repeatedly interrupt the group discussions with tangential topics. Some members may be off in a corner carrying on a side conversation during the group discussion, while another appears disengaged and lost in daydreaming. All these examples detract from the group's effective functioning and the benefits the individual members can realize. When the group norms and guidelines feel violated or cease to be enforced, the group is no longer a space where the members trust the process and feel safe.

Over or under-participation, resistance, distracting or disruptive behaviors, storytelling, sarcasm, help rejecting, excessive socializing or side talk, self-absorption, difficulty connecting to others, or becoming easily triggered or overwhelmed with emotions can disrupt the group process.

The challenge for the group leader is how to redirect these behaviors, avoid discounting the needs of the individual, and provide a safe space to address experiences that, at their core, may have been unsafe, unpredictable, and inconsistent. Trust grows when the participants feel physically and emotionally secure enough to share their experiences without fear of judgment, being discounted, dismissed, or re-traumatized.

The kind of support the group offers, the quality of empathic attunement, the group norms and guidelines, boundaries and limits, and facilitator characteristics and skills affect each member's experience (Brown, 2004, 2007; Griffin et al., 2023). The nature of each member's trauma, the similarity of the shared experience, the composition of the group (heterogeneous/homogeneous; gender composition), and the identification and degree of fit with other members all influence the success and effectiveness of the group. Insufficient attention to any of these factors could engender emotional dysregulation, ranging from angry outbursts to dissociation and trauma-related feelings such as shame, guilt, and stigma, challenging the therapist's ability to respond effectively. A thoughtful understanding of these challenges helps the leader provide a supportive, healing, and empowering space in which to address the consequences of complex trauma.

Empathic Attunement

Empathic attunement and emotional sensitivity are the very essence of successful groups. More than being kind and supportive, empathy is the ability to look beyond one's perspective through the eyes of the other to understand how that person (or the group) experiences the situation. Empathic attunement, a key component of empathy, is the process of tuning into the emotional experiences of others, understanding their feelings, and responding in a way that validates their experiences. It is stepping "into the patient's skin, to attempt to understand (in a felt way) their emotional reactions and behaviors vis a vis the backdrop of their personal narratives" (Behary, 2020, p. 227). People feel felt when they sense that they exist in the heart and mind of another and that they are not alone (Fosha, 2000; Siegel, 2010). Empathic attunement, being tuned in to one's own *and* others' vulnerability and needs, and being emotionally available to the child mode are the essence of the HA mode (Simpson & Smith, 2020).

Empathic attunement should be distinguished from sympathetic reassurance. Sympathetic reassurance, while well-intentioned, often involves problem-solving or telling others what to do or feel. It can minimize the person's problems, ignore their feelings, and be experienced as invalidating. The focus on being rational and logical and what "should" have been done or achieved conveys a message that the normal feelings and needs that every child experiences are unacceptable (Simpson & Smith, 2020).

Empathic Failures

Empathic failures arise when the client's emotional needs are misperceived, misunderstood, or responded to ineffectively. Misinterpreting a client's emotional state or reaction to group discussions, failing to recognize when a group member is becoming distressed or overwhelmed or invalidating their feelings, allowing certain members to dominate conversations at the expense of quieter members, not addressing hostile or disruptive behavior or insensitivity to cultural backgrounds, providing sympathy or giving advice are all examples of empathic failures. Failures can also occur when there is a lack of clear structure for the group or inadequate support during challenging discussions or conflicts. Empathic failures can be minimized or avoided in a supportive group environment through active listening, avoiding interruptions, paying close attention to verbal and non-verbal cues, and confirming understanding of what is said. Ensuring equal participation and attention for all members, promptly addressing disruptive or dominating behaviors, and facilitating productive discussions and interactions reduce the potential for empathic missteps.

Ruptures occur in any relationship, however attuned. Empathic failures can provide the opportunity for repair, and for new relational experiences (corrective emotional experiences) that increase insight and challenge the behaviors that often have resulted in problematic relationship patterns. When empathic failures occur, it is essential to acknowledge the failure openly, encourage the group to express their feelings about the rupture, and work collaboratively to repair it (Lonczak, 2020).

Strengthening the Healthy Adult Mode

Strengthening the Healthy Adult (HA) is a central component of a schema-informed group for complex trauma. This means helping each member develop a more balanced, compassionate, and effective way of managing their emotions and their relationships. The group leaders play an important role in modeling "good parent" qualities and facilitating "corrective experiences" as they demonstrate openness, authenticity, caring, compassion, empathic attunement, limit setting, and respect for personal boundaries. Group interactions and experiential exercises (imagery, chair work) afford members opportunities to practice HA behaviors as they are guided to meet core emotional needs more effectively by challenging maladaptive critical modes and nurturing child modes. Group participants gradually begin to internalize these corrective experiences as they learn to care for themselves and others in the group with empathy and compassion.

Empathy and compassion foster a connection and sense of shared understanding that allows the maladaptive coping patterns to be challenged. Schema-driven responses can be addressed collaboratively in the group, as the participants observe their reactions and those of other group members, identifying the schema and labeling the coping modes as the members come to understand how their early experiences influence their current behaviors and relationships. For example, consider the member who reacts angrily and with hostility during a group discussion. If the leader and the group empathically understand the member's hostility as a coping mode developed from the patient's early experiences, the triggering event, core underlying need, and survival mode can be explored. The empathically attuned "corrective experience" addresses the ruptures, repairs the relationships, and restores the trust, safety, and connection within the group. It is also a model for dealing with ruptures and repairs in relationships that extend beyond the group.

The group leader helps strengthen the HA mode by facilitating an atmosphere that allows members to confront their maladaptive patterns, provide and receive empathy and feedback, tolerate difficult emotions, and increase acceptance of their vulnerability. When ineffective models of relationships and limiting beliefs about self and others are empathically confronted, new behaviors can develop (Burlingame et al., 2001; Marmarosh et al., 2013; Behary, 2020). Attacking, blaming, and other hostile interactions decrease when one can become sensitive to one another's internal experiences and underlying intentions (Yalom & Leszcz, 2005). A group climate that is "safe, positive and supportive ... can withstand highly charged emotions, challenges and interactions between group members" (Riva & Haub, 2004, p. 41).

> Abigail is a 50-year-old woman who experienced family violence, abuse, and neglect as a young child. Her experience in the group provides an example of how hostile interactions can be sensitively addressed within the group when linked to early experiences. When memories of early violence and neglect were triggered during group discussions, Abigail repeatedly lashed out at other members. At those times, her combative and defensive "fight" part (Scolding Overcontroller or Bully Attack modes) emerged to protect her from the feelings of loneliness, helplessness, and fear she experienced when her parents left her in the care of her violent and aggressive siblings. She got angry at the group leaders, calling them "quacks" who didn't know what they were talking about, and felt that no one understood her or protected her (angry child). The group was able to gently confront these behaviors as they emerged in the group. They expressed the understanding that her anger served to protect her from feeling frightened, helpless, and alone when triggered in the group. At the same time, members shared that the anger also pushed them away from her, further perpetuating her loneliness and the belief that no one cared. Over time, the group's empathic attunement to these patterns allowed Abigail to recognize her reactions and allowed her to respond differently when these intense emotions arose.

Emotional Contagion

Emotional contagion is the quick spread of shared emotions and other behaviors between individuals or through the group that can either strengthen or weaken the group dynamic. The ability to reflect on personal feelings may be hijacked as members are gripped by "groupthink." Positive emotional contagion can strengthen cohesion and cooperation and boost motivation when, for example, the group leader or member uplifts the entire group by expressing understanding, enthusiasm, and excitement. An expression of warmth, caring, and concern when listening to another member's story or diffusing anger through empathic attunement can spread a sense of calm and comfort throughout the group. Conversely, negative emotions can increase stress and conflict within the group. The spread of negative emotions like anger or frustration can hinder communication and collaboration, ultimately undermining the group's effectiveness. Judgmental, critical, and rejecting reactions might spread through the group. Members whose behaviors do not align with the group may be scapegoated. Addressing the individual and the group's reactions when contagion occurs helps differentiate the individual's feelings from those of the group.

Group Norms and Guidelines

Norms, the unwritten standards guiding behaviors within the group, are heavily influenced by clearly defined group guidelines. The guidelines help shape the development of norms and rules that steer interactions and foster cohesion in the group. The consistency and predictability of the norms and guidelines help modulate affect, define the group's purpose, and outline the desired outcomes, providing a clear sense of direction for participants.

One of the most critical curative factors is group cohesion, or the "we" of the group. The sense of belonging, the relationships members form within the group, and the degree to which they experience the group as a secure base contribute to the "we." Norms develop from the initial group formation through the ongoing interactions and the development of emotional intimacy in the group. Leaders facilitate cohesion and "we"ness by guiding these interpersonal exchanges and modeling active engagement and active listening, ways to provide constructive feedback, and practicing respectful, open, and empathic communication (Mikulincer & Shaver, 2007). However, rigid norms or excessive cohesion, such as when dissenting opinions are suppressed or when group members feel pressured to conform, can lead to groupthink. It is worth noting that some members who avoid close connections may be more challenged by the group norms and growing cohesion. The impulse to drop out of the group may arise.

Diversity

Each group member brings their unique style, needs, and level of functioning. Overt and indirect differences influence group cohesion and functioning. Ethnicity, race, gender, age, and language are observable demographic differences, while religion, sexual orientation, disability, values, personal systems of meaning, or skill level are less visible but equally important concerns. Openness to and transparency about different cultural influences and individual differences promotes trustworthiness and inclusion, shows respect and consideration, reduces alienation and isolation, and facilitates the smooth functioning of the group. Identifying individual goals and boundaries based on personal needs empowers members to be true to themselves as they cope with the vulnerability inherent in sharing intense traumatic experiences. Therapists can manage this by emphasizing that everyone's needs and healing journey are unique.

> *Neurodivergence is a type of individual difference that is recognized more and more in therapy. Abby is a 35-year-old neurodivergent client diagnosed with dissociative identity disorder who struggled to stay present and articulate her thoughts verbally during group sessions. She was highly motivated to find a way to share her thoughts and contribute to the group's discussion. She discovered an app that could serve as her voice when she typed in her responses. Typing into the app helped her organize her thoughts and functioned as a grounding tool. The group validated this unique need by slowing down enough to allow space for Abby's contributions. Typing into the device helped Abby "find her voice." The collective understanding and supportive atmosphere afforded her the same opportunity as other group members to engage in discussions, share personal experiences and insights, and provide and receive feedback.*

It may sometimes be confusing to decide when and how to intervene when group members present with different behavior styles. The pressure to be vulnerable, as well as the pressure to protect oneself, creates a pattern of approach and avoidance that often plays out in the group. Some group members may become hyperaroused, easily activated, agitated, and disorganized during group interactions. In contrast, others may shut down, dissociate, and become hypoaroused when activated, or there may be a combination of the two strategies that reflect fear and avoidance. The timing and means of intervention may differ depending on whether there is a tendency to avoid/deny or become flooded by painful emotions. Openly identifying these patterns can enlist the collaboration of the group members in developing effective interventions. For example, it may be necessary to upregulate the hypoaroused member (e.g., physical movement, change of posture, and reorienting to the present moment) or downregulate the hyper-aroused member (e.g., soothing breathing, relaxation imagery, and calming music). Regulation within their Window of Tolerance is a priority for each. This is also true at the group level. Interpretations that tend to stir up intense emotions (e.g., anxiety and anger) in a dysregulated group will not be helpful. At the same time, they may serve to engage a detached and shut-down group (Mikulincer & Shaver, 2007).

Feedback

Supportive, nonjudgmental, honest, and constructive feedback allows group members to challenge old patterns of relating and responding that may no longer work. Clear guidelines for giving and receiving constructive feedback begin from the first interactions with potential group members. The distinction between empathy and sympathy can be explored with the group as they learn to provide feedback. How does empathy enhance connection? How might sympathetic reassurance result in an empathic failure? How does the experience differ? How can members provide validating and attuned feedback rather than giving advice or problem-solving? The therapist models the empathic, active, and non-judgmental approach to providing constructive feedback.

Members anxious to be heard may overshare before safety and trust are established. The group can discuss the experience and timing of sharing personal experiences, explore what is relevant to share, and learn ways to ask for the kind of feedback they need. The leader can remind the group that feedback is based on what has been shared by the other person rather than focusing on their own experience. The difficulty in giving feedback, empathic failures, and insensitivity to what is being shared can also be discussed (Mendelsohn et al., 2011). Specific techniques, such as using "I" statements to express observations and feelings or asking questions, allow room for greater exploration of what is being shared.

Constructive feedback acknowledges the group member's feelings and experiences and provides validation and empathy ("Thank you for sharing; I know that must have been very difficult for you"). It helps reduce feelings of isolation and shame when group members understand that their reactions are common and valid ("Given what you experienced, it makes so much sense that you feel this way"). Positive reinforcement boosts self-esteem and encourages continued participation and openness ("It took a lot of courage to challenge yourself the way you did; I admire that"). Constructive feedback offers practical suggestions while showing support and understanding of the participant's struggles ("Have you noticed what helps calm you when you are overwhelmed? I wonder if any of the techniques we have practiced in the group might be helpful. It sometimes helps reorient me when I name objects in the room"). Sharing personal experiences and strategies can provide other group members with new perspectives and coping mechanisms ("Talking to my best friend helped when that happened to me. I did not feel so alone. Maybe that could work for you too"). Highlighting progress motivates group members and reinforces their sense of achievement and personal development ("I noticed that you share so much more in the group than when you first joined. I appreciate what you have to say").

Therapy Interfering or Therapy Destroying Behaviors

Proactively addressing therapy interfering or destroying behaviors minimize potential disruptions to the group. Emotion dysregulation, persistent negativity, offensive behaviors, aggression and conflict, impulsivity, dissociation, side conversations, interrupting others, dominating the discussion, appearing to have all the answers, or going off-topic can be frustrating and disruptive to the group process. A silent group can be equally disconcerting and anxiety-provoking, perhaps reflecting that a topic is not working or that there is some problem that the group is reluctant to raise.

Empathic Confrontation

Empathic confrontation addresses group behaviors that interfere with participants getting their needs met (e.g., missing sessions, extreme detachment, or aggressive or risky behaviors). Farrell and Shaw (2012) describe an approach to empathic confrontation designed to address maladaptive, therapy-interfering behaviors in groups. The process begins by ensuring that the member feels supported, understood, and connected. The empathic confrontation clarifies the concern that the member's emotional needs won't be met in the session due to ... (the therapy-interfering behavior being addressed). The therapy-interfering behavior or coping mode is clearly identified to help the individual recognize their patterns without feeling attacked:

> I can understand you feel misunderstood and angry, but I'm worried that when you get angry and lash out, it frightens the group and pushes them away from you. It gives us the message that you don't want to connect, while we know the vulnerable part needs that connection.

The group/therapist identified that the behavior was a survival mechanism during childhood when other options were not available; it now interferes with them getting what they need:

> I understand that in your childhood when you got angry and fought back, you protected yourself from getting hurt further. Even though it may still feel safer for you to cope that way, the problem is that when you get angry in the group, we retreat from you. While it may have served a purpose in the past, it is no longer effective or healthy.

A correction is offered to allow them to get their needs met in the group:

> I know that in the past there was so much criticism that it would have been too risky to show any vulnerability. You had to fight back. But it would help us to know what you need and what you are feeling; we really want to know you and understand you. This is one of the goals of ST–to learn to be vulnerable with others who are safe. As a child, you

learned that you would be hurt or shamed for having needs, but this message was unhelpful. You're allowed to connect and to ask for what you need.

The individual is encouraged to reflect on the pros and cons of the mode.

Can we think about how this mode affects other relationships and how easy or hard it is to get what you need? Although it has helped you in the past, could you think about how it might feel to let it go for a short time?

Finally, support is offered: "This old way of coping is totally understandable, but it is not working for you. How can we better support you to get what you need from now on?".

Naming and acknowledging the problem, identifying any concerns, opening the discussion to the whole group, making space for everyone to share their views, and inviting the group to suggest ways to move forward when stuck can help clarify misunderstandings and avert more severe ruptures. ("I am noticing that the group is very quiet today and wonder what is going on. Has anyone else noticed this?" "Jo, you seem frustrated that Mary does not understand you. Would it be ok if we helped find a way to clear up the misunderstanding?"). Group guidelines set the framework for respectful behaviors and norms for taking turns, limiting side or cross-talking, and welcoming all contributions ("What you have shared is so important, and I wonder if some of the others can respond as well").

Chairwork can also be used to confront coping modes empathically. A chair can be allocated to all of the main coping modes represented in the group, and also one chair to represent the collective child modes. Group leaders help participants identify ways in which their coping modes urge them to avoid, and thereby sabotage, their ability to get their needs met. Participants are invited to say something to their own coping mode ("You helped me in the past, but while you are there, I can't connect with and trust other people. I need you to help me learn new healthy ways to trust others and meet the needs of Little X"). Participants are encouraged to finish by saying one thing to all of the Vulnerable Child modes on the chair ("I am here for you; You matter; Your feelings are important to me; Others do want to hear what you feel and to connect to you").

Sometimes, a group member may need more support, and allowing their concerns to take over temporarily may be necessary. At other times, taking a short break, shifting the conversation, or engaging in an activity that settles members in the present moment can re-engage the group. If a particular member's therapy-interfering patterns persist, speaking with that member privately may be necessary.

Emotional Dysregulation

Emotional overwhelm and dysregulation are significant challenges in trauma-focused groups. Revisiting traumatic experiences in a group can trigger intense emotional reactions or memories of trauma that may be overly distressing and dysregulating, even as this is considered a key component in the treatment of Post Traumatic Stress Disorder (PTSD). The intensity of fear and shame-based responses may heighten emotional distress and dysregulation if one member feels that their experience is less legitimate or severe when comparing their trauma to others (Beck & Coffey, 2007; Courtois & Ford, 2013). Defensive measures (fight/flight/freeze/submit/attach) may be elicited to protect against those feelings, increasing conflict, or negative dynamics within the group.

Increased distress and emotional activation during group discussions can be acknowledged as related to PTSD. Pacing interventions, teaching distress tolerance skills (Linehan, 1993) and practicing grounding with the whole group may help minimize dysregulation (Mendelsohn et al., 2011). Group members are encouraged to practice their grounding and coping resources as they learn to manage the intensity of their activated emotions.

Structure, consistency, and predictability also help reduce the anxiety and uncertainty that exacerbate emotional distress. Outlining the session's agenda and goals, incorporating an opening mindfulness exercise at the beginning of each group, and regular check-ins/check-outs reduce uncertainty. Mindfulness can help manage emotional responses and reduce reactivity as participants' awareness of their emotional state increases. However, some clients may become more dysregulated if asked to focus on internal sensations or their bodies. These clients may need an external intervention (e.g., counting the blue items in the room) to help them regulate. Checking in with the group with specific questions about what they are experiencing can help each member monitor their level of distress/regulation.

When a traumatic memory or system is activated (triggered), without being understood or processed, the pathological impact of the trauma is magnified. When there is therapeutic help, empathy, and recognition of the nature of the triggering, emotional processing (identifying, labeling, and understanding the function of activated emotions) can start to heal the memory system. Members learn to deescalate their distress and increase control over their emotional experiences. Enhancing interpersonal skills, such as assertiveness and direct communication, empowers group members to express their needs, manage conflicts, and reduce the helplessness and frustration that exacerbate emotional dysregulation. Educating members about trauma helps normalize and validate their experiences and helps them appreciate that their reactions are common and understandable.

The group leader models an atmosphere of mutual respect and validation by emphasizing that all trauma experiences are valid and that the group is a non-competitive space. Having a co-facilitator or a designated support person available to support a group member in crisis and providing a quiet "safe space" where the member can self-regulate with grounding and mindfulness exercises before rejoining the group can also facilitate emotion regulation for the individual and the group.

Dissociation

Dissociation is a specific response that interferes with the ability to engage with others. Intense emotional distress, traumatic memories, or flashbacks may be triggered within the group, causing a member to withdraw and isolate, space out, and become confused, sometimes losing contact with the present moment. Severe dissociation makes group participation difficult for the dissociative individual and challenges the group. Group therapy has, however, been found effective even for dissociative members when affective intensity is carefully modulated (Boon et al., 2011; Chu, 2011).

Sometimes, a member may refrain from participating or being quiet. Paying attention to the silence can help identify its root cause. Is the client upset, disinterested, or dissociating? Focusing on the possible causes can help reengage the client. Addressing dissociative symptoms promptly ensures individual's safety and well-being and reestablishes the connection to the group. Dissociative responses, stigma, and negative judgments decrease when the individual is reassured that their feelings are valid and understandable given their past. Educating the group about dissociation as a response to trauma and a response we all experience to some degree (e.g., highway hypnosis), helps them better understand, observe, and identify the changes that occur when someone dissociates (spacing out, blank stare, physical stilling, changes in style, behavior, eye contact, voice tone that reflects switching of self-states, etc.)

Pacing and titrating participation, providing trigger warnings when discussing potentially sensitive topics, and introducing coping strategies for managing those triggers respect the dissociative member's boundaries and enhance their ability to manage their dissociative reactions. Teaching grounding and reorienting, somatic strategies, sensory-based grounding exercises, breathing exercises, and self-soothing techniques to all members helps them support the dissociative member to regain a sense of safety and awareness of self and environment (Fisher & Ogden, 2009). Acknowledging dissociative coping gently challenges the dissociated parts of the personality (in the form of flashbacks or intrusive memories).

Developing ground rules and specific protocols for managing dissociative episodes when they occur helps alleviate the helplessness often experienced by the group.

Imagery and mindfulness can be complicated for clients with dissociation. Kathy described one of her most challenging experiences while conducting an opening mindfulness exercise. Intending to lead the group into a calm, contained internal space, she guided them down a "staircase into a deep well." It soon became evident that one of the group members had dissociated into a younger self. The frightened little girl had "gotten stuck," did not know where she was, and could not escape the image. Her adult self was no longer "driving the bus." Kathy related that in that moment, she, too, felt like a little child, alone, panicked, and out of control. She was flooded with self-judgments:

I do not know how to help the client. I do not know what I am doing. This is my fault because I chose this exercise. How do I get out of this? I am going to get in trouble. I need someone to help me.

After her initial panic, Kathy was able to tuck her vulnerable child and inner critic modes away as she assessed what the dissociated member needed (support to reorient to the present moment). Kathy helped guide the client back up the stairs, reminding her of where she was and that she was safe. She also moved the group outside for a change of scene. Movement and the change of place helped ground the dissociated client and the distressed group.

Conflict

Conflict, power imbalances, and adverse dynamics (inappropriate expression of anger or rage, dominance, rebellion, dissociation, therapy interfering/destroying behaviors) are natural but disruptive parts of group dynamics that arise when members have different opinions or coping styles. Refusing to engage in a power struggle, finding a compromise, refocusing the discussion on some other topic, allowing time to cool off, or firmly enforcing the guidelines and rules are different ways to respond when conflict arises. Assessing the group's needs at that moment may determine the choice of intervention and can be framed as an opportunity for growth and learning. It is essential not to ignore conflict or engage in no-win situations; maintaining a sense of humor may diffuse the conflict.

Normalizing conflict reduces anxiety around disagreements and validates the experiences of those involved by openly acknowledging that their conflict is being taken seriously. Revisiting ground rules and group norms provides the framework where participants can address disagreements constructively, perhaps meeting in the middle or agreeing to disagree. Emotional support and reassurance can help de-escalate the situation and make clients feel heard and understood. In situations where there is an immediate threat to safety, such as violence or self-harm, the physical safety of all participants is prioritized. Aggressive or abusive behaviors are immediately stopped. A member may need to leave the group to return to their Window of Tolerance or enlist other professionals' aid or emergency services if necessary.

When intense emotions erupt, a group leader should directly facilitate "working through" these emotions. Open communication, empathy, active listening, and understanding others' perspectives can help de-escalate tensions when participants are assured that everyone's feelings, needs, and perspectives are welcome when expressed in non-threatening ways. Pacing controls emotional stimulation and prevents emotional flooding and possible re-traumatization. Regular check-ins can address any lingering issues and monitor group members' feelings once the conflict has been resolved. Helping the members take responsibility for and ownership of the therapy-interfering (or destroying) behaviors can help reduce defensiveness and escalation of the conflict. Using "I" statements to express feelings and perspectives reduces blame and helps repair any ruptures. The leaders also need to be aware of their reactions to the anger, conflict, and intense emotion expressed in the group.

Mary and Beth were members of an art therapy group within a trauma-focused treatment program. A disagreement arose between them when working on their respective art projects. Suddenly, Beth raised a pair of scissors, gesturing angrily toward Mary. The group leader intervened immediately to reestablish the safety and smooth functioning of the group, setting a clear limit on hostile expressions of anger and intimidating behaviors. Group norms and guidelines were reviewed and enforced in a nonjudgmental or punitive manner.

> *Beth, I want to remind you that threatening or intimidating behavior is not tolerated in this group. We can see you are feeling very angry right now. Can you help us understand what set you off and tell us why you are angry? I know that you've shared with us that your anger helped you in the past, especially when you felt unsafe....*

Group members explore how behaviors that once helped them survive overwhelming experiences (anger/fight response in this example) often interfere with their ability to function effectively in present relationships. Beth and Mary's early experiences were linked to their preferred survival strategies. Beth identified feelings of threat, fear, and shame arising from the disagreement that triggered the hostile fight response, while Mary shared the impact Beth's threat had had on her. More effective ways of tolerating disagreement or resolving conflict were explored. A repair of the rupture created by Beth's hostility began with her apology to the group and Mary and their acceptance of that apology. A group grounding exercise helped all members calm down and return to their Window of Tolerance. (Dysregulated group members could also have been offered individual support and a "time out" to get back into their Window of Tolerance. Beth's removal from the group may have been necessary if entrenched defensiveness or hostility continued to threaten group safety and cohesion).

Louise, in the role of group leader, used the image of loud red fireworks to capture the rage expressed by another client during an altercation in the group. While reviewing a handout, the member suddenly erupted in rage at the feedback offered by Louise. She started yelling at Louise, her intensity frightening the group. Louise felt paralyzed with fear and uncertainty about handling this outburst, recognizing her desire to avoid conflict. The client could not calm down and rejected Louise's efforts to intervene. She eventually left the group to get support elsewhere and returned when she was back in her Window of Tolerance. Louise, however, knew that she had to ensure that all group members felt safe in the face of the member's rage. She checked in with each member to assess their reaction and what they needed, leading the group in a grounding exercise. When the client returned to the group, she was able to take responsibility for her outburst and acknowledge how frightening that was for all. The group explored the defensive function of the anger and how the outburst affected them. They were able to troubleshoot ways to manage these reactions in the future and discuss how expressing anger can be used more effectively to get needs met.

Transference

Transference is the "unconscious repetition in a current relationship of patterns, thoughts, feelings, expectations and responses that originated in important early relationships" (Pearlman & Saakvitne, 1995, p. 100). Schema Therapy understands transference as the activation of early maladaptive schemas and schema modes. Early childhood experiences and relational patterns are often reenacted in the group setting when group interactions trigger emotional responses related to early traumatic experiences. Idealization and devaluation, sexualization, or seeing the other person as a victim, omnipotent rescuer, or perpetrator are common reactions that emerge in trauma-focused groups (Pearlman & Saakvitne, 1995). They can occur between group members, towards the group as a whole, towards subgroups within the larger group, or toward the therapist.

Transference reactions, a common occurrence in trauma-focused groups, can significantly influence group cohesion and dynamics. Members may echo sibling dynamics as they vie for the therapist's attention. Some may develop romantic feelings towards the therapist or another group member, stemming from unmet needs for love and affection. Others may become distrusting, critical, or confrontational when faced with situations that trigger maladaptive schema. The Schema Therapy model provides a valuable framework for understanding these experiences as the result of the activation of early maladaptive patterns resulting from unmet needs in infancy and childhood, underscoring the need for a comprehensive understanding of the group's dynamics.

Activation of schema modes and early maladaptive schemas is exemplified by the following brief excerpt from a letter the therapist Michelle received after a group had ended. Elizabeth's central issues concerned her relationship with her mother, whom she perceived as a wealthy, uncaring, vain woman who was unable to nurture her as a child:

> *Michelle, I hope the following comment will not hurt you. I can't speak for the other group members, but your wardrobe was very off-putting. You are clearly in a position of authority, and your choice of clothes emphasizes that you are privileged compared to the rest of us (i.e., other group members). I don't think I am unusual in distrusting people who are different from me, and your shoes and clothes make you seem different. I have read that a therapist is well advised to dress inconspicuously, and I think that is true...*
> (Margolin, 1999).

Elizabeth's expression of distrust and criticism towards the therapist's appearance suggests activation of her Angry Child mode and the Mistrust/Abuse schema, perhaps activated by feelings of vulnerability or threat. Her attempt to "advise" the therapist on proper attire suggests an activation of the internalized inner critic messages that she projected onto the therapist. Her critical and somewhat confrontational approach in pointing out perceived flaws in the therapist's appearance and conduct is an overcompensation coping response designed to gain control and reduce feelings of vulnerability. Her statement, "I don't think I am unusual in distrusting people who are different from me," reveals the underlying Mistrust/Abuse schema and the expectation that others will intentionally harm, abuse, humiliate, or take advantage of her. Finally, the focus on the therapist's "privileged" status compared to the group members may indicate an activation of a Defectiveness/Shame schema, reflecting feelings of inferiority and shame. These examples of "mode flipping" would allow for exploring Elizabeth's underlying schemas and modes. The therapist might empathically confront her concerns while helping her recognize how past experiences and unmet emotional needs influence her current perceptions and reactions in the therapeutic relationship.

Countertransference

Countertransference refers to the activation of maladaptive schemas in the therapist. The therapist's personal history, attitudes, beliefs, and training influence how they respond to the group and the individual members. The therapist's unresolved maladaptive schema and modes may interfere with their ability to guide the healing process or run the group effectively. A therapist with an avoidant coping pattern might avoid addressing difficult topics that come up during the session or empathically confronting maladaptive behaviors that arise. A therapist with an overcompensating mode might become patronizing or too confrontational, critical, or judgmental. They may have difficulty setting limits or setting too many. A therapist with a compliant surrender mode may take on too much responsibility and try to rescue clients. A demanding critic mode will exacerbate this, leading more quickly to burnout.

In the earlier example, the therapist Michelle's early maladaptive schema and schema modes may have been activated when she received Elizabeth's letter. She might have felt attacked, triggering a defensive Angry Protector Mode, or she might have felt hurt, inadequate, ashamed, or a failure (Defectiveness Schema; Failure Schema; Vulnerable Child Mode). She might have internalized the criticism, believing she was incompetent (Surrender Coping Mode), or might argue or justify her clothing choices, attempting to prove her competence (Overcompensation Coping Mode). She might have dismissed or minimized Elizabeth's concerns, suppressing her emotional reaction to her comment (Emotional Inhibition Schema) as she ignored or downplayed the comment to avoid dealing with it (Detached Protector). By recognizing when the experiences in the group activate her schemas and modes, Michelle can model healthy responses to criticism, demonstrate appropriate boundary-setting, and use the situation as a therapeutic opportunity to explore the group dynamics and individual members' schemas and modes.

Helping clients understand their personal histories as they rebuild a fulfilling life can be rewarding, and it can also be overwhelming. Schema activation, ineffective coping, vicarious traumatization, empathic withdrawal, or empathic enmeshment can create difficulties for the therapist. When leading trauma-focused groups, the therapist might experience PTSD-like symptoms such as intrusive thoughts, emotional exhaustion, and a diminished sense of safety and trust (Mistrust/Abuse Schema; Vulnerable Child Mode) (McCann & Pearlman, 1990; Pearlman & Saakvitne, 1995; Quitangon, 2019). They may detach emotionally from clients (Detached Protector Mode) to protect against burnout (from overwhelming feelings of helplessness, anger, and disillusionment) or over-identify with clients, blurring boundaries, rescuing, or taking on too much responsibility (Self-Sacrifice Schema) (Phillips, 2004).

A group facilitator might become overprotective of a vulnerable member, feel exhausted when overinvested, or feel guilty when disengaging (Rescuer/Self-Sacrifice). The therapist may unconsciously favor certain group members who remind them of positive figures from their past (Vulnerable Child), become frustrated with a challenging group member who triggers anger reminiscent of their past (e.g., a member who is disruptive or non-compliant), or avoid confronting certain behaviors due to their discomfort with conflict (Detached Protector). The therapist must identify any issues that might arise and monitor their emotional reactions to the intense emotion, anger, or conflict expressed in the group. Self-care practices, supervision, peer support, and personal therapy help the therapist manage stress, burnout, and vicarious traumatization that often accompanies trauma-focused work.

Summary

Facilitating trauma-informed groups is both an art and a science where the therapist becomes a teacher, a model, a mediator, an interpreter, a container, and a "good parent" to the group. The art involves relating in a warm, empathic, attuned manner, with an awareness and sensitivity to individual and cultural differences the members bring into the group. Empathic attunement and emotional sensitivity are the very essence of successful groups. The science of facilitation involves planning, structure, predictability, consistency, targeting the audience's needs, understanding group dynamics and therapeutic factors, and understanding the primary and fundamental principles of trauma-informed care.

It is important to remember that there is not always a roadmap.

> Textbook recommendations and clinical care are not necessarily the same, and the path you would like to take may not always be possible. Being present with patients often means thinking on your feet, being flexible, and making modifications. Improvision and instinct can help therapists meet patients where they truly are
>
> (de Groh, 2024, p. 3).

Leading a trauma-informed group has its challenges. Flexibility, attunement, and the ability to remain present with the group help the leader manage fluctuating feelings and behaviors that can unsettle the group. Consistent reinforcement of group norms and guidelines enables the group to keep its focus on safety. The group remains strong and cohesive as emotional dysregulation, schema activation, reenactments of trauma-based patterns of behavior, dissociation, conflict, and other therapy-interfering or destroying behaviors are addressed with warmth, understanding, flexibility, and humor. Understanding the role of the therapist and the challenges inherent in running these groups increases the likelihood of their success.

References

Beck, J. G., & Coffey, S. F. (2007). Assessment and treatment of posttraumatic stress disorder after a motor vehicle collision: empirical findings and clinical observations. *Professional Psychology: Research and Practice*, 38(6), 629–639. https://doi.org/10.1037/0735-7028.38.6.629

Behary, W. (2020). The art of empathic confrontation and limit setting. In G. Heath & H. Startup (Eds.), *Creative Methods in Schema Therapy: Advances and Innovation in Clinical Practice*. London: Routledge.

Boon, S., Steele, K., & Van Der Hart, O. (2011). *Coping With Trauma-Related Dissociation: Skills Training For Patients And Therapists (Norton Series On Interpersonal Neurobiology)* (1st ed.). New York: W.W. Norton.

Brown, N. (2004). *Psychoeducational Groups: Process and Practice*. New York: Brunner-Routledge.

Brown, N. (2007). *Curriculum for Psychoeducational Groups*. New York: AGPA.

Burlingame, G. M., Fuhriman, A., & Johnson, J. E. (2001). Cohesion in group psychotherapy. *Psychotherapy: Theory, Research, Practice, Training*, 38(4), 373–379. https://doi.org/10.1037/0033-3204.38.4.373

Chu, J. A., Dell, P. F., Van Der Hart, O., Cardeña, E., Barach, P. M., Somer, E., Loewenstein, R. J., Brand, B., Golston, J. C., Courtois, C. A., Bowman, E. S., Classen, C., Dorahy, M., , Sar, V., Gelinas, D.J., Fine, C.G., Paulsen, S., Kluft, R. P., Dalenberg, C. J., Jacobson-Levy, M., Nijenhuis, E. R. S., Boon, S., Chefetz, R.A., Middleton, W., Ross, C. A., Howell, E., Goodwin, G., Coons, P. M., Frankel, A. S., Steele, K., Gold, S. N., Gast, U., Young, L. M., & Twombly, J. (2011). Guidelines for treating dissociative identity disorder in adults, third revision. *Journal of Trauma & Dissociation*, 12(2), 115–187.

Courtois, C., & Ford, J. (2013). *Treatment of Complex Trauma: A Sequenced, Relationship-Based Approach*. New York: Guilford Press.

De Groh, R. (2024). "Am I enough and other therapist thoughts?" *Princeton House Behavioral Health TODAY Newsletter*. Princetonhouse.Org.

Farrell, J. M. & Shaw, I. A. (2012). *Group schema therapy for borderline personality disorder—A step-by-step treatment manual with patient workbook*. West Sussex, UK: Wiley-Blackwell.

Fisher, J., & Ogden, P. (2009). Sensorimotor psychotherapy. In Courtois, C. & Ford, J. (Eds.), *Treating Complex Traumatic Stress Disorders: An Evidence-Based Guide*. New York: Wiley & Sons.

Fosha, D. (2000). *The Transforming Power of Affect: A Model for Accelerated Change*. New York: Basic Books.

Griffin, S. M., Lebedová, A., Ahern, E., McMahon, G., Bradshaw, D., & Muldoon, O. T. (2023). Protocol: group-based interventions for posttraumatic stress disorder: a systematic review and meta-analysis of the role of trauma type. *Campbell Systematic Reviews*, 19(2), E1328. https://doi.org/10.1002/cl2.1328

Hubbs Ulman, K. (2004). *Group Interventions for Treatment of Psychological Trauma Module 1: Group Interventions for Treatment of Trauma in Adults*. New York: American Group Psychotherapy Association, 13.

Johnson, D. W. & Johnson, F. P. (2006). *Joining Together: Group Theory and Group Skills*. Boston: Pearson (Allyn & Bacon).

Linehan, M. M. (1993). *Cognitive-behavioral treatment of borderline personality disorder*. New York: Guilford Press.

Lonczak, H. S. (2020). 34 counseling mistakes that therapists should avoid. *Positivepsychology.Com*. https://positivepsychology.com/things-therapists-should-not-do

Margolin, J. (1999). *Breaking the Silence: Group Therapy for Childhood Sexual Abuse, A Practitioner's Manual*. New York: The Hawthorn Maltreatment and Trauma Press.

Marmarosh, C. L., Markin, R. D., & Spiegel, E. B. (2013). *Attachment in Group Psychotherapy*. Washington, D.C.: American Psychological Association.

McCann, I. L., & Pearlman, L. A. (1990). Vicarious traumatization: a framework for understanding the psychological effects of working with victims. *Journal of Traumatic Stress*, 3, 131–149. https://doi.org/10.1007/BF00975140

Mendelsohn, M., Herman, J. L., Schatzow, E., Kallivayalil, D., Coco, M., & Levitan, J. (2011). *The Trauma Recovery Group: A Guide for Practitioners*. New York: Guilford Publications.

Mikulincer, M., & Shaver, P. R. (2007). Boosting attachment security to promote mental health, prosocial values, and inter-group tolerance. *Psychological Inquiry*, 18, 139–156.

Pearlman, Laurie A., & Saakvitne, Karen W. (1995). *Trauma and the Therapist: Countertransference and Vicarious Traumatization in Psychotherapy with Incest Survivors*. New York: W.W. Norton,

Phillips, S. B (2004). *CGP Group Interventions for Treatment of Psychological Trauma Module 7: Countertransference: Effects on the Group Therapist Working with Trauma*. American Group Psychotherapy Association, 194. https://www.agpa.org/docs/default-source/practice-resources/countertransference--effects-on-the-group-therapist-working-with-trauma.pdf

Quitangon, G. (2019). Vicarious trauma in clinicians: fostering resilience and preventing burnout. *Psychiatric Times*, 36(7), 18–19.

Riva, M. T., & Haub, A. L. (2004). Group counseling in the schools. In J. L. Delucia-Waack, D. A. Gerrity, C. R. Kalodner, & M. T. Riva (Eds.), *Handbook of Group Counseling and Psychotherapy*. Thousand Oaks, CA: Sage, 309–321.

Siegel, D. (2010). *The Mindful Therapist: A Clinician's Guide to Mindsight and Neural Integration*. New York: W. W. Norton & Company.

Simpson, S. & Smith, E. (2020). *Schema Therapy for Eating Disorders: Theory and Practice for Individual and Group Settings*. London: Routledge.

Yalom, I. D., & Leszcz, M. (2005). *The Theory and Practice of Group Psychotherapy* (5th ed.). New York: Basic Books/Hachette Book Group.

Chapter 6

Trauma, Mindfulness, and the Healthy Adult

Recovering from trauma, while often overwhelming and emotionally taxing, can be a journey of empowerment. The most significant damage after an experience of neglect or abuse may be the child's distorted interpretations of early events that continue to inform the meaning of present experiences. Mindful awareness sheds light on past interpretations and conditioned patterns so they no longer frame current experiences (Gabor Maté, 2018). Mindfulness, a potent tool, allows the individual to distance themselves from maladaptive interpretations and empowers them to reconnect with their bodies and surroundings as they navigate the path of trauma recovery.

Mindfulness is a present-centered, non-judgmental mode of awareness that emerges through purposively paying attention to the unfolding moment-to-moment experience (Kabat-Zinn, 2003; Follette et al., 2015; Tempone-Wiltshire, 2024). It is a mental state that involves observing and allowing one's thoughts and feelings as they arise in the present. It is considered a bottom-up and top-down intervention because it engages the conscious mind in regulating thoughts, feelings, and physical sensations in the body. Many body-focused practices are described as mindfulness techniques (Chiesa et al., 2013).

> Central to the practical implementation of mindfulness is developing the ability to recognize old, engrained, and automatic emotional response patterns as they occur. This process requires focused attention on the body's response to emotional patterns. The repeated bringing to awareness and allowance of these patterns gradually leads to acceptance and creates room for behavioral adjustment. With practice, patients can learn to apply this skill to their psychological symptoms
>
> (van Vreeswijk et al., 2014, p. 14).

Mindfulness and the Healthy Adult

The Healthy Adult mode is necessary for psychological well-being and effective functioning. This mode represents an individual's integrated, adult

DOI: 10.4324/9781003462958-7

self that can manage emotions, solve problems, take responsibility for choices and actions, engage in pleasurable activities, and maintain healthy relationships. The Healthy Adult can validate emotions, provide reasoning, build limits, give hope, and combat critical and demanding voices. Healthy Adult functioning is connected to positive emotions, defined as desirable adaptive experiences that subjectively feel good and signal and produce optimal functioning (Fredrickson, 2013).

The Healthy Adult mode can be considered the internal "good parent" that allows a person to balance their emotional needs for attachment and autonomy. Yakin and Arntz (2023) identified the three functions of the Healthy Adult – bond (through compassion and nurturance, emotional attunement and encouragement), balance (by setting boundaries and providing space, self-reflection and expressing emotions), and battle (hope and faith, embracing challenges and self-empowerment). These functions mediate between other schema modes, nurturing and regulating child modes, moderating inner critic modes, and adjusting unhealthy coping modes.

Strengthening the Healthy Adult mode is particularly relevant in trauma treatment. A more robust, Healthy Adult mode increases the individual's sense of safety and control, comforts and supports vulnerable parts of self that often hold traumatic memories, and moderates intense emotional responses that are usually sequelae of trauma. The Healthy Adult mode can reevaluate maladaptive schema and interrupt self-defeating beliefs and coping methods.

The Healthy Adult mode correlates with mindfulness, flexibility, self-compassion, self-regulation, and valued living (Wieczorek & Brockman, 2016). Increasing self-awareness is the first step toward changing self-defeating behaviors and moving away from maladaptive coping modes. When one can identify situations that trigger automatic thoughts, feelings, and behaviors, automatic reactivity is reduced. Awareness develops from mindful attention to what is happening in the here and now—mindfulness distances from the autopilot responses when schemas are activated. The Healthy Adult mode fosters curiosity while reducing automatic reactions or coping modes that lead to the avoidance of maladaptive schemas and impede adaptive functioning (van Vreeswijk et al., 2014).

Mindfulness is also connected to acceptance of reality, a key capacity of the Healthy Adult. The paradox is that avoiding difficult realities by wishing things were different, such as wishing a traumatic event never happened, makes us suffer more. Healthy Adults are compassionate to their pain, and the practice of self-compassion can counteract the messages of inner critic modes. The nurturing aspect of the Healthy Adult fosters a self-compassionate, kind, and understanding attitude towards oneself, making you feel cared for and understood.

Schema Therapy recognizes the importance of the capacity to step back and reflect on one's own experience and that of others as a key quality of the Healthy Adult mode. The capacity to distance oneself or diffuse from distorted or irrational thought patterns directs attention toward the inner experience of schema and mode activation. The Healthy Adult mode embraces a detached mindfulness that allows a "meta-awareness" without autopilot reactions and enables one to recognize and differentiate their schema and modes, self compassionately and without judgment. This creates a space for schema change as new response patterns emerge (van Vreeswijk et al., 2014; Haeyen, 2019; Edwards, 2022).

Mindfulness enhances the well-being of a healthy adult by cultivating self-regulation, emotional clarity, and adaptive resilience, enabling individuals to navigate challenges with greater balance and self-compassion. It decreases rumination and avoidance by grounding attention in the present, diminishing the grip of past traumas or future anxieties. Non-judgmental present-moment awareness fosters compassionate bonding and kindness toward oneself, countering critical inner voices and nurturing self-acceptance. Mindfulness enhances decision-making by integrating emotional and rational perspectives, enabling boundary-setting, goal-aligned actions, and adaptive conflict responses. By anchoring individuals in their present experience, mindfulness empowers the Healthy Adult to mediate between conflicting internal states, sustain emotional equilibrium, and engage with life's challenges from a place of clarity and agency.

The Pain Paradox

Two sources of distress are often associated with traumatic experience: the event and the emotional pain it produces and the suffering related to the attempts to avoid the pain and unwanted reality. Post Traumatic Stress Disorder (PTSD) is typified by first avoiding symptoms and then ruminating obsessively about them. This unproductive, ruminative thinking mode is "the repetitive rehearsal of thoughts and/or images in a manner that does not result in productive planning or problem-solving, and that perpetuates or even exacerbates problems" (Edwards, 2022, p.11).

The parable of the two arrows from Buddhist teachings highlights the difference between the pain of trauma and the suffering it engenders. A person is pierced by two arrows in rapid succession. The first arrow is the objective pain when encountering adversity and the loss incurred from the trauma. The second arrow is the extent to which the pain challenges rigid and inaccurate expectations and needs, resulting in resistance and avoidance of reality. The attachment to inaccurate assumptions and what was or should be increases suffering. The paradox is that *it is necessary to experience, accept, and process difficult emotions to relieve the pain.* In simpler terms, it means that to heal from trauma, one must face and accept the pain rather than avoid it (Briere, 2015). Trauma-informed mindfulness seeks to avoid emotional overwhelm while strengthening a person's ability to face the pain.

Lang et al. (2012) noted three components of mindfulness that help break this pattern. These include *attention, a mindful cognitive style,* and *nonjudgment.* Intentional *reorientation of attention* reduces the bias to trauma-related stimuli. A *mindful cognitive style* shifts attention away from distressing symptoms and supports clients in disengaging from ruminative or overwhelming thoughts, anxious arousal, and anhedonia. A *non--judgmental approach* encourages self-monitoring of spontaneous thoughts and body sensations. It may increase willingness to approach rather than avoid fear-provoking stimuli. This reassurance of mindfulness's role in recovery can instill confidence in its application. It can be learned through directed attention exercises and integrated with existing therapy methods and training programs for use with many psychological problems.

Challenges to Mindfulness

While mindfulness and body-oriented practices contain many elements that are helpful in the remediation of post-traumatic difficulties, the reduced avoidance of and increased exposure to traumatic memories and emotional states can be a concern for some clients. Clinical challenges of teaching and practicing mindfulness may arise due to the PTSD symptoms of avoidance, re-experiencing, and reactivity. While everyone can benefit from mindfulness practice, it can be activating for trauma survivors. Individuals may struggle with physical sensations, emotions, and the present moment. There may be greater attachment to a negative storyline that reinforces self-judgment and feelings of unworthiness, self-doubt, hopelessness, and a sense of failure. Rather than being present in their experiences, the fear that PTSD symptoms will be triggered leads to emotional numbing, emotional reactivity, and dissociation. Instead, individuals with significant dissociative tendencies seek to escape from overwhelming experiential flashbacks, ruminations, or the triggering of embodied memories (Briere, 2015). There is little willingness to practice mindfulness of the sensory and emotional material that can arise during meditation (Magyari, 2015).

Reminders of trauma live on in the mind and body in the form of intrusive thoughts, traumatic memories, or painful sensations that do not dissipate. Trauma-informed mindfulness is designed to increase tolerance of physical sensations, improve self-regulation, and relieve the experience of the trauma. Paying attention to the breath is often a starting point for a meditation practice, as it helps bring stability to the mind. The breath may not be the best place for trauma survivors to begin a meditation practice, however. The breath connects to the sympathetic nervous system, which may be chronically activated after trauma (Treleaven, 2018). Mindfulness and embodiment (body-focused work) are essential tools to help individuals increase their meta-awareness as they regulate their emotions and reconnect with their bodies and surroundings.

Grounding, anchoring, and self-regulation techniques supplement traditional mindfulness to maintain balance in the nervous system, help people manage their symptoms and feel safer in their bodies. This might involve choosing a place other than the breath to focus attention on, such as the sensations of the feet on the ground or sound (Treleaven, 2018).

Zerubavel and Messman-Moore (2015) suggest that, despite these concerns, mindfulness can address dissociation. The potential of mindfulness to address dissociation can motivate clients to incorporate it into their practice. Mindfulness can help reduce the person's detachment by encouraging them to tolerate aversive internal experiences and minimize the total immersion of attention to "nothing," i.e., going blank. Frewen and Lanius (2015) suggest that mindfulness may facilitate the reintegration and connection to the self as it increases awareness of internal and external experiences among individuals with prominent dissociative symptoms.

Practicing Mindfulness Within the Group

Group settings offer unique opportunities to strengthen and practice mindfulness and Healthy Adult skills. For example, group role plays can expand reflective capacities and meta-awareness. Peer feedback strengthens the awareness of one's behaviors and fosters perspective-taking and reciprocity. It enhances the capacity to "read," access, and reflect on mental states (e.g., thoughts, emotions, desires, attitudes) in ourselves and others. Hearing how other group members have dealt with their difficulties can normalize experiences and make room for change, encouraging and motivating individuals in their practice.

Incorporating mindfulness and body-focused exercises into trauma-focused group therapy can help individuals regulate their emotions and stay in the present moment. However, it may need to be modified from traditional meditation practices. Physical activity and present moment awareness (a stillness in thought and external stimuli that allows complete observation of the here and now) may be preferred to sitting still in meditation. Grounding activities such as observing objects, colors, or the space around you or listening attentively to music are also mindful practices. Guided breathing, body scanning exercises, or mindful movements such as yoga or tai chi anchor each member to their present moment-to-moment experiences and encourage them to connect with their surroundings, body, and breath. These practices have a calming effect, helping group members feel reassured and at ease, which in turn helps them engage more effectively in the therapy session. Breath focus may not work for all patients, and these modifications can help avoid nervous system dysregulation.

Incorporating brief mindfulness or body-focused exercises at the start of each group session is a practical way to increase present-centered practices. Briere (2015) suggests that mindfulness can be used as a form of affect regulation or "settling skills" to regulate distress when encountering painful emotions or triggers. Attending to the breath and body, engaging in the here and now, and noticing thoughts and feelings non-reactively facilitate the "settling in." Avoidance decreases in the "settled state" as the person is gradually exposed to emotionally laden memories and trauma-related thoughts. When seen as the mind's response to trauma, implicit trauma memories and beliefs can be differentiated from the current reality. They can be reframed as "just" memories or products of the mind that are not necessarily accurate information about self/other/environment.

Mindful awareness of triggers helps reduce reactive behaviors. Certain smells or images could potentially activate past traumatic memories and emotions. Things that are calming for some may have the opposite effect on others. Trauma-focused mindfulness aims to increase awareness of emotional activation by utilizing resources that differentiate the past from the present moment, reduce that activation, and create a sense of safety.

What triggers an individual's trauma reaction (e.g., rejection, criticism, facial expressions, interactions with authority figures)? What states are activated when triggered (intrusive thoughts, dissociative episodes, urges to use, self-harm, dysregulated emotions)? The individual can become mindful of triggers without reacting; avoidance behaviors (such as leaving the situation, distracting oneself, or denying the trigger) can be managed until the need to run away dissipates. For example, when urges to engage in distress reduction (such as substance use or self-harm) are triggered, mindfulness can help the individual "ride the wave" or "surf the urge" as they accept but do not react to the triggered state. The Healthy Adult's ability to notice inner experiences without identifying with them facilitates affect regulation and empowers individuals to respond more flexibly, compassionately, and value-driven.

Mindfulness and grounding resources can be used throughout the session as needed. For example, if mindfulness activities pull clients out of their Window of Tolerance, grounding exercises help them reconnect with the present moment. Mindful movement practices can be interwoven into the group to allow individuals to maintain the connection with their body and breath, release tension and trauma held within the body, and promote relaxation and safety. For example, the therapist can guide the group in a brief grounding or reorienting exercise when the group's discussion becomes particularly emotional or distressing. This can help minimize the feeling of being overwhelmed, allowing participants to tolerate their experience in the present moment better.

Clear communication, a safe, trusting space with good boundaries, and anticipating challenges in the group can help moderate some of the distress felt by the clients. Offering choice and control by inviting the clients' participation ("If you are ready, would you like to begin the check-in?"), pacing, staying within the Window of Tolerance, and using short practice periods help to lower the level of discomfort and allow exploration of the client's present moment experience. Clients begin to honor their inner wisdom as they master mindfulness skills. The therapist can guide them by asking questions such as "What is happening right now in your body? What do you notice you are feeling? Can you be with your emotions in a friendly way for this moment?".

Examples of Mindfulness Meditations

1 **Breathing Meditation**: Sitting upright in a relaxed and alert position, attention is focused on the physical sensation of breathing. The breath is used to anchor observations of one's thoughts, feelings, and impulses without judgment and as the principal object of attention. This is an exercise in turning off the automatic pilot and granting the freedom and space to react differently to whatever happens. Patients are encouraged to practice this skill in daily life as often as possible, especially when dysfunctional emotional patterns threaten to surface.

2 **Body-focused meditations** focus on one's perception of physical sensations, such as the body's contact with the seat, or somatic emotional responses, such as tension around the chest. There are two variants of this exercise. In the body scan meditation, awareness is progressively moved through parts of the body. The other variant is based on a broad, open form of attention to the body as a whole. If one particular physical sensation is in the foreground, it remains the point of focus until another sensation attracts attention. The instruction is to continually observe and allow perceptions to arise without discussing them.

3 **Mountain Meditation** is a grounding and empowering meditation that builds the Healthy Adult self by boosting self-confidence, strength, and feelings of stability. Like a mountain in a winter squall, this meditation reminds us that we can remain calm and stand tall and strong as the vagaries of life swirl around us.

   a *Picture a majestic mountain, any mountain that you can imagine. As you visualize the mountain, paint the picture with as much detail as possible. Notice the tall mountain, firmly rooted in the ground for thousands of years. The weather changes from sunny skies to hurricane-force winds to snow and ice all around the mountain. The mountain remains strong as the weather swirls around it, unaffected daily.*

   b *Now, sit quietly and focus on your breath going in and out. Relax and breathe. As thoughts come in and out of your mind, sit up or stand with your shoulders back, your chest open, and your feet firmly planted on the ground. Picture yourself as the tall, strong mountain, steadfastly grounded to the earth. Let the thoughts and stress and the anxiety whirl around you without affecting you. The thoughts that are pressuring you are just thoughts. You are a mountain, sitting strong. You are who you are and have always been, regardless of the "weather" around you. Breathe in and out slowly and deeply as you enjoy this feeling of power, strength, and majesty.*

4 **Meditations Focused on Various Objects:** Attention can be focused on sounds, thoughts representing words or phrases (internal speech), or thoughts in images (memories and fantasies). Another meditation exercise is choiceless awareness (or mindfulness without an object), in which no focal point exists, and anything goes. Whatever appears in awareness also disappears and does so without intervention. (This lack of structure may be too diffuse for participants who tend to dissociate).

5 **Meditation in Movement** directs attention toward the soles of the feet and gradually expands to the rest of the body while walking. These kinds of exercises are an effective way of involving mindfulness techniques in day-to-day life.

6 **Three Minute Breathing Space** is a specialized mindfulness application developed by Segal et al. (2016). The breathing space allows patients to step out of automatic pilot mode when situations require conscious consideration. The exercise is made up of three steps, each taking approximately one minute to complete: (1) bringing into awareness any bodily sensations, thoughts, or feelings coming into being (2) attention is focused as much as possible on the experience of breathing (3) attention is expanded to the whole physical presence, with the breath remaining in background awareness. A phrase that may be recited is "It is okay … whatever it is, it is already here: let me feel it" (Williams et al., 2007).

7 **Mindfulness to Strengthen the Healthy Adult** (van der Wijngaart, 2015, pp. 8–9):

a **Visualizing the HA** (Therapist): The therapist self-discloses a time she dealt with a difficult situation in a healthy way, describing the emotional, cognitive, and behavioral aspects of her response. (E.g., "When I asked my boss for a raise, I felt confident and strong with my feet firmly on the ground. I felt connected to a sense of calm in my belly despite facing this difficult problem. I visualized myself standing solid and erect like a mountain. I can draw on that image when facing an upset situation".) **Visualizing the HA** (Clients): The clients close their eyes and imagine a time they felt connected to their HA self. This can be in a non-challenging situation. The clients describe this in a way similar to the therapist's. They can practice visualizing this image as a homework assignment.

b   Ask group members to acknowledge the suffering of their Vulnerable Child, allowing them to connect soothingly ("I see you are upset; This is so painful. It is understandable; I never learned to feel safe"). Next, ask them to offer hope and a different perspective ("This will go away. Things will change. It feels overwhelming now, but it will not stay that way"). Finally, ask them to deal with the present moment's reality (challenging the inner critic or coping modes, identifying why they were triggered, and choosing healthy ways to solve the problem).

Summary

Mindfulness practices and developing the Healthy Adult mode in Schema Therapy synergistically support trauma recovery by fostering self-regulation, emotional awareness, and adaptive functioning. Mindfulness, character-ized by non-judgmental present-moment attention, enhances the Healthy Adult's capacity to observe schema-driven patterns without reactivity, cre-ating psychological space to challenge maladaptive beliefs and nurture self-compassion. The Healthy Adult mode utilizes mindful awareness to balance emotional needs, set boundaries, and mediate between trauma-related child modes and critical inner voices through three core functions: compassionate bonding, behavioral balance, and empowered battling of challenges. Trauma-informed mindfulness adaptations—such as grounding techniques, body-focused meditations, and environmental anchoring—help survivors stay within their window of tolerance while processing difficult memories. This integration allows individuals to reframe traumatic memo-ries as past events rather than current realities, reducing avoidance and rumination while increasing distress tolerance. Group therapy applications demonstrate how shared mindfulness practices strengthen meta-awareness and peer-supported growth, enabling survivors to reclaim agency over their healing process through embodied present-moment experiences.

References

Briere, J. (2015). Pain and suffering: a synthesis of Buddhist and western approaches to trauma. In V. M. Follette, J. Briere, D. Rozelle, et al., (Eds.) *Mindfulness-Oriented Interventions for Trauma: Integrating Contemplative Practices*. New York: Guilford Press.

Chiesa, A., Serretti, A., & Jakobsen, J. C. (2013). Mindfulness: top–down or bottom–up emotion regulation strategy? *Clinical Psychology Review*, 33 (1), 82–96.

Edwards, D. J. A. (2022). Using schema modes for case conceptualization in schema therapy: an applied clinical approach. *Frontiers in Psychology*, 12, 763670. https://doi.org/10.3389/fpsyg.2021.763670

Follette, V. M., Briere, J., Rozelle, D., et al., (Eds.) (2015). *Mindfulness-oriented Inter-ventions for Trauma: Integrating Contemplative Practices*. New York: Guilford Press.

Fredrickson, B. L. (2013). Updated thinking on positivity ratios. *American Psychologist*, 68, 814–822. https://doi.org/10.1037/A0033584

Frewen, P., & Lanius, R. (2015). *Healing the Traumatized Self: Consciousness, Neuroscience, and Treatment.* New York: W. W. Norton.

Haeyen, S. (2019). Strengthening the healthy adult self in art therapy: using schema therapy as a positive psychological intervention for people diagnosed with personality disorders. *Frontiers in Psychology*, 10, 445514. https://doi.org/10.3389/fpsyg.2019.00644

Kabat-Zinn, J. (2003). Mindfulness-based interventions in context: past, present, and future. *Clinical Psychology: Science and Practice*, 10, 144–156.

Lang, A. J., Strauss, J. L., & Bomyea, J., (2012). The theoretical and empirical basis for meditation as an intervention for PTSD. *Behavior Modification*, 36, 759–786.

Magyari, T. (2015). Teaching mindfulness-based stress reduction and mindfulness to women with complex trauma. In V. M. Follette, J. Briere, D. Rozelle, et al., (Eds.) *Mindfulness-Oriented Interventions for Trauma: Integrating Contemplative Practices.* New York: Guilford Press, 140–156.

Maté, G. (2018). *In the Realm of Hungry Ghosts: Close Encounters with Addiction.* Canada: Vermilion Press.

Segal, Z. V., Williams, J. M., & Teasdale, J. D. (2002). *Mindfulness-based Cognitive Therapy for Depression: A New Approach to Preventing Relapse.* New York: Guilford Press.

Segal, Z.V. (2016). The Three-Minute Breathing Space Practice. *Mindful.* https://www.mindful.org/the-three-minute-breathing-space-practice/

Tempone-Wiltshire, J. (2024). The role of mindfulness and embodiment in group-based trauma treatment. *Psychotherapy and Counselling Journal of Australia*, 12(1), 1–27 https://doi.org/10.59158/001c.94979

Treleaven, D. A. (2018). *Trauma-Sensitive Mindfulness: Practices for Safe and Transformative Healing.* New York: W. W. Norton & Company.

Van Der Wijngaart, R. (2015). The healthy adult mode: ways to strengthen the healthy adult of our patients. *Schema Therapy Bulletin*, May 2015, 7–10.

Van Vreeswijk, M., Broersen, J., & Schurink, G. (2014). *Mindfulness and Schema Therapy: A Practical Guide* (1st ed.). New York: John Wiley & Sons, Ltd.

Wieczorek, M., & Brockman, R. (2016). *The Schema Model and Core Emotional Needs: A Self-Determination Theory Perspective.* Master's Thesis, University of Technology Sydney.

Williams, M., Teasdale, J., Segal, Z., & Kabat-Zinn, J. (2007). *The Mindful Way Through Depression: Freeing Yourself from Chronic Unhappiness.* New York: Guilford Press.

Yakın, D., & Arntz, A. (2023). Understanding the reparative effects of schema modes: an in-depth analysis of the healthy adult mode. *Frontiers in Psychiatry* 14, 1204177. https://doi.org/10.3389/fpsyt.2023.1204177

Zerubavel, N., & Messman-Moore, T. L. (2015). Staying present: incorporating mindfulness into therapy for dissociation. *Mindfulness*, 6, 303–314.

Chapter 7

Trauma, Substance Use Disorders, Eating Disorders, and Behavioral Addictions

Substance abuse, eating disorders, and behavioral addictions continue to be problematic in society and remain serious health problems. While not the primary focus of this group program, the intricate interrelationship of these disorders with the experience of early childhood trauma and adverse childhood experiences like abuse, neglect, or household dysfunction cannot be overlooked. Trauma significantly increases the risk of developing these disorders, while addictions may expose the user to high-risk situations that increase the chance of revictimization. This complex web of connections underscores the need for a comprehensive understanding and approach.

The high rates of co-occurrence between PTSD, substance use disorders, and eating disorders have been well documented (Khoury et al., 2010; Haller, 2014; Trottier & MacDonald, 2017). A review of the literature on the relationship between trauma and eating disorders highlights a clear association between trauma exposure, particularly in childhood, and eating disorders. A study of over 5,000 participants from the National Comorbidity Survey-Replication found that both men and women with eating disorders had experienced most forms of traumatic events at a significantly higher rate than the general population, particularly for interpersonal traumas such as sexual assault (Mitchell et al., 2012). Multiple studies have shown an association between a history of childhood abuse and bulimia (Fichter et al., 1994; Wonderlich et al., 2001). Up to 59% of young people with PTSD subsequently develop substance abuse problems (NCTSN); 75% of women and men in substance abuse treatment report histories of abuse and trauma; up to 50% of people with eating disorders use illicit drugs or alcohol and approximately 75% of women in residential treatment for eating disorders report experiencing some form of trauma, and 50% have a history of PTSD (Khoury et al., 2010). Addictive disorders are also highly comorbid with personality disorders (PD) (Boog et al., 2018), with comorbidity tied to poorer treatment outcomes, failure to respond to treatment, or relapse. The rates of full diagnostic criteria for PD diagnoses

DOI: 10.4324/9781003462958-8

are estimated as high as 60–65% among patients suffering from addictions (Casadio et al., 2014; Roncero et al., 2019, cited in Lacy, 2024).

Trauma, Emotion Regulation Deficits, and Addiction

Trauma interferes with the body's ability to self-regulate. Many individuals who have experienced trauma turn to substances, disordered eating, or other addictive behaviors to "self-medicate" to manage the PTSD symptoms. Early learning milieus shape the way a child learns to cope. Childhood experiences characterized by neglectful, absent, or abusive caregiving hinder the development of secure attachments that model ways to regulate and tolerate difficult emotions. In the absence of effective models for co- and self-regulation, the individual finds ways to rapidly relieve and avoid their emotional pain, including abusing substances, disordered eating, or engaging in other behavioral addictions such as masturbation, shopping, or gaming (Lacy, 2024). These solutions may be used to escape the pain of anxiety or depression, help block intrusive traumatic memories, or escape the messages of a harsh internal critic (Tatarsky & Kellogg, 2011).

Addictive behaviors begin as survival strategies that help facilitate self-regulation by temporarily helping manage trauma symptoms, decreasing the need to depend on others, and maintaining a sense of control. Chemical dependency is an example of an attempt to escape, cope with, or numb the emotional pain and symptoms associated with trauma; disordered eating may help a person control one aspect of their lives when they feel powerless in other areas due to the trauma. Dysfunctional emotional processing and regulation are proposed to underpin many psychological disorders, including eating disorders (Oldershaw et al., 2019). Eating disorder behaviors are posited as mediating mechanisms for emotion dysregulation, dissociation, and maladaptive core beliefs (e.g., about defectiveness and abandonment) resulting from childhood abuse (Trottier & MacDonald, 2017).

Increased vulnerability and susceptibility to addictive behaviors may result from this failure to develop the ability to effectively regulate emotions, as well as from changes that occur in the structure or chemistry of the brain (e.g., in areas related to reward processing and impulse control) (Center for Substance Abuse Treatment, 2014). Early trauma has specific effects on the neurotransmitter systems involved in the positive reinforcing effects of alcohol and drugs, food, exercise, and sex, particularly the dopamine system (Meaney et al., 2002; Olsen, 2011).

These behaviors are theorized to enable the avoidance of trauma-related thoughts and feelings. Intrusive memories, flashbacks, nightmares, and body memories that trigger relapses are kept at bay by the addictive behaviors as they down-regulate hyperarousal or up-regulate hypoarousal, reducing chronic fear or mitigating the effect of numbing and dissociation. The addiction occurs as continual increases in dosage are necessary to achieve the same self-regulating effect (Fisher, 2000).

This "self-medication" interferes with trauma processing when used as a coping mechanism and may exacerbate PTSD symptoms, increasing negative affect and cognitions and high-risk behaviors. Substance use, disordered eating, or behavioral addictions themselves may facilitate reenactment of the trauma. They often involve secrecy, danger, and shame while temporarily helping decrease the shame and guilt associated with the trauma. The short-term relief undermines self-worth and self-respect as it perpetuates isolation, secrecy, and loneliness, leaving the basic underlying needs for love, nurturance, and acceptance unmet (Najavits, 2002, 2012).

Treatment

A significant challenge is knowing how to prioritize and integrate treatment components for both trauma and addiction. Clinicians often struggle with deciding whether to address trauma or the co-occurring behaviors first or how to combine treatments for both conditions effectively. It is crucial to remember that a balanced approach, considering all aspects of the individual's experience, is key. In the past, treatment programs have been reluctant to address trauma and addictions concurrently due to concerns that addressing trauma may lead to an escalation in substance use, disordered eating, repeated suicidal crises, self-injury, or interpersonal problems. This concern can lead to hesitation in using trauma-focused therapies despite their proven effectiveness (Krejci et al., 2008).

High dropout rates are a significant challenge in treating these populations, regardless of the intervention used. A history of childhood trauma was associated with a greater likelihood of treatment dropout (Mahon et al., 2001). It is believed that restricting substance use and reducing disordered eating without alternative ways of coping may leave individuals more emotionally vulnerable to their trauma symptoms. This may partially explain the greater dropout rates.

In the past, traditional addiction or eating disorder programs may have been inappropriate for individuals with comorbid PTSD symptoms. These programs, particularly programs for substance abuse, relied on confrontational interventions, rigid 12-step involvement, an emphasis on powerlessness, abstinence, and the assumption that psychiatric symptoms would resolve with abstinence from substances or refeeding (Krejci et al., 2008). It was believed that trauma work was inappropriate until after a patient had been abstinent and in control of their behaviors for a sustained period (e.g., three months). This model, known as the "sequential" model, posited that continued use of substances or disordered eating impedes therapeutic efforts to address and process the trauma and that if trauma work is begun before an individual has achieved sustained abstinence, there will be an increased risk of relapse. However, studies conducted by several investigators in the USA and Australia show that substance-dependent patients who engage in integrative Cognitve Behavior Therapy (CBT) interventions typically experience significant improvements in both conditions, and rates of relapse are not increased by the introduction of trauma work (Najavits, 2002; Hien, 2004; Audrain-McGovern et al., 2009). Brewerton (2023) noted the importance of integrated treatment in which the functional connection between trauma history/PTSD and subsequent eating disorder is identified and processed cognitively (e.g., bingeing and purging serve to avoid and numb). Integrated, concurrent approaches that understand the interrelationship between trauma and addiction are often the most effective treatments.

Schema Therapy (ST) is an effective model for the treatment of patients with maladaptive behaviors, PDs, and complex trauma (Ball & Young, 2000; Sempértegui et al., 2013; Bamelis et al., 2014; Arntz, 2015; Arntz & Simpson, 2020). Addiction and Eating Disorders are conceptualized in ST as dysfunctional coping modes (Simpson, Morrow, Van Vreeswijk & Reid, 2010; Simpson, 2020; Lacy, 2024). The model's use of the therapy relationship to meet core needs and implement evidence-based interventions has been shown to keep patients engaged longer than other treatment models (Sempértegui et al., 2013). A strong and positive alliance between the patient and the clinician facilitates positive treatment outcomes, retention, and completion (Bethea et al., 2008). It allows the therapist the opportunity to model and teach self-regulation or self-management skills, provides the safety for the patient to practice these skills, and the opportunity to address the interpersonal aspects of the pain that addictions and eating disorders have helped to avoid (Triffleman, Carroll & Kellogg,2010; Tatarsky & Kellogg, 2011; Kellogg & Tatarsky, 2012).

ST distinguishes itself in the treatment of addictions and eating disorders by targeting deep-rooted emotional patterns, unmet childhood needs, addiction-driven modes, and the unique psychological functions of disordered eating behaviors that fuel these disorders. Compared to other therapies, these treatments emphasize long-term schema transformation over symptom management, with distinct advantages for complex cases involving co-occurring disorders or trauma.

In chronic, complex addiction cases, ST's developmental lens and mode-based interventions offer a nuanced alternative to standard approaches, mainly when substance use masks unmet attachment needs or identity fragmentation. Schema Therapy for Addictive Treatment (STAT, Lacy, 2024) is a model for the integrative treatment of addictive disorders that addresses many of the shortcomings of existing treatment options. This model focuses explicitly on the interconnection of addictive and co-occurring colluding behaviors (e.g., avoidance/surrender) with the early and continued frustration of core developmental needs. Lacy (2024) illustrates how the addiction cycle is perpetuated through the process of schema reinforcement and the operation of schema modes (addictive protector, avoidant colluding mode, compliant surrender). Treatment focuses on integrating recovery behavior change, healing dysfunctional schemas and modes, and preventing relapse. STAT shows promise in meeting the need for a comprehensive treatment approach to help patients achieve long-term recovery from addictions.

For patients with a support system built around their addictive behaviors, group therapy, in particular, offers a unique opportunity for corrective emotional experiences and the development of new attachment skills (Dingle et al., 2015; Tirandaz & Akbari, 2018). The supportive and therapeutic space allows individuals to address not only their addictive behaviors but also the underlying attachment issues, social skills deficits, and feelings of shame (Flores, 2001; Farrell et al., 2009; Moeller et al., 2022). Group treatment lends itself to the ST model by providing *in vivo* exposure to situations that trigger schemas and modes (especially in terms of interacting and forming close bonds with others). Members can benefit from the supportive context of the group as they link their early experiences with here-and-now schema processes as they arise in the group. Group members become therapists to each other, thereby increasing opportunities for both evidence-based and vicarious learning, taking risks with new behavior, and experiences of self-efficacy (Farrell & Shaw, 2012; Lacy, 2024). Group ST (GST) was also found effective in enhancing psychological well-being and resilience in a sample of patients with substance dependence under treatment with methadone and buprenorphine (Pourpashang & Mousavi, 2021).

In ST for eating disorders, distorted body perception and memories linked to body image/social rejection schemas are challenged with body-oriented imagery and reprocessed through guided visualization. Childhood humiliation narratives contributing to restrictive eating are rewritten (Simpson, 2020). GST (Farrell & Shaw, 2012) has been specifically adapted for the eating-disordered population (Simpson, 2020). This program demonstrated improvement in eating-disordered symptoms, as well as schema severity, shame, anxiety, and quality of life.

The complex interplay between co-occurring issues of trauma and substance abuse, eating disorders, and behavioral addictions can be addressed in the trauma-focused group as they arise, even though this manual has not dedicated specific sessions to these topics. Therapists are referred to Lacy (2024) and Simpson (2020) for comprehensive reviews of ST for addictions and eating disorders. The mind-altering properties of addictive behaviors, be it substance abuse, disordered eating, or behavioral addictions, impair recovery from trauma, and trauma symptoms and maladaptive schemas and modes equally impair the ability to stay clean and sober. As the group understands these interconnections and the role of substances, food, or other behaviors in the avoidance of painful emotions, they can replace maladaptive coping patterns that may once have been lifesaving but have now become dangerous. Recovery is enhanced as participants gain a sense of mastery and control through the acquisition of new skills to replace the short-term relief provided by substances, disordered eating, or behavioral addictions. Healthy coping is a prerequisite for safety, stability, and self-care.

Summary

There is a complex relationship between trauma and addictive disorders, including substance abuse, eating disorders, and behavioral addictions. Trauma survivors frequently develop these conditions as maladaptive coping mechanisms to manage unresolved psychological pain, creating a cyclical pattern where behaviors temporarily alleviate symptoms like hyperarousal or dissociation while exacerbating long-term distress. These behaviors act as emotional regulators, helping survivors avoid trauma-related memories and shame while perpetuating isolation.

Up to 75% of individuals in substance abuse treatment report trauma histories, with 50–59% developing PTSD. Eating disorder patients show similar patterns, with 75% experiencing trauma and 50% meeting PTSD criteria. Early trauma disrupts brain development, particularly in dopamine regulation and regions governing impulse control, increasing addiction vulnerability.

Modern treatment has shifted from traditional sequential models that required sustained abstinence prior to trauma treatment to evidence-based integrated approaches. Sustainable recovery requires concurrent trauma/addiction treatment focused on replacing maladaptive coping with healthy self-regulation strategies. Integrated trauma-informed treatment such as ST simultaneously addresses addictions and eating disorders through schema mode work and core developmental need repair. Group therapy offers a unique opportunity for corrective emotional experiences and the development of new attachment skills, especially for patients whose support system has been built around their addictive behaviors. Group therapy yields improved outcomes, fewer dropouts, and lower relapse rates, which are essential for long-term recovery and stability. These approaches show particular promise for breaking the trauma-addiction cycle.

References

Aaron, D. J. (2013). Early maladaptive schemas and substance use. *Addictive Disorders & Their Treatment, 12*(4), 193–200. https://doi.org/10.1097/ADT.0b013e31827d8763

Arntz, A. (2015). Imagery rescripting for posttraumatic stress disorder. In B. B. Thoma& D. McCay (Eds.), *Working with Emotion in Cognitive Behavioral Therapy: Techniques for Clinical Practices*. New York: Guilford Press, 203–215.

Arntz, A., & Simpson, S. (2020). Core principles of imagery. In G. Heath & H. Startup (Eds.), *Creative Methods in Schema Therapy*. London, New York: Routledge.

Audrain-Mcgovern, J., Rodriguez, D., & Kassel, J. D. (2009). Adolescent smoking and depression: evidence for self-medication and peer smoking mediation. *Addiction*, 104(10), 1743–1756. https://doi.org/10.1111/j.1360-0443.2009.02617.x

Ball, S. A., & Young, J. E. (2000). Dual focus schema therapy for personality disorders and substance dependence: case study results. *Cognitive and Behavioral Practice*, 7(3), 270–281.

Bamelis, L. L., Evers, S. M., Spinhoven, P., & Arntz, A. (2014). Results of a multicenter randomized controlled trial of the clinical effectiveness of schema therapy for personality disorders. *American Journal of Psychiatry*, 171, 305–322. https://doi.org/10.1176/appi.ajp.2013.12040518

Bethea, A. R., Acosta, M. C. & Haller, D. L. (2008). Patient versus therapist alliance: whose perception matters. *Journal of Substance Abuse Treatment*, 35, 174–183.

Boog, M., Van Hest, K. M., Drescher, T., Verschuur, M. J., & Franken, I. H. (2018). Schema modes and personality disorder symptoms in alcohol-dependent and cocaine-dependent patients. *European Addiction Research*, 24, 226–233. https://doi.org/10.1159/000493644

Brewerton, T. (2023). The integrated treatment of eating disorders, posttraumatic stress disorder, and psychiatric comorbidity: a commentary on the evolution of principles and guidelines. *Frontiers in Psychiatry*, 14, 1149433. https://doi.org/10.3389/fpsyt.2023.1149433

Brewerton, T., & Dennis, A. B. (2014). *Eating Disorders, Addictions and Substance Use Disorders: Research, Clinical and Treatment Perspectives*. Heidelberg: Springer Berlin.

Casadio, P., Olivoni, D., Ferrari, B., Pintori, C., Speranza, E., Bosi, M., Belli, V., Baruzzi, L., Pantieri, P., Ragazzini, G., Rivola, F., & Atti, A. R. (2014). Personality disorders in addiction outpatients: prevalence and effects on psychosocial functioning. *Substance Use: Research and Treatment*, 2014, 17–24. https://doi.org/10.4137/SART.S13764

Center for Substance Abuse Treatment (2014). *Trauma-informed care in behavioral health services*. Treatment Improvement Protocol (TIP) Series 57. HHS Publication No. (SMA) 13–4801. Rockville, MD: Substance Abuse and Mental Health Services Administration. https://arcr.niaaa.nih.gov/volume/34/4/childhood-trauma-posttraumatic-stress-disorder-and-alcohol-dependence

Dingle, G. A., Cruwys, T., & Frings, D. (2015). Social identities as pathways into and out of addiction. *Frontiers in Psychology*, 6, 153612. https://doi.org/10.3389/fpsyg.2015.01795

Farrell, J. M., Shaw, I. A., & Webber, M. A. (2009). A schema-focused approach to group psychotherapy for outpatients with borderline personality disorder: a randomized controlled trial. *Journal of Behavior Therapy and Experimental Psychiatry*, 40, 317–328.

Farrell, J. M., & Shaw, I. A. (2012). *Group Schema Therapy for Borderline Personality Disorder: A Step-by-Step Treatment Manual with Patient Workbook*. United Kingdom: Wiley.

Fichter, M. M., Quadflieg, N., & Rief, W. (1994). Course of multi-impulsive bulimia. *Psychological Medicine*, 24(3), 591–604. https://doi.org/10.1017/S0033291700027744

Fisher, J. (2000). Addictions and trauma recovery. Paper Presented at the International Society for the Study of Dissociation, November 13, 2000, San Antonio, TX.

Flores, P. J. (2001). Addiction as an attachment disorder: implications for group therapy. *International Journal of Group Psychotherapy*, 51, 63–81. https://doi.org/10.1521/ijgp.51.1.63.49730

Haller, M. (2014). Risk pathways among traumatic stress, posttraumatic stress disorder symptoms, and alcohol and drug problems: a test of four hypotheses. *Psychology of Addictive Behaviors*, 28(3), 841–851.

Hien, D. A. (2004). Promising treatments for women with comorbid PTSD and substance use disorders. *American Journal of Psychiatry*, 161, 1426–1432.

Kellogg, S. H., & Tatarsky, A. (2012). Re-envisioning addiction treatment: a six-point plan. *Alcoholism Treatment Quarterly*, 30(1), 109–128. https://doi-org.proxy.libraries.rutgers.edu/10.1080/07347324.2012.635544

Khoury, L., Tang, Y. L., Bradley, B., Cubells, J. F., & Ressler, K. J. (2010). Substance use, childhood traumatic experience, and posttraumatic stress disorder in an urban civilian population. *Depress Anxiety*, 27(12), 1077–1086. https://doi.org/10.1002/Da.20751

Krejci, J., Margolin, J., Rowland, M., & Wetzell, C. (2008). Integrated group treatment of women's substance abuse and trauma. *Journal of Groups in Addiction and Recovery*, 3(3–4), 263–284.

Lacy, E. (2024). STAT: Schema therapy for addiction treatment, a proposal for the integrative treatment of addictive disorders. *Frontiers in Psychology*, 15, 1366617. https://doi.org/10.3389/fpsyg.2024.1366617

Mahon, J., Bradley, S., Harvey, P. K., Winston, A. P., & Palmer, R. L. (2001). Childhood trauma has a dose-effect relationship with dropping out from psychotherapeutic treatment for bulimia nervosa: a replication. *International Journal of Eating Disorders*, 30(2), 138–148.

Meaney, M. J., Wayne Brake, W., & Gratton, A. (2002). Environmental regulation of the development of mesolimbic dopamine systems: a neurobiological mechanism for vulnerability to drug abuse? *Psychoneuroendocrinology*, 27(1–2), 127–138. https://doi.org/10.1016/s0306-4530(01)00040-3

Mitchell, A. L., Lacroix, S., Weiner, B. S., Imholtz, C., & Goodair, C. (2012). Collective amnesia: reversing the global epidemic of addiction library closures. *Addiction*, 107, 1367–1368. https://doi.org/10.1111/j.1360-0443.2012.03813.x

Moeller, S. J., Stoops, W. W., & King, A. C. (2022). Shame and addiction treatment outcomes: a scoping review. *American Journal on Addictions*, 31, 71–79. https://doi.org/10.1111/ajad.13241

Najavits, L. M. (2002). *Seeking Safety: A Treatment Manual for PTSD and Substance Abuse*. New York: Guilford Press.

Najavits, L. M. (2012). Dissociation, PTSD, and substance abuse: an empirical study. *Journal of Trauma Dissociation*, 13(1), 115–126.

Oldershaw, A., Startup, H., & Lavender, T. (2019). Anorexia nervosa, and a lost emotional self: a psychological formulation of the development, maintenance, and treatment of anorexia nervosa. *Frontiers in Psychology*, 10, 219. https://doi.org/10.3389/fpsyg.2019.00219

Olsen,R.W. (2011). Extrasynaptic GABAA receptors in the nucleus accumbens are necessary for alcohol drinking, *Proc. Natl. Acad. Sci.* U.S.A. 108(12), 4699–4700, https://doi.org/10.1073/pnas.1102818108.

Pourpashang, M., & Mousavi, S. (2021). The effects of group schema therapy on psychological wellbeing and resilience in patients under substance dependence treatment. *Journal of Client-Centered Nursing Care (Online)*, 7(2), 159–166. https://DOI:10.32598/JCCNC.7.2.366.1

Roncero, C., Daigre, C., Gonzalvo, B., Valero, S., Castells, X., Grau-López, L., Eiroa-Orosa, F. J., & Casas, M. (2019). Personality disorders in cocaine and opioid addicts: influence of socio-demographic factors and consumption characteristics. *Adicciones*, 31, 66–76. https://doi.org/10.20882/adicciones.927

Sempértegui, G. A., Karreman, A., Arntz, A., & Bekker, M. H. (2013). Schema therapy for borderline personality disorder: a comprehensive review of its empirical foundations, effectiveness, and implementation possibilities. *Clinical Psychology Review*, 33, 426–447. https://doi.org/10.1016/j.cpr.2012.11.006

Simpson, S. G., Morrow, E., Van Vreeswijk, M., & Reid, C. (2010). Group schema therapy for eating disorders: a pilot study. *Frontiers in Psychology*, 1, 182. https://doi.org/10.3389/Fpsyg.2010.00182

Simpson, S. (2020). Manual of group schema therapy for eating disorders. In S. Simpson & E. Smith (Eds.), *Schema Therapy for Eating Disorders: Theory and Practice for Individual and Group Settings*. London: Routledge, 136–184.

Tatarsky, A., & Kellogg, S. H. (2011). Harm reduction psychotherapy. In G. A. Marlatt, M. E. Larimer, & K. Witkiewitz (Eds.), *Harm Reduction*, 2nd ed., New York, NY: Guilford Press, 36–60.

Tirandaz, S., & Akbari, B. (2018). The effectiveness of group schema therapy on adjusting the early maladaptive schemas of the drug-dependent women. *Avicenna Journal of Neuropsychophysiology*, 5, 123–130. https://doi.org/10.32598/ajnpp.5.3.123.

Triffleman, E., Carroll, K., & Kellogg, S. (1999). Substance dependence posttraumatic stress disorder therapy: an integrated cognitive-behavioral approach. *Journal of Substance Abuse Treatment*, 17(1), 3–14.

Trottier, K., & Macdonald, D. E. (2017). Update on psychological trauma, other severe adverse experiences and eating disorders: state of the research and future research directions. *Current Psychiatry Reports*, 19, 45. https://doi.org/10.1007/s11920-017-0806-6

Wonderlich, S. A., Crosby, R. D., Mitchell, J. E., Thompson, K. M., Redlin, J., Demuth, G., & Smyth, J. (2001). Eating disturbance and sexual trauma in childhood and adulthood. *International Journal of Eating Disorders*, 30(4), 401–412.

Chapter 8

Theoretical Underpinnings and Treatment Considerations

A Summary

Integrating Schema Therapy (ST) with Trauma-Focused Group Therapy (TFGT) offers a nuanced framework for addressing the multifaceted impact of early childhood trauma and Complex Post-Traumatic Stress Disorder (CPTSD). It yields enduring benefits that extend beyond immediate symptom reduction, fostering sustained healing for individuals with complex trauma histories. This synergy addresses both surface-level trauma responses and the deep-seated schemas perpetuating distress, creating a foundation for long-term resilience.

Group Schema Therapy

Group Schema Therapy (GST) has evolved into diverse applications tailored to specific populations and clinical contexts, demonstrating flexibility while maintaining core principles of addressing unmet needs, maladaptive schemas, and modes. It was first developed as a comprehensive treatment for Borderline Personality Disorder (BPD) (Farrell et al., 2009). GST combines the central components of process/interpersonal groups with cognitive, experiential, and behavioral pattern-breaking.

Specific factors inherent in a group format augment and catalyze ST interventions. The closer analog to the family in the group allows corrective experiences through reparenting and experiential learning. The emphasis on authenticity, understanding, acceptance, and care within the group provides corrective emotional experiences that allow schema change to occur. The group as a healthy surrogate family helps heal disorganized attachment representations through validation by and relationships with other group members. The therapeutic power of the group is used strategically to help patients change dysfunctional life patterns and get their basic needs met. The group process becomes a powerful vehicle for change, providing opportunities for connection, validation, and corrective experiences crucial for complex trauma recovery. Opportunities abound to observe others, get feedback, benefit from the experience of peers, and practice skills in the

DOI: 10.4324/9781003462958-9

group's safe environment. Empathic confrontation becomes more powerful when delivered by the group members. Group members can risk being vulnerable.

Research into GST has demonstrated higher remission rates and lower dropout rates in outpatient and inpatient settings than treatment alone (Farrell et al., 2009). When combined with individual ST, GST effectively reduces BPD symptoms and improves quality of life (Arntz et al., 2022; Fassbinder & Arntz, 2021). Since GST for BPD was first introduced in 2009, other GST formats have been developed and tailored to offer effective treatment for multiple patient populations. These include eating disorders (Simpson, 2019); group schema cognitive–behavioral therapy (SCBT-g) for heterogeneous psychiatric populations (Van Vreeswijk et al., 2014); mixed personality disorders (Skewes et al., 2015; Koppers et al., 2021); anxiety (Staarup et al., 2022); online GST during the COVID-19 shutdown (Van Dijk et al., 2020); premenstrual dysphoric disorder (Mohtadijafari et al., 2019); and divorce (Nameni et al., 2022). GST is successful in reducing personality disorder symptomology, global symptom severity, anxiety and depression, quality of life, and functional capacity. Integrating cognitive, behavioral, experiential, and relational techniques allows GST to facilitate recovery beyond symptomatic remission while reducing maladaptive behaviors.

Group Therapy for Complex Trauma: A Schema-Informed Approach

Group Therapy for Complex Trauma: A Schema-Informed Approach (GTCT-SI) represents a specialized adaptation of GST that shares many of the foundational elements with the original model of GST for BPD. There is a significant overlap between BPD and Complex Trauma, with a majority of BPD clients having a history of trauma (Cloitre et al., 2013). These individuals struggle to regulate their emotions, maintain a coherent sense of self, and sustain healthy relationships. Rapid mode shifts can be compared to dissociated states, with modes such as the abandoned child mode reflecting the reexperiencing of traumatic past events (Farrell & Shaw, 2012; Arntz et al., 2022).

Central to the current model is its emphasis on the six D's, which capture the systemic fragmentation caused by chronic trauma (dysregulation, disruption, distortion, disorientation, disconnection, and defensiveness). Combining ST with a wide range of contemporary trauma research offers a CPTSD-specific framework that expands the initial groundwork in GST (Farrell & Shaw, 2018). It bridges gaps in treating complex trauma's systemic impacts while retaining ST's fundamental strengths in schema/

mode work. Combining ST's focus on challenging maladaptive schemas and modes and strengthening the Healthy Adult with trauma education and trauma-informed group dynamics further facilitates healing and recovery from early childhood trauma. Prioritizing safety and stabilization within a supportive "corrective family" environment and using strategies like limited reparenting, empathic confrontation, and experiential exercises help group members develop resources and capabilities that promote self-regulation and healthy relational dynamics.

GTCT-SI diverges from traditional GST in several ways. It expands GST's reach by incorporating a wider range of trauma-specific psychoeducation, making it distinct from BPD-focused models while maintaining schema mode analysis as a unifying thread. Both demonstrate GST's versatility in treating disorders rooted in unmet childhood needs. However, the tailored interventions of GTCT-SI more directly address population-specific vulnerabilities and the systemic effects rooted in chronic adversity (identity disruptions, somatic and emotional dysregulation, fear-based defensive coping, cognitive distortions, and attachment disconnections). The interventions are tailored to reduce fragmentation and rebuild self-identity, interpersonal relationships, and self-regulation coherence. The systematic effects of trauma are contextualized through psychoeducation on themes such as the nature of CPTSD, the neurobiology of trauma, trauma and memory, trauma and the body, attachment, relationships, dissociation, and emotion regulation. Flexible protocols blend structured ST techniques with unstructured sessions to address emergent trauma themes. The group replicates family dynamics, offering a relational laboratory to process maladaptive schemas and coping modes as they manifest in real time. Relational repair occurs through limited reparenting, peer validation, and therapist modeling as the group replicates family dynamics in the "group-as-microcosm" of the "corrective family" (Farrell & Shaw, 2018).

Integrating trauma-focused interventions into ST leverages the strengths of each modality, offering multifaceted benefits. Trauma-focused interventions help reduce avoidance behaviors and process traumatic material, while ST addresses early maladaptive schemas rooted in childhood adversity. Exposure to traumatic material paired with ST's imagery rescripting and restructuring associated schemas (e.g., replacing helplessness with empowerment) creates a synergistic approach to healing trauma. ST's focus on replacing maladaptive coping modes while strengthening the Healthy Adult mode enhances emotional regulation and resilience as it helps clients manage trauma-induced emotional dysregulation. These combined approaches improve overall emotional resilience as they widen the window of tolerance, reduce PTSD dysregulation, and strengthen the Healthy Adult mode.

Integrating Current Literature

Findings from the broader trauma literature have been integrated into GTCT-SI. This program aligns with the triphasic model of trauma-informed treatment (safety/processing/reconnection) described by Herman (1992). Safety and stabilization (e.g., widening the Window of Tolerance) are prioritized alongside the schema/mode work. The incorporation of trauma's impact on the nervous system, memory, the body, and attachment reflects modern trauma research (Ogden et al., 2008; van der Kolk, 2014). The focus on trauma-specific schemas (e.g., Mistrust/Abuse, Emotional Deprivation, and Defectiveness/Shame) and modes (e.g., the Abused Child, the Helpless Surrenderer, and the Avoidant Protector) mirror the traditional ST framework (Young et al., 2003) but with trauma-informed adjustments. Mindfulness, self-compassion, and somatic resourcing (e.g., weighted blankets and grounding objects) are woven into sessions, reflecting the inclusion of third-wave strategies in trauma therapy. ST's experiential techniques (e.g., imagery rescripting and chairwork) are combined with somatic interventions (e.g., grounding, pendulation, orienting, and focusing) to address the understanding that "the body keeps score" (Gendlin, 1982; Ogden et al., 2006; van der Kolk, 2014; Payne et al., 2015).

The literature also supports ST groups tailored for specific disorders (Younan et al., 2018; Simpson, 2020; Lacy, 2024). The trauma-focused group can effectively address co-occurring schema-related issues with its flexible structure (e.g., unstructured sessions for emergent themes) and its attention to the broad symptom overlap (e.g., shame that arises in both trauma and multiple other disorders). By targeting shared mechanisms (e.g., emotional dysregulation and shame), this integrated approach diminishes the long-term burden of comorbidities like substance use, eating disorders, or depression.

The integrated schema-informed approach to group therapy for complex trauma, emphasizing safety, phased processing, self-regulation, and relational repair, can holistically address intersecting schema patterns. Research comparing TFGT and GST reveals sustained long-term outcomes, particularly in symptom durability, schema modification, and treatment adherence with GST. In a comparison of long-term outcomes, TFGT showed modest, long-term effects in long-term reduction in PTSD symptoms. A symptom-specific focus demonstrated a moderate rate of symptom relapse (40–50%), modest short-term improvement in relational stability, and self-reported well-being (Bamelis et al., 2014; Bever-Philips et al., 2023). Patients with high CPTSD risk experienced sustained reductions in emotion dysregulation and relational difficulties due to group-based skill-building (e.g., mindfulness and social support) (Bever-Philips et al., 2023). Initial increases in somatoform symptoms (linked to trauma reactivation) were resolved by a six-month follow-up (Bamelis et al., 2014). Higher dropout rates (e.g., 23–30%) (Sloan &

Beck, 2016) were noted, potentially due to difficulty tolerating exposure techniques (Schnurr et al., 2023). TFGT is effective for normalizing trauma reactions and fostering social support and may have cost-effective benefits for symptom management in non-complex cases.

Integrating GST into treatment evidenced a further reduction in comorbid symptoms (50–60%) and a low rate of relapse (15–20%), significant improvement in relational stability (+70%), and high sustained gains in self-reported well-being when integrated with ST. GST significantly reduces early maladaptive schemas (e.g., defectiveness and mistrust) and dysfunctional modes (e.g., Avoidant or Overcompensating modes, Inner Critic). PTSD symptom reduction appears to occur indirectly via schema change with longer-lasting effects for complex trauma symptoms with long-term improvements in emotional regulation and self-worth (Younan et al., 2018; Arntz et al., 2022). GST combined with individual therapy for complex trauma with comorbid BPD achieved 52–70% recovery rates at three-year follow-up, outperforming treatment-as-usual (Arntz et al., 2022). GST enhances psychosocial functioning and quality of life by addressing interpersonal deficits with sustained relational and self-efficacy improvements (Bamelis et al., 2014; Arntz et al., 2022). Participants maintain gains through continued use of schema-focused skills and group-based social support. Lower attrition (11–27%) was attributed to structured schema work and group cohesion (Younan et al., 2018).

TFGT stresses the normalization of trauma responses and skill-building (e.g., mindfulness). However, the lack of schema-focused work limits the durability of recovery from complex trauma. Integrating trauma-focused treatments (e.g., exposure) into ST targets the root causes of trauma, addressing both trauma symptoms and underlying maladaptive schemas. This enhances emotional processing, fosters deeper cognitive-emotional restructuring, and reduces avoidance and relapse risk, leading to significant and lasting improvements in mental health (Bamelis et al., 2014; Younan et al., 2018; Bay Area CBT Center, 2025). TFGT is successful for symptom stabilization in non-complex PTSD but may require adjunctive therapies for lasting change (Weber et al., 2021). GST, with combined individual and group formats, is preferred for complex trauma (e.g., CPTSD and BPD) due to its dual focus on symptoms and schemas (Arntz et al., 2022).

Multiple examples have demonstrated that the combined approach yields sustained outcomes, long-term symptom reduction, and schema change by modifying the schemas that perpetuate trauma responses (Giesen-Bloo et al., 2006; Arntz et al., 2022). Different factors appear to drive this long-term success. Core schemas (e.g., Emotional Deprivation) are not just managed but are restructured and "digested" differently, preventing trauma re-enactment. For example, PTSD symptom recurrence is reduced by resolving underlying schemas that fuel hypervigilance or avoidance. Pairing ST's imagery rescripting with trauma-focused exposure or trauma-focused mindfulness and mode dialogues helps rewire maladaptive neural pathways linked to flashbacks. It reinforces neuroplasticity by jointly strengthening prefrontal cortex regulation over limbic reactivity. ST's focus on limited reparenting and attachment repair cultivates healthier interpersonal patterns, reducing long-term relational conflicts, improving trust and boundary-setting, and replacing maladaptive schemas with secure relational templates. Integrated therapy also addresses fragmented self-identity that results from chronic trauma by strengthening the Healthy Adult mode (Brockman et al., 2023). The trauma-focused group aligned with ST principles (e.g., Healthy Adult role-modeling) consolidates schema change. The key lies in balancing structured psychoeducation with a secure relational base for exploring trauma-specific and broader schema-driven challenges (Brockman et al., 2023).

Unique Challenges

Integrating ST techniques into TFGT presents unique challenges that require careful navigation of emotional, structural, and systemic factors. While ST's emphasis on maladaptive schemas and schema modes offers a robust framework for addressing trauma's systemic effects, its application in group settings demands adaptations to ensure safety, efficacy, and inclusivity.

ST experiential techniques like imagery rescripting and mode dialogues can reactivate traumatic memories, leading to emotional dysregulation in group participants. Trauma survivors often grapple with hyper or hypoarousal, requiring therapists to balance experiential interventions with grounding strategies to prevent overwhelm. Unlike schema groups for non-trauma populations, trauma-focused groups must prioritize safety stabilization in the pacing of therapeutic work. Additionally, trauma groups frequently face disruptions due to avoidance behaviors and fluctuating engagement (e.g., no-shows or dropouts), particularly in populations with comorbid conditions.

Managing interpersonal dynamics, such as comparisons between members triggering shame-based schemas (e.g., Defectiveness), requires skilled facilitation to prevent relational ruptures. Effective integration demands clinicians proficient in trauma-informed care and ST's cognitive-experiential techniques. Many therapists lack training in experiential methods or struggle with approaches that may not accommodate trauma's complexity. Another layer of complexity is added when interventions are tailored to address cultural, social, or physical diversity.

Summary

Integrating ST with trauma-focused interventions offers transformative, lasting benefits. While disorder-specific groups optimize acute symptom targeting, this trauma-focused schema-informed group, with its multifaceted emphasis on safety, trauma-specific themes, and deep emotional restructuring, provides a scaffold healing both the wounds of trauma and the schemas that bind them for enduring recovery, particularly when tailored to cultural and systemic contexts. *Group Therapy for Complex Trauma: A Schema Informed Approach* fills a critical niche by addressing disintegration and fragmentation through phased stabilization, balancing processing traumatic material with schema restructuring, and leveraging group cohesion for attachment repair, a priority in the treatment of Complex Trauma.

References

Arntz, A., Jacob, G. A., Lee, C. W., Brand-de Wilde, O. M., Fassbinder, E., Harper, R. P., Lavender, A., Lockwood, G., Malogiannis, I. A., Ruths, F. A., Schweiger, U., Shaw, I. A., Zarbock, G., & Farrell, J. M. (2022). Effectiveness of predominantly group schema therapy and combined individual and group schema therapy for borderline personality disorder: a randomized clinical trial. *JAMA Psychiatry*, 79(4), 287–299. https://doi.org/10.1001/jamapsychiatry.2022.0010

Bamelis, L. L. M., Evers, S. M. A. A., Spinhoven, P., & Arntz, A. (2014). Results of a multicenter randomized controlled trial of the clinical effectiveness of schema therapy for personality disorders. *American Journal of Psychiatry*, 171(3), 305–322. https://doi.org/10.1176/appi.ajp.2013.12040518

Bass, J. K., Murray, S. M., Lakin, D. P., Kaysen, D., Annan, J., Matabaro, A., & Bolton, P. A. (2022). Maintenance of intervention effects: long-term outcomes for participants in a group talk-therapy trial in the Democratic Republic of Congo. *Global Mental Health*, 26(9), 347–354. https://doi.org/10.1017/gmh.2022.39

Bay Area CBT Center (2025). Integrating Prolonged Exposure into Schema Focused Therapy: Techniques and Benefits. https://bayareacbtcenter.com/prolonged-exposure-into-schema-focused-therapy

Bever-Philipps, A., Silbermann, A., Morawa, E., Schäflein, E., Stemmler, M., & Erim, Y. (2023). Long-term follow-up of a multimodal day clinic, a group-based treatment program for patients with very high risk for complex posttraumatic stress disorder and patients with non-complex trauma-related disorders. *Frontiers in Psychiatry*, 14, 1152486. https://doi.org/10.3389/fpsyt.2023.1152486

Brockman, R. N., Simpson, S., Hayes, C., van der Wijngaart, R., & Smout, M. (2023). Working with complex trauma and dissociation in schema therapy. In R. Brockman, S. G. Simpson, C. Hayes, R. van der Wijngaart, & M. F. Smout (Eds.), *Cambridge Guide to Schema Therapy*. Cambridge: Cambridge University Press, 266–278.

Cloitre, M., Garvert, D. W., Brewin, C. R., Bryant, R. A., & Maercker, A. (2013). Evidence for proposed ICD-11 PTSD and complex PTSD: a latent profile analysis. *European journal of psychotraumatology*, 4, 10.3402/ejpt.v4i0.20706. https://doi.org/10.3402/ejpt.v4i0.20706.

Drozdek & Rodenberg J. (2024). Healing wounded trees: clinicians' perspectives on treatment of complex posttraumatic stress disorder. *Frontiers in Psychiatry*, 9(15), 1356862. https://doi.org/10.3389/fpsyt.2024.1356862

Edwards, D. J. A. (2022). Using schema modes for case conceptualization in schema therapy: an applied clinical approach. *Frontiers in Psychology*, 12:763670. https://doi.org/10.3389/fpsyg.2021.763670

Farrell, J.M., Shaw, I. A., & Webber, M. A. (2009). A schema-focused approach to group psychotherapy for outpatients with borderline personality disorder: a randomized controlled trial. *Journal of Behavior Therapy and Experimental Psychiatry*, 40(2), 317–328. https://doi.org/10.1016/j.jbtep.2009.01.002

Farrell, J.M & Shaw, I.A (2012). *Group schema therapy for borderline personality disorder—A step-by-step treatment manual with patient workbook*. West Sussex, UK: Wiley-Blackwell.

Farrell, J. M., & Shaw, I. A. (2018). *Experiencing Schema Therapy from the Inside Out a Self-Practice/Self-Reflection Workbook for Therapists* (1st ed.). New York: Guilford Press.

Fassbinder, E., & Arntz, A. (2021). Schema therapy. In A. Wenzel (Ed.), *Handbook of cognitive behavioral therapy: Overview and approaches* (pp. 493–537). American Psychological Association. https://doi.org/10.1037/0000218-017

Gendlin, E.T. (1982). *Focusing*. New York: Bantam Books.

Giesen-Bloo, J., van Dyck, R., Spinhoven, P., van Tilburg, W., Dirksen, C., van Asselt, T., Kremers, I., Nadort, M., & Arntz, A. (2006). Outpatient psychotherapy for borderline personality disorder: randomized trial of schema-focused therapy vs transference-focused psychotherapy. *Archives of General Psychiatry*, 63(6), 649–658. https://doi.org/10.1001/archpsyc.63.6.649

Herman, J. L. (1992). Trauma and Recovery. New York: Basic Books.

Koppers, D., Van, H., Peen, J., & Dekker, J. J. M. (2021). Psychological symptoms, early maladaptive schemas and schema modes: predictors of the outcome of group schema therapy in patients with personality disorders. *Psychotherapy Research*, 31(7), 831–842. https://doi.org/10.1080/10503307.2020.1852482

Lacy, E. (2024). Stat: schema therapy for addiction treatment, a proposal for the integrative treatment of addictive disorders. *Frontiers in Psychology*, 15:1366617. https://doi.org/10.3389/fpsyg.2024.1366617

Mohtadijafari, S., Ashayeri, H., & Banisi, P. (2019). The effectiveness of schema therapy techniques in mental health and quality of life of women with premenstrual dysphoric disorder. *Iranian Journal of Psychiatry and Clinical Psychology*, 25(3), 278–291.

Nameni, E., Saadat, S. H., Keshavarz-Afshar, H. and Askarabady, F. (2022). Effectiveness of Group Counseling Based on Schema Therapy on Quality of Marital Relationships, Differentiation and Hardiness in Women Seeking Divorce in Families of War Veterans. *Journal of Military Medicine*, 21(1), 91–99.

Ogden, P., Pain, C., & Fisher, J. (2006). A sensorimotor approach to the treatment of trauma and dissociation. *Psychiatric Clinics of North America*, 29(1), 263–279, xi–xii. https://doi.org/10.1016/j.psc.2005.10.012

Payne, P., Levine, P. A., & Crane-Godreau, M. A. (2015). Somatic experiencing: using interoception and proprioception as core elements of trauma therapy: corrigendum. *Frontiers in Psychology*, 6, 423.

Reiss, N., Lieb, K., Arntz, A., Shaw, I. A., & Farrell, J. (2014). Responding to the treatment challenge of patients with severe bpd: results of three pilot studies of inpatient schema therapy. *Behavioural and Cognitive Psychotherapy*, 42(3):355–367. https://doi.org/10.1017/S1352465813000027

Schnurr, P. P., Friedman, M. J., Foy, D. W., TracieShea, M., Hsieh, F. Y., Lavori, P. W., Glynn, S. M., Wattenberg, M., & Bernardy, N. C. (2023). Randomized trial of trauma-focused group therapy for posttraumatic stress disorder. *Archives of General Psychiatry*, 60, 481–489.

Simpson, S. (2019). **Manual of group schema therapy for eating disorders.** In Simpson, S. & Smith, E. (Eds.). Schema Therapy for Eating Disorders: Theory and Practice for Individual and Group Settings (1st ed.). Oxford: Routledge. https://www.taylorfrancis.com/chapters/edit/10.4324/9780429295713-10/manual-group-schema-therapy-eating-disorders-susan-simpson

Skewes, S. A., Samson, R. A., Simpson, S. G., & van Vreeswijk, M. (2015). Short-term group schema therapy for mixed personality disorders: a pilot study. *Frontiers in psychology*, 5, 1592. https://doi.org/10.3389/fpsyg.2014.01592

Sloan, D. M., & Beck, J. G. (2016). Group treatment for PTSD. *PTSD Research Quarterly*, 27(2), 1–9.

Straarup, N. S., Renneberg, H. B., Farrell, J., & Younan, R. (2022). Group schema therapy for patients with severe anxiety disorders. *Journal of Clinical Psychology*, 78, 1590–1600. https://doi.org/10.1002/jclp.23351

Tan, Y. M., Lee, C. W., Averbeck, L. E., Brand-de Wilde, O., Farrell, J., Fassbinder, E., Jacob, G. A., Martius, D., Wastiaux, S., Zarbock, G., & Arntz, A. (2018). Schema therapy for borderline personality disorder: a qualitative study of patients' perceptions. *PLoS One*, 13(11), e0206039. https://doi.org/10.1371/journal.pone.0206039

van der Kolk, B. A. (2014). *The Body Keeps the Score: Brain, Mind, and Body in the Healing of Trauma*. New York: Viking.

van Dijk, S. D. M., Bouman, R., Folmer, E. H., den Held, R. C., Warringa, J. E., Marijnissen, R. M., & Voshaar, R. C. O. (2020). (Vi)-rushed Into Online Group Schema Therapy Based Day-Treatment for Older Adults by the COVID-19 Outbreak in the Netherlands. *The American journal of geriatric psychiatry : official journal of the American Association for Geriatric Psychiatry*, 28(9), 983–988. https://doi.org/10.1016/j.jagp.2020.05.028

van Vreeswijk, M. F., Spinhoven, P., Eurelings-Bontekoe, E. H., & Broersen, J. (2014). Changes in symptom severity, schemas and modes in heterogeneous psychiatric patient groups following short-term schema cognitive-behavioural group therapy: a naturalistic pre-treatment and post-treatment design in an outpatient clinic. *Clinical psychology & psychotherapy*, 21(1), 29–38. https://doi.org/10.1002/cpp.1813

Weber, M., Schumacher, S., Hannig, W., Barth, J., Lotzin, A., Schäfer, I., Ehring, T., & Kleim, B. (2021). Long-term outcomes of psychological treatment for posttraumatic stress disorder: a systematic review and meta-analysis. *Psychological Medicine*, 51(9), 1420–1430. https://doi.org/10.1017/S003329172100163X

Younan, R., Farrell, J., & May, T. (2018). 'Teaching me to parent myself': the feasibility of an in-patient group schema therapy programme for complex trauma. *Behavioral and Cognitive Psychotherapy*, 46(4), 463–478. https://doi.org/10.1017/S1352465817000698

Young, J. E., Klosko, J. S., & Weishaar, M. E. (2003). *Schema Therapy: A Practitioner's Guide*. New York: Guilford Press.

Zona, K., Hsiang Huang, H., & Spottswood, M. (2025). Implementing group therapy for posttraumatic stress disorder within a primary care setting: A pilot study. *Journal of Affective Disorders Reports*, 19, 100856.

Part 2

Session Protocols

Chapter 9

Group Structure and Framework

Complex Post Traumatic Stress Disorder (CPTSD) is conceptualized here as a disorder of dysregulation characterized by a failure of integration of core functions resulting from some combination of the six D's—dysregulation, disruption, distortion, disorientation, disconnection, and defensiveness. From this perspective, daily functioning and the ability to manage the onslaught of *disorienting* and *dysregulating* emotions and physical sensations is *disrupted*. What one knows and believes about oneself becomes *distorted* and contributes to *disconnection* and *distancing* from others. Survival *defenses* are activated to protect when the world seems so threatening. Impaired integration impacts people's sense of who they are, their place in the world, and how they relate to others after what happened. Their brain, their body, their emotions, their relationships, and their narrative are all shaped by their trauma.

Group therapy, a potent tool for healing, recovery, and growth, is particularly empowering for individuals who have endured early childhood trauma. With its unique strength-based approach, this model harnesses the individual's existing resources to replace behaviors driven by debilitating emotions. Incorporating a Schema Therapy-informed approach helps the participants recognize and gradually accept their internalized beliefs, messages, and personal vulnerability and distinguish their different "sides" or modes to facilitate a healthy integration of a coherent self. The concepts of maladaptive schemas and coping modes provide an additional lens through which group members better understand their emotional and behavioral responses to triggering situations and intrusive material. It empowers participants to confront their trauma and its impact on their lives, inspiring hope and resilience.

This program combines a structured orientation with planned activities that emphasize the experiential and affective nature of the group. It includes a range of topics to address the diverse needs and experiences of the participants. Specific psychoeducational topics provide information

DOI: 10.4324/9781003462958-11

about trauma and its effects on the mind, body, and relationships. They are intended to increase understanding of the impact of early childhood trauma, personal reactions and behaviors, and those mirrored by others in the group. Participants link the didactic material with their individual experiences through exercises related to the different themes.

The group is structured to be a haven where members can challenge the secrecy, silence, and isolation that often accompany early trauma. The sharing and support of other survivors within this safe, predictable, consistent, empathetic space fosters a sense of reassurance and safety that allows them to remove the "mask" that hides their true selves. As group members share their experiences, they can begin to recognize their strengths and resilience, further reinforcing the supportive nature of the group.

The group provides resources to help individuals better manage their symptoms and reactions to trauma and replace self-defeating coping strategies with more effective methods. Discussions about the impact of trauma on trust, safety, intimacy, roles, and boundaries guide group members as they navigate their relationships and interactions with others. The group is expected to be a space where all members can feel accepted and differences are respected. Constructive and non-judgmental feedback is emphasized, and advice-giving or problem-solving is discouraged. Resources, strengths, and progress are highlighted as members are encouraged to assert their needs and take responsibility for their healing. The focus is on emotional processing and the group process as it unfolds in the moment. Titrating the emotional intensity of the group teaches the members how to manage their symptoms as they heal and recover.

Goals: Through participation in this group, participants will:

1 Increase their understanding of the impact of early childhood trauma on the brain, body, self-regulation, beliefs about self, and relationships.
2 Decrease *dysregulation* and *disruption* by increasing their ability to regulate emotions and manage stress.
3 Decrease *disconnection* and *defensiveness* by reducing the isolation, stigma, and secrecy surrounding early childhood trauma and by establishing safe social and emotional connections that increase the capacity for healthy relationships.
4 Decrease *disorientation* by increasing mindful awareness and cognitive flexibility.
5 Decrease *distortion* by reducing feelings of shame, guilt, self-blame, and other maladaptive beliefs while increasing self-compassion and self-acceptance.

Structure and Format

Target Population: Adults with histories of early childhood trauma, with or without the formal CPTSD diagnosis, 18 years of age or older, who are not actively psychotic or at imminent risk of suicide or homicide. Chronic suicidal ideation, substance abuse, and disordered eating are often comorbid with complex trauma. These are not definitive exclusion criteria but must be assessed carefully to determine whether the person can tolerate the material discussed in the group without exacerbating symptoms. Intoxicated members will not be allowed to participate in the group. It may also be necessary to determine the heterogeneity or homogeneity of the group based on demographic characteristics such as gender or age.

Group Structure: The group is structured for twenty 90-minute sessions. The 20-week curriculum addresses different themes and allows time for follow-ups on prior sessions or unstructured sessions if desired. Each session follows a similar format, with the didactic theme varying weekly. This model can adapt to open or closed formats depending on the setting. The curriculum can repeat on a revolving schedule in an open group as new members enter at different points. The open format may be more applicable at higher levels of care, while a closed, 20-week group may be a better fit in the traditional outpatient setting.

Group Size, Therapist Number, and Physical Space: Group size depends on the number of therapists co-leading the group, its composition, and the member's level of functioning. Eight clients with two therapists are optimal, but one can facilitate a group with six or fewer members. The physical space should be free from distractions, ensure confidentiality, and be large enough to accommodate all members comfortably. It should allow room for movement, which is part of some experiential exercises. Farrell and Shaw (2012) suggest using a "safety corner" as a place for clients to take a brief time out from the intensity of the group. This can be an alternative to clients leaving the group when dysregulated.

Screening: A complete intake is necessary before inviting prospective members to join the group. Addressing their motivation for joining and their needs, goals, and expectations can help determine their readiness for the group and if it can adequately meet their needs. Trauma history, prior therapy experience, the stability of their current life situation, relevant problems, symptoms, strengths, and relational functioning are reviewed as the group's suitability is assessed. Group goals, expectations, guidelines, attendance and safety commitments, structure, and contact with outside providers are thoroughly discussed during the intake (**Handout 1.1 Sample Group Guidelines**). Initial paperwork and fee setting can be completed during the intake, and relevant consents (e.g., informed consent; authorization to release/obtain information) can be obtained.

Potential members are also introduced to Schema Therapy during the initial intake. The Young Schema Questionnaire (YSQ) (Young, 2003) and The Schema Mode Inventory (SMI) (Young et al., 2007) may be administered and reviewed with prospective members before the group starts to identify their profiles (Farrell and Shaw (2018) offer condensed versions of the YSQ and the SMI). It is recommended that group members read *A Client's Guide to Schema Therapy* (Bricker & Young, 2012 https://www.davidbricker.com/client-resources), *An Introductory Guide to Schema Therapy: Adapted for Use with the YSQ-R* (Created by Bricker & Young, modified by Yalcin (2023) https://anima.com.au/schema, *Reinventing Your Life: The Breakthrough Program To End Negative Behaviour And Feel Great Again* (Young & Klosko, 2019) or *Disarming the Narcissist* (Behary, 2021) for a comprehensive introduction to Schema Therapy and Schema Modes.

Session Format: Sessions follow a consistent format, beginning with a mindfulness exercise and then a brief check-in or "temperature check." During check-in, the member identifies whether they are within their Window of Tolerance, assessing their degree of risk, activation of schema modes, internal alarms or defensive action urges, resources they can use during the group, and whether they need anything from the group that day. The leader then introduces the day's theme and opens the topic for discussion and practice. (Group members can be asked to complete handouts in the group or as homework. Sufficient time should be allowed to discuss the member's responses to the handouts and exercises.) As the group winds down, key points from the discussion are summarized, each member checks out, and the group ends with a grounding/centering exercise before leaving for the day (**Handout 1.2 Sample Group Format**).

Session Outline: The proposed order for the group sessions follows a logical progression based on best practices in trauma treatment, particularly the three-phase approach of stabilization, trauma processing, and integration. The first phase focuses on establishing group cohesion and safety, building coping skills, and providing psychoeducation. Grouping coping skills (Window of Tolerance and Emotional Regulation) early in the program equips clients with tools to manage distress during later, more intense sessions. This aligns with the recommendation that the first phase should be central and foundational. The middle phase takes a more in-depth look at the impact of trauma on the nervous system, the body, and memory. This corresponds to the second phase of trauma treatment when clients are better equipped to address aspects of the traumatic material. The final phase focuses on applying new insights and preparing for termination. Ending with relationship-focused sessions and termination helps clients apply their learning to current situations as they integrate their experiences and consolidate treatment gains. Three unstructured sessions are included in the program to allow completion of previous core topics and flexibility to dive deeper into issues relevant to the particular group. These open sessions can be used at any time during the group at the leaders' discretion. While this is the recommended progression, each session can be a separate unit. This may be relevant for open groups at higher levels of care when new members enter at different points in the program.

Sessions

Session 1:   Beginning the Group (Safety and Stabilization)

Session 2:   Schema Therapy (Psychoeducation)

Session 3:   Post-Traumatic Stress Disorder and Complex Post-Traumatic Stress Disorder (Psychoeducation)

Session 4:   The Window of Tolerance (Stabilization/Emotion Regulation)

Session 5:   Emotion Regulation (Stabilization/Emotion Regulation)

Session 6:   The Neurobiology of Trauma (Psychoeducation)

Session 7:   Trauma and the Body (Psychoeducation/Physiological Regulation).

Session 8:   Trauma and Memory (Psychoeducation)

Session 9:   Intrusive Symptoms of PTSD: Flashbacks, Nightmares, and Intrusive Memories (Symptom Management/Emotion Regulation)

Session 10:   Trauma and Dissociation (Symptom Management/ Emotion Regulation)

Session 11:   Trauma and Attachment (Relationships)

Session 12:   The Trauma Triangle (Relationships)

Session 13:   Shame and the Inner Critic (Challenging Maladaptive Schema and Coping Modes)

Session 14:   Self-Compassion (Integration and Consolidation)

Session 15:   Developing Healthy Relationships (Integration and Consolidation)

Sessions 16–17: Making Sense of it All: Recovery, Reconnection and Integration (Integration and Consolidation)

Summary

This group program provides a comprehensive treatment framework for individuals with CPTSD resulting from early childhood trauma. Psychoeducation on trauma and its effects, together with experiential and affective activities, help to increase the participant's understanding of the impact of their early childhood experiences, improve their ability to regulate their emotions, and manage stress. The group's focus on emotional processing and group dynamics helps reduce isolation, establish safe connections, enhance mindful awareness and cognitive flexibility, decrease shame, guilt, and self-blame, and increase self-compassion. The program emphasizes strength-based healing and recovery within a safe, supportive environment for sharing experiences.

References

Behary, W. (2021). *Disarming the Narcissist: Surviving and Thriving with the Self-Absorbed* (3rd ed.). New York: New Harbinger Publications.

Bricker, D. & Young, J. E. (2012). *A Client's Guide to Schema Therapy*. https://www.davidbricker.com/client-resources

Farrell, J. M. & Shaw, I. A. (2012). *Group Schema Therapy for Borderline Personality Disorder: A Step-by-Step Treatment Manual with Patient Workbook*. New York: Wiley-Blackwell & Co.

Farrell, J. M. & Shaw, I. A. (2018). *Experiencing Schema Therapy from the Inside Out: A Self-Practice/Self-Reflection Workbook for Therapists*. New York: Guilford Press.

Yalcin, O. (2023). *An Introductory Guide to Schema Therapy: Adapted for Use with the YSQ-R* (Created by Bricker & Young, modified by Yalcin, 2023). https://anima.com.au/schema

Young, J. (2003). *Young Schema Questionnaire: Long Form*. https://www.schematherapy.com/id53.htm

Young, J. E & Klosko, J. S (2019). *Reinventing Your Life: The Breakthrough Program to End Negative Behavior and Feel Great Again: The Breakthrough Program to End Negative Behavior and Feel Great Again*. UK: Scribe.

Young, J. E., Arntz, A., Atkinson, T., Lobbestael, J., Weishaar, M. E., & van Vreeswijk, M. F. (2007). *The Schema Mode Inventory*. New York: Schema Therapy Institute.

Beginning the Group

The first session sets the stage for success by establishing safety, building initial rapport, and providing members with a basic understanding of what to expect in the coming weeks. The members are welcomed into a prepared space equipped with proper lighting and temperature, large enough to accommodate all, including the group leaders comfortably, is conducive to open discussion, safeguards confidentiality, meets special needs, and minimizes distractions.

The initial welcome sets the tone for the group and helps put participants at ease. The group begins to coalesce around its unifying purpose of understanding and healing from the effects of early childhood trauma. Discussing this objective and reviewing the structure, content, and process provides clarity and manages expectations for the group.

Goals

1 Outline the group's organization, including its structure, content, and process.
2 Review group guidelines and the importance of commitment to the process.
3 Identify members' individual goals, expectations, and concerns.
4 Understand the development of Maladaptive Schema and Schema modes and their relationship to unmet core needs (introduced during intake session).
5 Address any questions and concerns.

Procedure

1 Introductions
2 Identify the group's shared purpose and goals.
3 Provide a brief overview of early childhood trauma
4 Review the group organization (structure, content, and process).

DOI: 10.4324/9781003462958-12

5 Identify group members' goals, expectations, and concerns.
6 Address Needs, Maladaptive Schema, and Schema modes. Discuss the importance of participants recognizing their emotional needs and learning to ask for them to be met within the group.
7 Discuss Needs: Share the story of Ella and the Thunderstorm and the analogy of The Orchid and the Dandelion (**Handout 1.3 Identifying Needs**).
8 Check out.
9 Introduce Coping and Grounding Skills. Grounding can be used throughout the session as needed but is a critical practice at the end of a session before the group disbands for the day. End today's session with the **Connecting Web Exercise** (Farrell & Shaw, 2012) to begin building cohesion within the group.

Main Themes

Introductions

The group leaders briefly welcome the group and acknowledge the common reason everyone is there. Leaders provide a basic overview of trauma and its impact, for example:

> Welcome to our group. This group is designed to increase your understanding of how early childhood trauma affects the developing child, the satisfaction of basic needs, the relationship with caregivers, and the impact on you today. The group will be a safe and supportive space to explore and understand these early experiences.

"Over the next 20 weeks, you will learn a great deal about trauma and its effect on physical and mental health, brain functioning, coping, beliefs, relationships, emotions, and your sense of self." (Share the topics that will be addressed). "You will develop a new lens through which to view your experiences and develop coping strategies and resilience-building techniques that will help break the cycle of trauma."

Introductions begin with the group leaders and continue around the group. "My name is...and..." (the leader briefly shares something with the group). Each member states their name, voluntarily sharing what brought them to the group and anything about their current life situation (marriage, children, employment, school, etc.) they would like the group to know. Emphasize that detailed trauma narratives are not expected. You can ask the group to consider how their early experiences have affected them as common reactions and symptoms are briefly reviewed and normalized.

Group Organization (Structure, Content, and Process)

Review the goals and purpose of the group, the meeting calendar and weekly themes, group guidelines, the daily check-in format, and the Feelings Wheel. (Necessary materials that the group will use during the duration of the group can be compiled in a notebook or digital file that each member can easily access during the group or at home. This may include a statement about the goals and purpose of the group, a calendar of meetings with an outline of the weekly themes, group guidelines, the daily check-in format, a feelings wheel, summaries of psychoeducational information, handouts and exercises, essential resources, and contact information). Distribute handouts for the daily Group Format, Group Guidelines, the Feeling Wheel, Ella and the Thunderstorm, and the Orchid and the Dandelion.

Guidelines (Handout 1.1 Sample Group Guidelines)

A primary goal for the group is to establish a safe space where you can explore the impact of your early experiences. To do so, it is necessary to establish some basic guidelines. We invite you to share your thoughts as we review these guidelines

You may have each member read one of the guidelines to begin active involvement. It is essential to reiterate the commitment to the group's safety. This includes discussing non-negotiable rules such as confidentiality, the substance-free nature of the group, zero tolerance for abuse or unsolicited physical contact of any kind, remaining in the group during the session unless informed of the need for time to self-regulate, the option to pass if they are not ready to share, and making a commitment to attend the entirety of the group. If appropriate, members may suggest guidelines or ground rules for discussion. There is room for flexibility, except for rules about confidentiality, the substance-free nature of the group, or anything that would threaten individual or group safety. Confirm that all members understand and accept all the guidelines.

Structure/Format (Handout 1.2 Sample Group Format)

The group will meet for 90 minutes weekly over the next 20 weeks. It has been designed to provide information about complex trauma and to normalize common reactions and symptoms to help you understand your experiences. This space will allow you to establish new connections and attachments and develop healthy ways to recognize and ask for what you need. We will work together to engage and strengthen the Healthy Adult side of you that can challenge critical messages, manage emotions, and care for vulnerable parts of yourself. Each week, we will address an important topic to help explain the effects of early childhood trauma and explore how it has impacted your life. After today, each group will begin with a mindfulness exercise. Mindfulness can reduce anxiety and hyperarousal, improve self-regulation, and increase tolerance of physical sensations. The ability to stay grounded and present will help you engage in the work necessary to heal from your early trauma. A brief check-in will follow the mindfulness practice as a 'temperature check' to address current needs and any residual issues arising after the prior group. The week's theme will be presented and discussed, exercises practiced, and handouts completed and reviewed. We will also 'check your temperature' when each session ends; the final grounding exercise will help ensure everyone feels safe before leaving the group.

Distribute **Handout 1.2 Group Format.** Using a **Feeling Wheel** (obtainable from the internet) can assist in labeling emotions.

Goals, Expectations, and Fears About the Group

Ask each member what they hope to get out of it. Discuss their expectations for and fears about the group. "What would you like to accomplish over the next twenty weeks? How will you know that you have achieved your goal (e.g., how will you know that you have improved your feelings about yourself)"?

> You have come here today with some ideas of what you would like this group to be. It can also be a scary and intimidating prospect. What are your hopes and wishes for the group? What are some of the concerns you may have?

Record the goals for later reference. Remember that it may be enough for some to attend each session.

Needs, Maladaptive Schema, and Schema Modes

Discuss the relationship between unmet needs and the development of maladaptive schema and schema modes (the lens through which we see the world, our emotional buttons, and how we learn to cope with them). This will be discussed in detail in the next session.

The group members may be significantly disconnected from the concept of needs. Their experience may have been that needs were only met at a price. They may have been told they were too needy or that it was wrong to have needs. Acknowledge that having needs met may be an alien concept for many. Explore what it means to have basic needs unmet.

Unsupported but common negative beliefs result from internalized implicit or explicit messages received when a young child's basic needs for safety and protection, secure attachment, autonomy and competence, and the freedom to express valid needs and feelings are unmet. The critical messages from external sources are internalized by our clients, reinforcing their feelings of worthlessness, shame, self-blame, and self-loathing.

What do we hear from clients when they come into therapy? ("I cannot cope." "This is too much for me to deal with." "I am hopeless." "I feel like I am crazy." "I'm bad." "I'm damaged." "It's my fault." "I'm a failure." "I do not deserve good things." "I'm worthless." "I hate myself."). These negative beliefs are not unique. Lloyd (2023) suggests that 100 people with Complex Post Traumatic Stress Disorder (CPTSD) will feel these things about themselves rather than about others with similar experiences. Ask them to imagine they are in a room with these 100 people and ask them, "How many deserved what happened? None. Did you deserve it? Yes—everything bad that happened is because of me."

A primary goal of therapy is to help people see themselves differently and to recognize that many of their current difficulties result from not having their basic needs met when they were young. Bad things happened TO them, but not because THEY are bad. The impact of trauma confirms their worst fears about themselves and prevents good things from happening to them. It gets in the way of them thriving and reaching their potential.

Discuss what every child needs for healthy development (safety, stability, loving and reliable relationships, competence, autonomy, limits, emotional expression, play, etc.). "Sometimes, these needs are met in affirmative ways that contribute to healthy development; other times, they are not. What happens when these needs are not met for whatever reason? The child finds a way to make sense of their world and begins seeing it through a particular lens, a schema. It is like seeing a world colored by cellophane glasses. We aren't always aware of or don't question the color we see through these glasses. What we experience becomes fact, our blind spots or emotional buttons. Schemas, the emotional buttons, are how we view ourselves, others, and the world, shaped by early experiences and relationships. Unfortunately, these beliefs may no longer hold in adult life and continue interfering with getting what is needed" (Simpson, 2019, p. 144).

Introduce the concept of schema modes as the way we respond and cope when these emotional "buttons" are pushed. "Schema modes are activated as we find ways to respond when our emotional 'buttons' are pushed. Coping modes helped us survive painful experiences." (Simpson, 2019, p. 144). The primary goal of a Schema Therapy-informed approach is to enable participants to recognize their emotional needs and to learn to ask for them to be met within the group. It is often difficult for people to identify their needs when they may have yet to have the opportunity to learn about needs and emotions or getting needs met. Parents may not have had their emotional needs met and did not have the skills or understanding to teach this to their children. Recognizing their emotional needs, asking for their needs to be met (which feels scary if they have been rejected in the past), and allowing others to meet their needs are essential skills to develop during the group (Simpson, 2019).

Share the story of Ella and the Thunderstorm (**Handout 1.3 Identifying Needs**). Introduce the concept of the Healthy Adult, or "Good Parent" self. Emphasize the importance of addressing unmet needs from early childhood and the goal of strengthening the Healthy Adult mode as part of our healing process. Explore members' reactions to the story. What would a good parent do?

Discuss the analogy of The Orchid and the Dandelion (**Handout 1.3 Identifying Needs**). The orchid-dandelion theory and the characteristics of orchids (highly sensitive) and dandelions (more resilient) (or a tulip, which is somewhere in between) can be introduced in the group to help normalize experiences, highlight individual differences in sensitivity and resilience, and reduce self-blame for heightened reactions to trauma. Sharing experiences in the group can highlight how different sensitivity levels affect trauma responses. Orchid's sensitivity may reflect an increased "neediness" and dependency on others. Therapy for orchids might focus on reframing their sensitivity to environmental factors as a strength and leveraging it to develop increased autonomy. Dandelions may reject the vulnerability associated with having needs and may not ask for or reject support. They may require approaches focusing on building awareness and acceptance of their needs and increasing responsiveness to environmental supports.

Coping Skills and Resource Development

Introduce the importance of developing strengths, resources, and coping skills to aid their healing journey. Introducing coping skills early provides participants with immediate tools to manage distress. Discuss how this will help strengthen their Healthy Adult mode. Grounding is designed to help group members regulate their emotions and return to their Window of Tolerance when they have transitioned (or "flipped") into a coping mode. Grounding can be used throughout the session as needed but is a critical practice at the end of a session before the group disbands for the day. Depending on the group's needs, the exercise can be upregulating (energizing—e.g., movement) or downregulating (calming—e.g., breathing). Encourage the group to notice what they feel in their body as they engage in this practice.

"The Connecting Web Exercise" (Farrell & Shaw, 2018) is a way to establish a felt sense of connection to the group. Just as a spider weaves her web, group members develop their web of connection as they toss a ball of yarn around and hold on to a piece each time it comes to them. They become aware of the strength of connection in the group as they tighten the pull on the yarn or the lack of connection when one or two members release the yarn. "The individual connections are identified as representing what is needed in the group, with each member offering what he or she needs (e.g., trust, acceptance, respect, etc.)" (Farrell & Shaw, 2018, p.55). (This exercise can be extended further as the yarn is used to make a bracelet that reminds the group of their connection). In between sessions, each member can visualize their connection to the group as they feel the pull of the string and experience how all are linked together. Discuss this experience with the group.

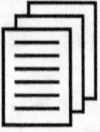

HANDOUT 1.1

Sample Group Guidelines

(Adapted from Courtois & Ford, 2013)

This group is intended to be a place to safely make sense of your past experiences and how they continue to impact you today. Consistent expectations and ground rules provide the stability and predictability necessary for the group to function well. We ask that you commit to following these ground rules throughout the group. They will be in effect until the group chooses to revisit them based on changing group needs.

- **Confidentiality**: Confidentiality is not just a rule; it is a commitment we all make to each other. It is the cornerstone of our trust and security within the group. *All sessions are confidential* so that every participant can feel comfortable and safe. Please do not reveal other patients' names or other identifying information. Any discussions with outsiders about the group should be strictly limited to your own experience and the skills you are learning.

  __ I understand that what happens in the group stays in the group.
  __ I agree not to share personal information about other participants outside the sessions. If I meet another member outside of the group, I will refrain from mentioning anything that would compromise confidentiality.
  __ While I may choose to share my personal information, I will protect the privacy of the other members.
  __ I understand that the group leaders will share information between themselves but can only release my private information with my permission.
  __ If the leaders learn of the abuse of a child, elder, or disabled individual, or if they believe that I am in danger of hurting myself or someone else, they are obligated to share this information with others for my protection. They may also maintain communication with my therapists when necessary.

- **Respect and Non-Judgment**: We are each responsible for making this group work.

  __ I commit to being kind, nonjudgmental, respectful, and supportive of everyone in the group. This commitment to respect and non-judgment is the foundation of our supportive and empathetic environment.
  __ Active listening is key. I will listen attentively when others speak, avoiding interruptions or dominating the conversation. This ensures that everyone has the opportunity to share their thoughts and experiences.

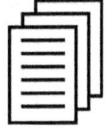

__ I will refrain from engaging in side conversations.

- **Feedback**: Please refrain from discussing any problems or matters unrelated to the group and refrain from side conversations that interfere with the group discussions.

  __ When providing feedback, I will focus on the needs of the person who is sharing. This ensures that my feedback is constructive and supportive, contributing to a positive group dynamic.

  __ I understand that opinions, advice-giving, and problem-solving limit discussion.

  __ I will offer observations and ask questions to help others explore their issues.

- **Boundaries:**

  __ I will not touch another member without their permission.

  __ I can decline any physical contact if I wish.

  __ I will maintain appropriate physical boundaries in the group and refrain from imposing on someone else's personal space.

- **Managing Emotions**: Intense emotions that arise during group discussions are sometimes challenging. As you expand your emotional tolerance, you may feel overwhelmed and out of your Window of Tolerance. Strategies used to survive difficult experiences in the past may be ineffective in the present.

  __ I will try to get myself grounded and calmer within the group. If I need to leave the room, I will take a short break to use my skills and return to the group independently. I will inform the group what I need, check in, and not leave abruptly.

  __ Group leaders and other patients will not follow me if I take a break, as it is expected that I will be responsible for managing my emotions.

  __ I will ask for assistance if I am unable to self-regulate and find myself reverting to ineffective ways of coping.

- **Conflict Resolution**: Conflict and disagreement are parts of all relationships and often cannot be avoided. They will be addressed promptly and directly in the group and used as opportunities to learn how to communicate respectfully amid disagreements and strong feelings.

  __ I understand that violence, threats, physical or verbal intimidation or manipulation, and other types of abusive behavior will not be tolerated. Physical or verbal abuse can lead to an immediate discharge from the program.

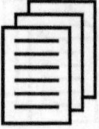

___ It is expected that I will remain in an adult state and be respectful of myself and others.

___ I will avoid aggressive, hostile, or intimidating behaviors, including cursing, yelling, threatening gestures, or physical altercations. If these behaviors remain problematic, I realize that I may be asked to leave the group.

- **Active Participation is a commitment** to the whole group process and is expected during each session. Participation will help you stay more present, focused, and engaged. It will help you learn more effectively, even when you feel intense. *The group is designed to draw on your strengths and help you master specific skills*. It will help you learn skills to improve your ability to handle difficulties.

  ___ I understand that my privacy and right to pass will be respected when I cannot participate and that I still may be encouraged to participate to help widen my Window of Tolerance.

  ___ I commit to fully engage in the group process throughout the group, even when it is uncomfortable.

  ___ I understand that the leaders may encourage us to share our thoughts and feelings with the group.

- **Attendance:** Ongoing and consistent attendance is required to gain the most significant benefit from the group. This enhances stability, security, and trust.

  ___ I will arrive on time to get the most out of the group.

  ___ I will inform the group leaders if I must leave early or cannot attend.

- **Weapons or instruments of self-harm** of any kind are not allowed in the program. Everyone, including yourself, deserves and needs to feel safe.

- **Substance-Free Group**: To ensure a safe and focused environment, the use of alcohol and drugs is not allowed during sessions. No one will be allowed to attend the group if they are under the influence of alcohol or drugs.

  ___ I understand that drugs or alcohol are not allowed, and I will be asked to leave the group session if intoxicated or high.

  ___ I will not attend the group while under either influence.

- **Developing a diverse support network beyond the group members.** Limiting support to and from those who may be struggling with self-harm, substance abuse, and suicidal thoughts decreases feelings of responsibility for their needs at the expense of your own.

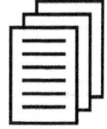

- **Outside relationships** with other group members impact group dynamics. It can create conflicts among group members, affecting what happens during the sessions. It is expected that contact outside the group will avoid over-involvement, special or exclusive friendships, or inappropriate caretaking demands that detract from my healing.

  __ I will share any outside contact with the group to avoid secrecy.
  __ I will not keep secrets related to relapse, self-injury, or suicidal ideation.
  __ Sexual contact is expressly prohibited throughout the group.
  __ I can decline outside contact with other group members.

- *The therapist plays a crucial role in setting and enforcing these ground rules. They model appropriate behavior, provide feedback and guidance, and address rule violations promptly and directly. Their role is to ensure that the group functions in a safe and supportive manner.*

*For a complete discussion of ground rules and a template for developing group guidelines, refer to
Courtois, C. & Ford, J. D. (2015). *Treatment of Complex Trauma: A Sequenced, Relationship-Based Approach*. New York: Guilford Press.

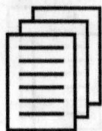

HANDOUT 1.2

Sample Group Format

1 **Mindfulness Exercise** (This can be a quiet, meditative, or active participatory exercise that helps ground the individual in their body and the present moment. *Meditative exercises may increase dissociation in some clients who may struggle to connect with their bodies. Explore what might be helpful to improve their ability to engage in this practice (e.g., leaving eyes open, external anchoring, physical movement).

2 **Check-In:** (Brief Temperature Check: Each group member briefly shares their current emotional status and any concerns/needs they want to share with the group. Minimal feedback is provided at this point to allow time for all members to check in).

   a Are they in their Window of Tolerance? (Refer to Window of Tolerance Chart) If not, are they hyper or hypoaroused? Can they identify what is pulling them out of their window? (Clients can use a feelings chart to better label the emotion).

   b Can they identify any action urge or activation of their internal alarms (fight/flight/freeze/submit/attach)? What mode are they in? What signs help them recognize this?

   c What is contributing to today's emotional state?

   d Are there any safety concerns, or have they engaged in unsafe behaviors (physical, emotional, mental)?

   e What skills/resources can they use today to help regulate their emotions?

   Encourage members to notice any signs of dissociation or dysregulation they may experience when sharing or listening to another member. Remind them to use coping resources to reorient and reengage with the group and ask for assistance when needed.

3 **Discussion of Session Topic:** Discuss key points of the topic.

   a Relate them to current problems in the member's life.

   b Review any handouts or worksheets.

   c Summarize the main points to close the discussion.

4 **Check Out** (The goal is to increase each member's awareness and regulation of their emotional state as the session ends. Group leaders can choose to check out after the closing grounding exercise if appropriate).

   a Ask each member to notice if they are in their Window of Tolerance, addressing what helped them stay in the window or pulled them out.

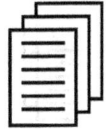

b Identify a skill or resource to help regulate their current emotions.

c Ask members to identify one takeaway from the group's discussion.

5 **Closing Grounding Exercise**: Grounding is designed to help group members regulate their emotions and return to their Window of Tolerance when they have transitioned (or "flipped") into a coping mode. Grounding can be used throughout the session as needed but is a critical practice at the end of a session before the group disbands for the day. Depending on the group's needs, the exercise can be upregulating (energizing—e.g., movement) or downregulating (calming—e.g., breathing). Encourage the group to notice what they feel in their body as they engage in this practice.

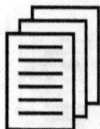

Identifying Needs

1 Ella and the Thunderstorm: A Story to Educate on Needs and Modes

A little child 4 years of age woke up from the crackling and banging sounds and loud rumbling of a thunderclap. It was so loud that she felt like it was shaking her bed. Bright flashes of lighting left behind scary images on the walls and were followed by loud noises. At the next thunderclap, she flew from her bed and ran to her parents' room, feeling so frightened that all she could do was shake and cry. Her crying turned into a scream at the next sound of thunder. One parent woke and started to yell at her. 'Stop crying,' the parent said, 'it is just a thunderstorm. Stop being such a big baby! Go back to bed before you wake the entire household.' Ella went back to her room but could not stop crying. She bit down on her blanket so no sound would escape. She covered her ears and closed her eyes to block out the thunder and the scary arms of the tree reaching out to grab her. After a while, she did not jump anymore, even though the thunder was louder, nor did she shake or duck when the creepy arms tried to get her. She just sat there staring off into space.
(Farrell & Shaw, 2018, p. 102)

Consider:

1 What does this child feel when lying in bed and running into her parents' room? (Afraid? Anxious? Alone?).
2 What do you think the child felt after leaving the parents' bedroom? What do you think this child needed from her parents? What would she have liked them to do? How would she have felt then?
3 What messages would Ella have taken away about herself, the world, and others?
4 What modes were triggered or began to develop from this experience? How might this affect her adult life if similar experiences occurred repeatedly?

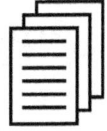

2 The Orchid and the Dandelion

The analogy of a dandelion and an orchid is another way to address needs and how different people may have different needs. This analogy often describes how people respond differently to stressors and trauma.

1 The "Orchid Hypothesis" (Boyce, 2020) suggests that some individuals, like orchids, are more susceptible to positive and negative environmental influences and are more sensitive and vulnerable to adverse experiences, including trauma.
2 Dandelions are hardy and can grow and flourish everywhere, even under challenging conditions. Dandelion people are highly resilient, capable of enduring stress, and adapting to adversity. They survive and even thrive, regardless of their life circumstances.
3 Orchids are sensitive and delicate and require the right, carefully maintained conditions (proper resources, sunny environment, proper care) to thrive. Orchid individuals, being more sensitive to their environment, are likely to be more strongly affected by whether their core emotional needs are unmet. For such individuals, unmet needs, a harsh environment, or a traumatic incident can potentially lead to issues like anxiety, depression, or post-traumatic stress disorder. Unmet emotional needs may more deeply impact orchids, who may develop maladaptive patterns that lead to greater emotional and behavioral challenges.
4 However, when their core needs are met, orchids can thrive exceptionally well, developing more adaptive schemas and greater emotional resilience. Should the orchid be given the specific conditions it needs, it too can flourish. Both "dandelions" and "orchids" possess immense potential for growth, healing, and exceptional outcomes. They can bloom into a lovely flower, much like an orchid, with the proper support, care, and conditions that address their unique needs.

References

Boyce, W. T. (2020). *The Orchid and the Dandelion: Why Sensitive Children Face Challenges and How All Can Thrive*. New York: Penguin Books.

Courtois, C. A., & Ford, J. D. (2013). *Treatment of complex trauma: A sequenced, relationship-based approach*. New York: Guilford Press.

Farrell, J.M & Shaw, I.A (2012). *Group Schema Therapy for Borderline Personality Disorder: A Step-by-Step Treatment Manual with Patient Workbook*. West Sussex, UK: Wiley-Blackwell

Farrell, J. M. & Shaw, I. A. (2018). *Experiencing Schema Therapy from the Inside Out: A Self Practice/Self-Regulation Workbook for Therapists*. New York: Guilford Press.

Lloyd, M. (2023). *CTAD Clinic*. Https//www.Cheshirepsychology.Com

Simpson, S. (2019). Manual of group schema therapy for eating disorders. In S. Simpson, & E. Smith (Eds.), *Schema Therapy for Eating Disorders: Theory and Practice for Individual and Group Settings* (1st ed.). London: Routledge, 136–184.

Schema Therapy

This session explores the central concepts of Schema Therapy (ST), including schemas and modes, and examines how they can be used to help heal from early childhood trauma. ST was first introduced during the intake process when members began to identify their schemas and modes. ST is particularly effective in treating complex trauma survivors as it helps make sense of traumatic experiences and develop self-compassion that counters the negative self-perceptions resulting from trauma. *Limited Reparenting* provides a framework for corrective emotional experiences that help meet unmet needs in childhood. *Empathic Confrontation* challenges self-defeating patterns that contribute to the disruptions in a person's life. *Experiential exercises* help increase awareness and change the self-defeating patterns that interfere with healthy functioning. Irrational beliefs connected to the early maladaptive schemas (EMS) are challenged and reframed, and maladaptive coping behaviors and beliefs can be replaced with healthier alternatives.

Goals

1 Identify how early childhood trauma shapes maladaptive schemas.
2 Connect past experiences to present behavioral patterns.
3 Recognize personal schemas and modes and their impact on current functioning.
4 Learn to challenge maladaptive schemas.
5 Recognize schema modes and their triggers in daily life.
6 Modify dysfunctional and self-defeating behavior patterns developed from unmet emotional needs.
7 Strengthen the Healthy Adult mode.
8 Develop healthier ways of meeting their emotional needs within a supportive group environment.

DOI: 10.4324/9781003462958-13

Procedure

1 Mindfulness Exercise: Introduce imagery to the group with **Exercise 2.1 Introducing Imagery: The Ice Cream Shoppe** (Farrell & Shaw, 2012).
2 Check in.
3 Introduce ST's core principles and interventions in treating trauma (schema, modes, limited reparenting, empathic confrontation, experiential exercises, etc.).
4 Explain the concept of limited reparenting and how it addresses unmet childhood needs.
5 Explore how the group can serve as a "corrective emotional experience" for past traumas.
6 Facilitate a conversation about how sharing personal experiences in the group setting can provide new perspectives on individual schemas and modes. Discuss how group support can challenge long-held beliefs and encourage new behaviors.
7 Explore how maladaptive modes affect daily functioning. Role-play **Exercise 2.2 Modes on the Bus** (Farrell & Shaw, 2018).
8 Summarize key points from the session, emphasizing how ST concepts relate to complex trauma.
9 Introduce the **Handout 2.1 Walking through My Modes** (Farrell & Shaw, 2018). Discuss the **Schema Diary** and the **Schema Flashcard** (Young et al., 2007) as tools for recording and reflecting on daily experiences related to maladaptive schemas and challenging and reframing the irrational beliefs connected to them.
10 Check out.
11 Grounding exercise. **Category game**. Choose a category (e.g., TV shows, songs, ice cream flavors, and favorite movies). Each member will name something in the category. Go around the group twice.

Main Themes

Schema Therapy (ST)

ST is an integrative approach developed by Dr. Jeffrey Young in the 1980s. It combines elements of cognitive-behavioral therapy, psychoanalysis, attachment theory, and experiential therapies to address deeply ingrained patterns of thought and behavior. It is particularly effective for complex trauma, as it addresses deep-rooted patterns formed in childhood. **Schema Healing** is gaining control over your thinking and behavior by modifying Early Maladaptive Schemas and fulfilling unmet core emotional needs (Young et al., 2007).

Schemas (Young et al., 2007) are enduring and stable core themes or patterns that are repeated and elaborated throughout our lives. They develop during childhood from an interplay between innate temperament and early experiences with parents, siblings, peers, and others. It is the lens through which we see the world, what we feel and think about ourselves, others, and the world. They are self-perpetuating, rarely challenged, and resistant to change, though we are not always aware of their influence. "The schema fights for its survival and is usually quite successful" (Yalcin, 2023, p. 2). When triggered, however, schemas dominate our feelings, thoughts, and behaviors. (Refer to Yalcin (2023) An Introductory Guide to Schema Therapy: Adapted for use with the YSQ-R for a comprehensive discussion of ST).

Core maladaptive schemas develop when primary needs for attachment and autonomy are unmet due to adverse experiences such as a *toxic frustration of needs, traumatization, overindulgence or overprotectiveness,* or an *overidentification with significant others* that lead to pervasive feelings of disconnection, rejection, helplessness, dependency, and inadequacy. Automatic and unconscious self-destructive beliefs and behavior patterns cause a confusing, emotionally distressing, and imbalanced view of self and others.

For example, a child may come to believe she is fundamentally flawed, unlovable, unsafe, and unwanted, that others will intentionally cause harm, that emotional needs will never be met, or that others will leave them (Mistrust/Abuse, Emotional Deprivation, Abandonment/Instability, and Defectiveness/Shame) (Young, 1990; Yalcin et al., 2022). The persistent fear of imminent disaster or harm, the belief that one needs significant help to handle daily responsibilities, and the pervasive feeling of loneliness and alienation can lead to schemas that significantly limit autonomy, independence, and competence. Other-directed schemas (e.g., self-sacrifice, unrelenting standards, or emotional inhibition) may develop as automatic, compensatory coping styles to avoid activating core maladaptive schema. Mistrust/Abuse, Vulnerability to Harm, and Emotional Deprivation schema are especially significant in the development of Post Traumatic Stress Disorder (PTSD) (Karatzias et al., 2016).

Young (1990) identified 18 EMS, reflecting attachment issues, as seen in a lack of expectation of reliability, support, empathy, and respect, impaired autonomy and performance, inadequate boundaries, low frustration tolerance, a focus on the needs of others at the person's expense, to receive love and acceptance, and suppression of spontaneity and emotional expression. These were further elaborated by Yalcin (2023) to include a fear of losing control and internalized/externalized punitiveness schemas. Trauma survivors often experience a generalized elevation of maladaptive schemas rather than a unique profile of specific schemas.

1 **Abandonment/Instability**: The expectation that one will lose anyone with whom an emotional attachment is formed, that close relationships

will end ("Eventually people I love will leave me"). This leads to clingy behavior or avoidance of close relationships.

2 **Mistrust/Abuse**: Suspicion of others' motives and expectation that others will hurt, abuse, humiliate, cheat, lie, manipulate, or take advantage (I can't let my guard down or trust anyone). This may interfere with intimate relationships, and individuals may remain emotionally distant. the expectation

3 **Emotional Deprivation**: Belief that others will not adequately meet one's need for healthy emotional support (nurturance, empathy, and protection) ("I don't matter, I can't rely on anyone to meet my needs")

4 **Defectiveness/Shame**: Feeling fundamentally flawed, unlovable, or unworthy of care and attention from others. ("I'm not good enough" "there is something wrong with me").

5 **Social Isolation/Alienation**: Feeling fundamentally different from others and isolated from the larger community. ("I do not belong; I'm different").

6 **Failure**: Believing that one has or will fail relative to others ("Nothing I do is as good as other people; I won't succeed no matter how hard I try").

7 **Dependence**: Difficulty handling everyday responsibilities without significant help from others. ("I am helpless; I can't cope on my own").

8 **Vulnerability to Harm and Illness:** An exaggerated fear that catastrophe could strike any moment and can't be prevented ("I'm not safe; I can't protect myself; I am vulnerable").

9 **Enmeshment/Undeveloped Self**: Excessive emotional involvement and closeness with significant others at the expense of complete individuation and normal social development ("I don't know who I am; I can't separate myself from others").

10 **Self-Sacrifice:** Excessive focus on meeting others' needs at the expense of their well-being to prevent causing pain, avoid guilt, and maintain connection. ("My own needs aren't important; It is selfish to do things for myself").

11 **Subjugation**: Excessive surrendering of control (of needs/emotions) because one feels coerced to avoid anger, retaliation, and abandonment ("I am powerless; If I say what I feel, I will be punished").

12 **Unrelenting Standards**: Striving to meet high internalized standards and avoiding criticism that results in significant impairment in pleasure, relaxation, self-esteem, and relationships (perfectionism, rigid rules, preoccupation with time/efficiency). ("I have to be perfect; I can't accept 'good enough'").

13 **Emotion Constriction**: The excessive inhibition or disconnection of spontaneous emotion, action, or expression due to underlying shame/embarrassment ("Showing emotions means I'm weak/vulnerable; It is foolish to be emotional").

14 **Fear of Losing Control**: The excessive inhibition or disconnection of spontaneous emotion, action, or expression due to a fear that one would otherwise lose control of their impulses (fear of being overwhelmed, fear of other's responses, fear of harming oneself/others, fear of overindulging). ("If I show how I feel, it will cause damage; I won't be able to stop; I won't be able to cope").

15 **Entitlement-Grandiosity**: The belief that one is superior to others, entitled to special rights and privileges, not bound by rules ("I deserve special treatment; I should be able to do whatever I want").

16 **Insufficient Self-Control**: Pervasive difficulty or refusal to exercise self-control and frustration tolerance to achieve one's goals—"discomfort avoidance."("I can't control my behavior; I can't tolerate discomfort").

17 **Approval-Seeking**: Excessive emphasis on gaining approval, recognition, or attention from others or fitting in at the expense of developing a secure sense of self. ("I only have value if others say so; I am only worthwhile if I am getting attention/praise").

18 **Negativity/Pessimism**: Pervasive focus on the negative aspects of life while minimizing or neglecting the positive aspects ("Bad things always happen to me; If things are good, it is only temporary").

19 **Punitiveness** (Attacking Self-Internalizing): Self-directed hypercriticalness toward one's mistakes, suffering, imperfection, the belief that one should be punished for failing to meet expectations that leads to self-blame, self-directed anger, and lack of forgiveness. ("I deserve to be punished; I should have known better").

20 **Punitiveness** (Attacking Others-Externalizing): Hypercriticalness toward others' mistakes, suffering, or imperfections; the belief they should be punished for their indiscretions; preoccupation with concepts of justice. ("There is no excuse for mistakes; It's all their fault").

Schema Modes are moment-to-moment emotional states and coping responses that we all experience. Schema modes can significantly perpetuate post-traumatic symptoms and maladaptive behaviors in trauma survivors. Research has shown that maladaptive schema modes are predictors of PTSD symptoms among trauma survivors (Edwards, 2022). The mildest form of a schema mode is a typical mood shift (lonely mood, angry mood). At the other extreme is Dissociative Identity Disorder, a term used to describe individuals who flip into schema modes that are at the end of the dissociative spectrum. Patients with Dissociative Identity Disorder may name each schema mode. (Refer group members to Edwards (2022). Using Schema Modes for Case Conceptualization in Schema Therapy: An Applied Clinical Approach for a comprehensive and easily understood breakdown of schema modes).

Common modes in trauma survivors include:

1 **Vulnerable Child (VC):** This is the traumatized part of the individual that often feels helpless, scared, or abandoned. In trauma survivors, this mode may be particularly intense, reflecting the overwhelming emotions experienced during traumatic events. In this mode, a person might experience heightened sensitivity to perceived rejection or criticism, difficulty trusting others, forming close relationships, or feeling overwhelmed by daily stressors. *A person in VC mode might become extremely distressed when their partner is late coming home, interpreting it as abandonment and reliving childhood feelings of neglect.*

2 **Angry Child (AC):** This part feels rage, frustration, or impatience as a response to unmet needs, mistreatment, perceived threats, or injustices. This mode can be controlling, demanding, indignant, or abusive of others with a temper-tantrum-like quality and intensity to their reactions. A person in this mode may have sudden outbursts of anger in response to minor triggers, difficulty regulating emotions in interpersonal conflicts, or tend to perceive threats in everyday interactions. *A person in the AC mode might react disproportionately to a coworker's constructive criticism, viewing it as a personal attack and responding with hostility.*

3 **Impulsive/Undisciplined Child (ImpC):** These modes display selfish or uncontrolled behaviors when their needs are not met. People in this mode may avoid "mundane" tasks as they seek more enjoyment and excitement. They may not respond well to limit setting.

4 **Inner Critic (IC-Punitive; IC-Demanding):** This mode is the critical or demanding voice that reflects the internalization of harsh, punitive, judgmental, or demanding messages heard as children. This mode places excessive pressure to meet high standards or shows up with self-critical and negative self-talk, self-sabotaging behaviors, reluctance to pursue goals, or difficulty experiencing positive events or emotions (calling oneself names like "stupid" or "worthless," placing unrealistic expectations on oneself). *People in this mode might constantly berate themselves for minor mistakes, believing they don't deserve affection or support.*

5 **Coping Modes** are individuals' defensive strategies to manage or avoid the pain caused by maladaptive schemas. They often operate unconsciously, and while initially protective, they may become self-defeating and reinforce underlying schemas. ST identifies three primary coping modes that develop in response to early childhood experiences and unmet emotional needs:

    a **Surrender (Freeze/Submit/Attach).** The **Compliant Surrenderer** (CS) mode is characterized by giving in to the schema, seen in compliant and submissive behavior, a passive acceptance of mistreatment, self-deprecating tendencies, and excessive reassurance-seeking. A person in this mode puts others' needs first, accepts abuse or criticism without protest, and is intent on people-pleasing for approval to maintain relationships. A subcategory of this mode is the Helpless Surrenderer, which can manifest as a frozen helpless surrender or as a "rescue me" surrender, where the individual is helpless and desperate, attracting rescuing or counterattacking rejection.

b **Avoidance (Flight)**—Often seen after traumatic experiences, the **Detached Protector** (DP) mode helps disconnect from and avoid the pain associated with traumatic memories. In an avoidant mode, a person is emotionally detached and withdrawn, disconnected from feelings. In this mode, the person appears engaged and responsive but is, in reality, walling off their feelings. They may engage in excessive TV watching, gaming, or workaholism to stay disconnected from their feelings. A Detached Self-Soother might use substances, self-harm, compulsive shopping, gambling, or emotional eating to fend off feelings. An Angry Protector uses anger to distance others. Dissociation is another example of a detached protector mode where the person shuts down and feels emotionally numb, foggy, or depersonalized.

c **Overcompensation (OC) (Fight)**—This mode fights against the schema, behaving in ways opposite to core beliefs to prove the schema wrong. This includes a Bully-Attack mode, the Perfectionistic Overcontroller, the Self Aggrandizer, and an Attention/Approval Seeking mode. A person in this mode may become controlling to avoid feeling vulnerable, seek perfection, approval, or "being special" to combat feelings of defectiveness, become aggressive or bullying to mask fear, or be excessively independent to counter dependency needs.

d **Repetitive, Unproductive Thinking**—this can be viewed as another form of a coping mode that is a significant factor in perpetuating PTSD. This form of rumination can include counterfactual thinking, social comparison rumination, and self-attacking.

6 **Healthy Adult (HA)** mode represents an executive, self-nurturing function with the capacity for "meta-awareness," the ability to step back and be aware of the bigger picture through mindfulness, distancing, or diffusion, and interrupt triggered responses to review situations realistically. The Healthy Adult can feel loved, connected, and joyful, self-soothe constructively, and demonstrate competence in managing daily stressors. Seen as the "Good Parent" mode, the HA nurtures and validates the VC part, builds psychological resources and coping skills, fosters self-development and inner exploration, and provides protection and safety to other parts of the self. The Healthy Adult engages in positive dialogue and challenges maladaptive behaviors.

7 **Happy/Contented or Authentic Child (HC)** mode emerges when an individual feels safe, loved, and capable. It is expressed through spontaneous and playful behaviors, joyful emotions, and natural contentment. This mode represents the natural state that emerges when core emotional needs are met, and other modes (particularly protective and critical ones) are not dominating the person's experience. The Authentic Child captures each individual's core self's spontaneity, creativity, energy, and uniqueness (Edwards, 2022).

The HA mode is strengthened through therapy and healing, while the IC modes are internalized from childhood experiences with caregivers. The HA mode nurtures and protects, while the IC modes often criticize and demand. The HA mode promotes healing and growth, while the IC modes perpetuate trauma-related schemas. The HA mode cares for the VC; the IC mode may attack or suppress the VC. Therapy is directed toward strengthening the often-undeveloped HA and HC modes to better care for the "Vulnerable Child" when triggered by trauma reminders, to reduce the impact of the dysfunctional inner critic modes, and to bring in more play, joy, and spontaneity.

Goals of Schema Therapy

The primary goal of ST is to strengthen the Healthy Adult mode so that a person can be a kind and gentle "good parent" to themselves and diffuse from irrational ways of being and thinking to enable an emotionally regulated life with fulfilling relationships and personal and professional satisfaction. The Healthy Adult meets the VC's need for care and comfort, and it substitutes maladaptive coping modes with more adaptive responses that reflect their adult experience rather than the past trauma. The Healthy Adult expresses emotions directly and assertively and makes wise decisions rather than resorting to self-defeating patterns that may have negative consequences. It replaces the messages of the inner critic modes with a self-compassionate voice.

Mode Flipping

Mode flipping refers to rapidly switching between different schema modes in response to emotional triggers. Mode flipping can lead to unpredictable emotional responses in various situations or difficulty maintaining consistent relationships. Mode flipping often occurs unconsciously, triggered by stimuli that the mind associates with past traumatic experiences. This can lead to seemingly disproportionate reactions to everyday situations, as the individual may be reliving trauma at a child's emotional level. A person might quickly move from feeling vulnerable and seeking comfort (VC mode) to becoming angry and defensive (AC mode) to shutting down and dissociating (DP mode) when their partner attempts to offer support. The rapid mode shifts can confuse the individual and those around them, causing difficulty in personal and professional relationships, neglect of personal needs and self-care, engaging in self-destructive behaviors, heightened sensitivity to stressors, and difficulty staying within the Window of Tolerance. Understanding these modes and the concept of mode flipping is crucial for trauma survivors. Mindfulness fosters the awareness and self-control necessary to recognize mode "flipping" and to resist the urge to self-soothe with maladaptive coping.

Working With ST in the Group

Group members can increase their awareness of schema modes, challenge maladaptive patterns, and develop healthier coping mechanisms through various techniques.

1 **Identifying triggers, emotional needs, and early warning signs** of different modes. Increasing attention to moment-to-moment emotional states, thoughts, and behaviors and noticing rapid shifts between different emotional states (mode flipping).
2 **Developing the Healthy Adult mode** to engage in positive dialogue and challenge maladaptive behaviors.
3 **Providing and receiving a corrective emotional experience** within the group helps meet unmet childhood needs.
4 **Chair Work** (a Gestalt-inspired technique): Various schema modes are represented in different chairs, facilitating direct access and work with the modes through dialogues that engage the different parts of self.
5 **Imagery/Imagery Rescripting:** Visualizing past events and linking them to current situations helps identify emotional responses and associated modes. Practicing healthier responses from the Healthy Adult mode challenges self-defeating patterns.
6 **Mode Tracking:** A daily log of triggers, emotional states, thoughts, and behaviors. Analyzing active schema mode patterns increases awareness of moment-to-moment shifts in emotional states (mode flipping).
7 **Mode Mapping:** Visually representing schema modes and their interactions helps identify triggers, emotional needs, early warning signs, and relationships between modes.
8 **Schema Diary:** The schema diary is a form that clients fill out between therapy sessions to organize their experiences when schemas or modes are triggered. The diary documents the triggering situations and activated schema. It captures how the individual responds when triggered and identifies the feelings and thoughts related to the event. The diary prompts them to identify genuine concerns versus overreactions, enabling healthier, more effective responses. Consistent diary use can show clients their progress throughout therapy.

9 **Schema Flashcard:** The schema flashcard (written or audio format) is a quick reference tool for clients to use when schemas are triggered. It prompts clients to identify their current emotions, triggers, and modes and links their reactions to past experiences. The flashcard encourages clients to challenge their negative thoughts with healthier perspectives and alternative behaviors (e.g., *"No one has called me in days, and I feel completely alone and lonely. This is probably Little Amy, my vulnerable child mode. I have felt all alone since I was a little girl. When this happens, I usually pull back, withdraw and isolate. I believe no one likes me or will ever be interested in me again, but I know this is no longer true. I know I have good friends who care, call, and visit regularly. Instead of withdrawing and being alone, I can contact them"*). Audio flashcards are handy as they can provide soothing messages in the therapist's voice that the client can listen to outside of the session, extending the reparenting aspect of therapy. As clients' Healthy Adult mode grows stronger, they can create or narrate their flashcards to counteract maladaptive schemas.

10 **Photographs:** Viewing photos from childhood can help facilitate the development of compassion and caring for the younger self, and diminish critical feelings such as shame, blame or disgust.

EXERCISE 2.1

Introducing Imagery: The Ice Cream Shoppe

(Farrell & Shaw, 2012)

> Our childhood memories are images that we have connected to child-hood events. Though they are not happening right now, when we bring them to mind, we can feel like they are happening right now, and it causes emotional pain. In imagery, we can change the ending of painful memories by creating an image of what would have happened if the strong "Good Parent" you deserved had been there. We can experience comfort, protection, and care when we create a new ending.
>
> (Farrell & Shaw, 2012, p. 170)

1 Ask group members to close their eyes (or direct their gaze to the floor if they are uncomfortable closing their eyes).
2 Enthusiastically describe the experience of visiting an ice cream shoppe, and the enjoyment of eating the ice cream treat in detail.

> *You just won an ice cream treat at your favorite shop. You can invite 10 of your friends to join you. Imagine the whole group going into the store. Take a deep breath and smell the aroma of the ice cream as you enter. Look at all the flavors you can choose from! You can choose whatever your heart desires. What flavors do you choose? What kind of cone do you want - a sugar cone? A waffle cone? Or do you prefer a cup? How many scoops do you take? Do you ask for any toppings? See yourself taking your first lick or spoonful of the cold, sweet ice cream. Feel the coolness in your mouth. Savor the flavor you chose. Imagine yourself eating all the ice cream. Perhaps you see all your friends enjoying their choices as well. Ummm. Yummy!* (This story can be spun with as much detail as possible to paint the image fully for the group).

3 Ask the group to open their eyes when finished. Ask, "How many were able to get a picture of eating the ice cream cone?" (Most people usually raise their hands).
4 Say to them, "You have just done imagery work! All of you could do it! You've had a chance to see how imagery brought your Happy Child alive! This gives you a sense of how we'll use imagery as the group progresses."

EXERCISE 2.2

Modes On the Bus Exercise

(Farrell and Shaw 2018)

This mode role-play exercise illustrates the relationship of the different sides/ modes within one person. The group members will play the different modes (two each): Healthy Adult "Good Parent" mode, Coping modes (Compliant Surrenderer, Detached Protector, Self Soother and/or Angry Protector, and Overcompensator) modes, Inner Critic (Critical and Demanding) modes, Angry Child, and VC modes. More than two people can represent each mode depending on the number of participants.

Present a triggering situation (e.g., group leaders have forgotten to check in with you and are focusing on other group members). Ask participants to generate a script based on the trigger for the mode they represent. Write the script down on a whiteboard. For instance, the Overcompensator mode might say, "Who needs them anyway? I can cope on my own. I've got everything under control." The Angry Child might say: "It's not fair, you don't care about me. You never listen. What about me?" while the VC mode laments: "I feel sad and hurt like I don't belong. No one cares about me." The Inner Critic modes respond to the VC: "No one cares about you–you're useless and lazy. You're a burden. You're bad/worthless; you have to do better, work harder." The Detached Self Soother might react: "I need to self-harm (cut, drink, eat, gamble, etc.) to block out these feelings," while the Detached Protector might say, "There is no need for me to pay attention to what is going on. I don't need to be part of this." The HA would say: "You're ok as you are; you deserve to get your needs met. You're worthwhile. I've got your back. I'll help you work through this. I'm here for you."

Place the necessary amount of chairs in rows to imitate a bus. Place the VC and Angry Child chairs together in the back row of the bus, with the coping modes (Compliant Surrenderer, Detached Protector/Detached Self Soother/, and Overcompensator) in the middle row. Sit the Inner Critics in the front seat, facing toward the child and coping modes. The Healthy Adult/Good Parent Modes are behind the Critic modes, facing the child modes, but blocked from reaching them.

Ask group members to notice their experience (including body sensations and urges) as the different modes play out. Participants are prompted to talk all at once in character (drawing on scripts on the whiteboard, e.g., Inner Critic is punitive or demanding toward the VC; the Coping modes try to protect the VC in their way, while the Healthy Adult sends validating messages). Allow this "cacophony" to go on for a minute or so, with all participants speaking from the perspective of their 'mode character'. After a minute, the HA modes (group leader and participant) call out, "Enough!"

Check-in with the participants (How did everyone feel about their roles?). Explain that this is happening within each of us–the voice of the Inner Critic is strong, and we are trying to block it by using coping modes. In order to reach the child modes, the Healthy Adult has to quiet the Inner Critic voices and move them outside the circle ("You aren't needed here–you belong in the past!") and validate the protective intention of coping modes while asking that they move to aside to give access to the child modes. When these modes move out of the way, the Healthy Adult "Good Parent" mode can reach the child modes, validate the unmet needs of the Angry Child (explain she can learn new ways to express her anger so that others understand her needs and comfort the VC ("How are you feeling? What do you need? We see you. You are not invisible to us. We will care for you").

This role-play demonstrates the primary goal of therapy–for our HA side to be the one driving the bus. For many, the coping modes are in the driving seat (trying to block out the feelings of the Child modes or Inner Critic messages). If our HA mode can be strengthened, it can take over from coping modes to validate and protect our emotional needs in healthy ways.

Discuss with the group how they can help each other detect the Inner Critic mode when it arises during the group, to make sure that it no longer "flies under the radar." Encourage group members to think about what it means to allow themselves to be vulnerable, to have emotions, and to recognize that their needs are valid. Present the VC mode as a healthy side that facilitates connection, warmth, love, and affection, and that despite what they may have been taught, it is important to accept and take care of this side of ourselves. Emphasize that for genuine connection and intimacy, we need to gradually learn to tolerate sharing vulnerability, to view it not as a weakness but as part of being human (Simpson, 2020).

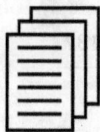

HANDOUT 2.1

Walking Through My Modes

(Farrell & Shaw, 2018)

The following are questions to check in with all of the modes you experienced today from your Healthy Adult Mode, which includes your Good Parent.

1 My Vulnerable Child Mode

What am I aware of when I connect to my VC Mode? What are my feelings, needs, thoughts, physical sensations? If there is distress–what was the triggering situation?

_____

_____

_____

_____

2 My Angry Child Mode

What am I aware of when I connect to my Angry Child Mode? What are my feelings, needs, thoughts, physical sensations? If there is distress–what was the triggering situation?

_____

_____

_____

_____

3 My_____(list your Maladaptive Coping Mode)

What am I aware of when I connect to my _____ Mode? What are my feelings, needs, thoughts, and physical sensations? If there is distress—what was the triggering situation?

_____

_____

_____

_____

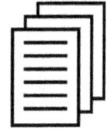

4 My Dysfunctional Critic Mode

What am I aware of when I connect to my Critic Mode? What are my feelings, needs, thoughts, physical sensations? (Limit your Critic Mode to no more than three statements. The Critic's comments are hurtful and serve no healthy purpose. As a child, you had no choice but to listen. You may still hear them today, but you have your Healthy Adult perspective to limit their effects.)

_____

_____

_____

5 **Healthy Adult Mode Management Plan**: I have checked in with all the modes I experienced today and utilized the information I derived from this awareness to make the following plans

a To meet the needs of my VC, my Good Parent will take the following acti ons:

_____

_____

_____

b To meet the need of my Angry Child to be heard and have his/her feelings validated, I will take the following actions

_____

_____

_____

_____

c Instead of allowing my _____ Coping Mode to take over, I will take the following healthy action to meet my underlying need

_____

_____

_____

_____

d To decrease the effect of my Dysfunctional Critic Mode, I will take the following action:

_____

_____

_____

_____

References

Edwards, D.J.A. (2022). *Definitions of Schema Modes*. South Africa: Schema Therapy Institute of South Africa. www.schematherapysouthafrica.co.za

Edwards D. J. A. (2022). Using Schema Modes for Case Conceptualization in Schema Therapy: An Applied Clinical Approach. *Frontiers in psychology*, 12, 763670. https://doi.org/10.3389/fpsyg.2021.763670

Farrell, J. M. & Shaw, I. A. (2012). *Group Schema Therapy for Borderline Personality Disorder: A Step-By-Step Treatment Manual With Patient Workbook*. New York: Wiley-Blackwell.

Farrell, J. M & Shaw, I. A. (2018). *Experiencing Schema Therapy From The Inside Out: A Self Practicing/Self Reflection Workbook for Therapists*. New York: Guilford Press.

Karatzias, T., Jowett, S., Begley, A., & Deas, S. (2016). Early maladaptive schemas in adult survivors of interpersonal trauma: foundations for a cognitive theory of psychopathology. *European Journal of Psychotraumatology*, 7, 30713. https://doi.org/7. 10.3402/ejpt.v7.30713

Lobbestael, J., Van Vreeswijk, M., & Arntz, A. (2007). Shedding light on schema modes: a clarification of the mode concept and its current research status. *Netherlands Journal of Psychology*, 63, 76–85.

Simpson, S. (2020). Manual of group schema therapy for eating disorders. In Simpson, S & Smith, E. (Eds.), Schema Therapy For Eating Disorders: Theory And Practice For Individual And Group Settings. London: Routledge, 136–184.

Yalcin, Ozgur & Marais, Ida & Lee, Christopher & Correia, Helen. (2021). Revisions to the Young Schema Questionnaire using Rasch analysis: the YSQ-R. Australian Psychologist. 57. 1-13. 10.1080/00050067.2021.1979885.

Yalcin, O. (2023). *An Introductory Guide to Schema Therapy: Adapted for use with the YSQ-R*. Created by Bricker, D. & Young, J. E. and modified by Yalcin, O.

Young, J. E. (1990). Cognitive therapy for personality disorders: A schema-focused approach. Philadelphia, PA: Professional Resource Exchange, Inc.

Young, J. E., Klosko, J. S., & Weishaar, M. E. (2007). *The Schema Therapy: A Practitioner's Guide*. New York: Guilford Press.

Post-Traumatic Stress Disorder and Complex Post-Traumatic Stress Disorder

Trauma is a complex and profound experience that can be so painful and shocking that it overwhelms an individual's ability to cope. It can be what has been described as a big "T" experience, such as war, devastating natural disasters, life-threatening illnesses or accidents, epidemics (COVID-19), terroristic acts (9-11), or physical or sexual abuse. Trauma is also much more than just the event. Little "t" experiences, such as emotional abuse, neglect, rejection, betrayal, loss, isolation, excessive criticism, and discrimination that cause a person to feel powerless, helpless, defective, damaged, unlovable, and alone, also have a profound effect.

Early childhood trauma, also known as complex or interpersonal trauma, develops from prolonged exposure to adverse experiences across different developmental stages within significant and intimate relationships meant to provide safety and security. These repetitive experiences compromise the person's identity, self-perception, ability to regulate emotions, physical self, and how they relate to the world.

Trauma is a disorder of connectedness that disrupts the connection with the self, others, and the world. It is a disorder of exclusion—from the community, social bonds, and safety. It is a disorder of memory that is disrupted as the nervous system responds to danger, and new memories cannot be consolidated. It is a disorder of information processing that disrupts the ability to take in new information and make meaning of the experience. Basic needs go unmet when you are left alone overwhelmed by an experience, when good things don't happen when you need them (Mate, 2018). Understanding the wide-ranging effects of trauma is the first step in the healing process.

Goals

1 Differentiate Post-Traumatic Stress Disorder (PTSD) and Complex Post-Traumatic Stress Disorder (CPTSD).
2 Understand that "Trauma survivors have symptoms instead of memories" (Fisher, 2022).

DOI: 10.4324/9781003462958-14

3 Appreciate the pervasive impact of traumatic stress across different domains of functioning that results in systemic dysregulation and a failure of integration.
4 Recognize the impact of early childhood trauma on participants' sense of self, relationships, physiology, mood regulation, etc.

Procedure

1 Mindfulness Exercise: **Exercise 3.1 Safe Place Imagery**
2 Check-In.
3 Review PTSD diagnostic criteria and the differences between PTSD and Complex Trauma (differences between a prolonged, repetitive, traumatic experience (CPTSD) or an acute or single incident trauma (PTSD); big "T," little "t" differences). (*This dichotomy is not exact as other variables such as temperament and degree of social support can influence the impact of the experience).
4 Discuss trauma as a disorder of dysregulation, integration, information processing, and memory.
5 Discuss how trauma may disrupt the individual's sense of self, beliefs, system of meaning, relationships, physical health, and ability to regulate emotions. Explore how this results in emotional dysregulation, distortion of the sense of self and system of meaning and belief, disconnection in relationships, avoidance, denial, and the activation of survival defenses.
6 Review **Handout 3.1 Understanding PTSD and Complex Trauma.** The *PCL-5 (2023, National Center for PTSD)* is a self-report questionnaire obtainable online that can also help identify PTSD symptoms.
7 Help the group members recognize the impact of trauma and the expression of CPTSD symptoms and behaviors in their lives, interpersonal interactions (increased impulsivity, anger, rage, and distrust in relationships), and feelings about themselves (low self-regard, the belief that they are permanently damaged, and cannot heal). Have members identify which PTSD/CPTSD symptoms they may experience.
   Discussing diagnoses, especially those related to trauma, can be emotionally challenging. Many people with complex trauma have been labeled with multiple diagnoses in the past. Some may find that diagnosing CPTSD helps develop a more cohesive understanding of their symptoms and that naming them increases their ability to communicate their experience to others. The discussion may trigger others. Discuss the different reactions.
8 Sample questions might include: How does the concept of dysregulation relate to their experience of trauma? What does CPTSD mean to them, and how is it different from their understanding of PTSD?

How do they cope with the symptoms that arise? How do they manage moments of intense emotion or distress? Does the diagnosis increase feelings of inadequacy and shame, or do they find it destigmatizing?

9 Explore if there are any aspects of the group members' routine or environment they have adapted to manage symptoms better. Do they avoid reminders of the trauma in daily life and routines? How have they learned to cope? How have their experiences influenced their feelings and beliefs about themselves? Relationships with others? What kind of support is most helpful when struggling with symptoms of complex trauma? What differences arise in the group members' experiences of trauma as a result of culture and diversity (gender, neurodiversity, race, etc.)? How might differences be reflected in the group? What adaptations might be necessary to address the different needs?

10 Summarize the main takeaways from the group discussion.

11 Check-out.

12 Grounding Exercise: **Exercise 3.2 The Safety Bubble** (Farrell & Shaw, 2018, p. 69)

Main Themes

Post-traumatic Stress Disorder (PTSD) describes the problematic aftereffects of living through "extremely threatening or horrific" events (ICD-11, 2022) that involve "actual or threatened death, serious injury, or sexual violence" (DSM-V, 2013). The brain's capacity to self-organize, regulate emotions, and integrate experiences becomes compromised. Core symptoms of PTSD explicitly related to reactions to the traumatic event include *reexperiencing intrusions* from the past (unwanted memories, nightmares, flashbacks, physical symptoms), *avoiding reminders of the trauma, marked alterations in arousal and reactivity, a heightened sense of threat* (startling easily, needing to stay hypervigilant and on guard) and *alterations in cognition and mood* (DSM-5R, 2022; ICD-11, 2022).

Complex Post Traumatic Stress Disorder (CPTSD; Complex Trauma) results from prolonged and inescapable traumatic experiences within a significant relationship that begins early and lasts through many developmental stages that occur (Herman, 1992; Courtois & Ford, 2009). It is also called Interpersonal, Relational, or Developmental Trauma. A serious relational injury results from the pervasive, persistent, chronic, and cumulative exploitation of a person less powerful than the abuser. The normative expectations of a close interpersonal relationship are betrayed, and the ability to trust is damaged. Survival becomes the primary goal when trapped, helpless, and unable to escape.

"Trauma survivors have symptoms instead of memories" (Fisher, 2022). The enduring consequences of childhood-onset interpersonal trauma symptoms appear as cognitive, emotional, or physiological responses rather than explicit memories. These reactions are common among trauma survivors as the brain and body develop protective survival mechanisms. They are not signs of personal failure. What many see as "symptoms" began as creative ways to cope with overwhelming situations. All these symptoms make it harder to move on from the trauma they have faced as they struggle to form relationships with the self and others, regulate emotions, and function in daily life (van der Kolk & d'Andrea, 2010).

Complex Trauma is a disorder of *dysregulation* and *lack of integration* (Lanius, et. al., 2010; van der Kolk, 2014; Baldwin & Korn, 2021; Siegel, 2023).

- **Self-dysregulation** drives the development of maladaptive beliefs and messages that are incorporated into an unpredictable and disjointed sense of self, poor body image, and low self-esteem. This may include a sense of defectiveness, inadequacy, feeling damaged, chronic guilt and feelings of responsibility, intense shame and feelings of worthlessness, hopelessness, despair, and feeling that "no one can understand me."
- **Cognitive dysregulation** shifts core beliefs and perceptions about self, others, and the world (loss of faith, hope, purpose, the inability to envision a future, and mistrust). The world becomes a dangerous, unsafe place where no one can be trusted. Life loses meaning or purpose, with no hope for the future, a rejection of spirituality, and a loss of previously sustaining beliefs.
- **Attentional dysregulation/dissociation** can result from overstimulation and difficulty filtering incoming information or an attempt to filter painful experiences from conscious awareness. Impairments in executive functioning, attention, concentration, self-integrity, and dissociative behaviors result. The person is left with a disrupted sense of reality and their sense of self, feeling that they or their surroundings are unreal (derealization and depersonalization). They experience difficulty remembering events (amnesia) yet have intrusive reexperiencing of the past (fragmentation of trauma-related sensations, feelings, thoughts, and memories).
- **Relational dysregulation** is often reflected in disorganized, insecure attachment patterns. A person may try to please others, subjugate or self-sacrifice their needs to maintain a relationship, or, conversely, distrust and avoid relationships with few expectations. These disturbances can be exhibited as an increased neediness and dependency on others, with boundary violations and difficulty setting appropriate limits, enmeshment, excessive caretaking, attempts to control others, increased vulnerability to subsequent trauma (revictimization), or victimizing others. Withdrawal and excessive self-sufficiency can result in isolation and

aloneness, alienation and detachment from others, a fear of intimacy, and an inability to trust.
- **Emotional dysregulation** results in difficulty managing overwhelming emotions within a too-narrow Window of Tolerance. Mood lability (anxiety, depression, anger/rage, and hyper/hypoarousal), difficulty tolerating distress, and a slow return to baseline characterize emotional dysregulation. This includes recognizing, labeling, accepting, modulating, and communicating emotions (fear, anxiety, anger, sadness, happiness, joy, and excitement). The individual often does not see emotions as a valuable part of a healthy self.
- **Behavioral dysregulation** occurs when efforts to avoid, defend, or protect against painful memories become the dominant mode of functioning. Ineffective ways of coping include substance abuse, disordered eating, self-destructive behaviors, impulsivity, and suicidality.
- **Somatic dysregulation** is caused by a chronic elevation of stress hormones that results in physical and medical issues across multiple bodily systems (Multiple unexplained physical symptoms (MUPS), sleep disturbance, chronic pain, irritable bowel syndrome (IBS), fatigue, autoimmune disorders, and disordered eating).

Culture, neurodiversity, and individual differences affect the experience of trauma. The subjective meaning of trauma and pain is culturally shaped, which directly influences symptom expression. Both cultural background and personal experiences shape individual responses. For example, research has found that in a sample group comprised of Hispanic, non-Hispanic Caucasian, and African American survivors of sudden physical injury, the Hispanic group reported higher levels of overall post-traumatic distress along with different patterns of symptoms (i.e., hypervigilance versus sleep disturbance and numbing) (Marshall et al., 2009; Javanbakht, 2019). Cultural beliefs also influence how significant others and the community respond to trauma survivors. Social support is perceived differently among populations that emphasize individuality than other cultures that may emphasize the community and their role in the family. Neurodivergent individuals may experience heightened vulnerability to trauma due to more reactive nervous systems and are up to four times more likely to develop PTSD compared to neurotypical individuals (Rumball et al., 2021). Understanding these individual differences is crucial for integrating treatment approaches into the group that acknowledge and respect culture and neurodiversity while promoting healing and recovery (Burback, et. al, 2024).

Case Example
The following case example demonstrates the pervasive and profound consequences of early childhood trauma:

Janie is a 52-year-old, married, Caucasian female and mother of three young children who has been in therapy since her early twenties. She is a college graduate and worked outside the home before she had children and in-home childcare as they grew up. Her central role today is as a homemaker and support to her family. She describes her relationship with her husband and extended family as invalidating and emotionally abusive.

Janie has received many diagnoses over the years, including Major Depression, PTSD, Dissociative Identity Disorder, and Eating Disorder NOS. She has a history of non-suicidal self-injury and chronic suicidal ideation, multiple suicide attempts, and disordered eating that resulted in frequent hospitalizations.

She described a chaotic early home environment. After her parents divorced when she was 10, Janie's mother left her in the care of her abusive father and violent siblings. Her trauma history includes prolonged verbal, emotional, and sexual abuse and neglect by family members beginning at age four and lasting until Janie left home for college. Abuse and neglect, alcoholism, conflict, aggression, and violence defined those early years.

Emotional dysregulation: Janie has difficulty tolerating distress, is often overwhelmed, and has difficulty regulating her emotions. She reacts intensely with feelings of depression (what she calls "the pit"), anxiety, shame, and guilt, and a high level of self-invalidation and self-blame. She sets high expectations for herself and others, shuts down, and inhibits feelings when these are not realized. She rarely identifies joy in her life. Janie is often outside her 'Window of Tolerance.' Self and environmental invalidation leads to a roller coaster ride with downward spirals into emotionally dysregulated states, with a sharp escalation of anxiety, panic, self-loathing, and agitation that then swings into a state of blunted emotions, dissociation, and collapse. Trying to avoid her feelings, she turns to overmedication, suicidal thoughts, and frequent self-injury. All these reactions can last for hours or days at a time.

Attentional and self-dysregulation: Janie has a chaotic and fragmented sense of self, with frequent episodes of dissociation. She is co-conscious with distinct "parts" (alters), each with personalities, needs, and functions. She displays a pattern of cognitive dysregulation and distortion, including rigid rule-bound behaviors *(showering only with very hot water; not drinking water), nega-tive ruminations, pessimism, high levels of shame, sensitivity to criticism, and a sense of aloneness.*

Relational dysregulation: Janie rarely leaves the home these days due to impaired physical health. Her social isolation is only in part due to her recent illnesses. She tends to avoid social interactions and trauma-related triggers (e.g., fear of men, avoidance of anger, and con-flict). Paradoxically, the isolation and loneliness are also triggers due to her early history of neglect. A push-pull is evident in her avoidance of social interaction and her yearning for it. She becomes very attached and, at times, dependent on relationships, fearing abandonment.

Janie has conflicted relationships with family members. Her hus-band and sons are both demanding of her time when they need something and neglectful, spending long hours away from home, even when she has been recovering from surgery and unable to care for herself. She is not sexually intimate with her husband. She has minimal contact with her male siblings and an unstable rela-tionship with her sister and mother. Her father is deceased but con-tinues to be idealized. She maintains sporadic contact with past friends, primarily through social media.

Cognitive dysregulation: Janie holds on to a sense of hopeless-ness and despair. She cannot envision a future for herself, believing she is too damaged. She frequently expresses suicidal communi-cations and the wish to die and maintains suicide-related expec-tancies, beliefs, and related effects. She can only briefly sustain thoughts of any long-term goals. She feels misunderstood by others and often accepts blame for the past abuse. Faith is essential to her, although she has no organized religious practice.

Somatic dysregulation: Janie has fibromyalgia and has also had a series of health setbacks (gynecological issues, cancer, severe back pain) over the past few years, resulting in multiple surgical treatments. She continues to experience severe chronic pain that severely impairs her ability to function. Physiologically destabi-lized results in a chronic state of hyperarousal, anxiety, fear, panic, depression, and irritability. Significant pain and nightmares inter-fere with sleep, which increases both her physical and emotional vulnerabilities. Trauma-related aversion to drinking fluids and dis-ordered eating result in restriction of fluid and food intake, dehy-dration, and a lack of proper nutrition. She reports that she feels like her brain is short-circuiting and, at times, takes more medica-tion than prescribed "in order to sleep."

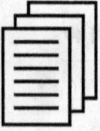

HANDOUT 3.1

Understanding PTSD and Complex Trauma

Check off the symptoms of PTSD/Complex Trauma that you may experience. How do you think these symptoms affect you today?

___ Sometimes, I feel as if I am reliving the trauma in this very moment (flashback).

___ I frequently have nightmares reminding me of my trauma.

___ I cannot stop thinking about what happened.

___ I do anything to distract myself from remembering my past.

___ I feel emotionally numb.

___ I avoid socializing.

___ I cannot seem to enjoy things in my life.

___ I often forget what I have done during the day.

___ I am often tense and on guard, waiting for something terrible to happen.

___ I feel worthless

___ I feel disconnected from my body.

___ I often think, "What is the point?"

___ I am frequently irritable or angry.

___ I have chronic pain.

___ I worry a lot and fear the worst will happen.

___ I do things to hurt myself.

___ I abuse substances.

___ I have an eating disorder.

___ I have trouble sleeping.

___ I cannot relax.

___ I feel disconnected from the world around me.

___ I feel sad all the time.

___ I do not trust people.

___ I am jumpy and startle easily.

___ I am often on edge around others

___ I freeze at times when I should act.

___ Life often overwhelms me.

___ I feel damaged and inadequate.

EXERCISE 3.1

Safe Place Imagery

Share ideas of your safe (or calming) place to help the group develop their image. I often share the image of being alone in my room in the afternoon. I see myself lying on my bed, bathed in a halo of the afternoon sunlight streaming into the room. The sun's warmth, the softness of my bed, and the quiet and solitude helped me feel safe and secure.

> *Anna describes an image she used to calm her dysregulated system: She imagines herself walking down a path into a wide-open field with a big shade tree. All modes are able to find respite in this image. A child mode burdened with sadness and hopelessness 'laid down his load' as he slept under the tree. The youngest vulnerable child modes played duck, duck, goose; the angry child expended his rage in a game of football. (Anna included me as a good parent and a healthy adult until she replaced me with the figure of her adult mode).*

People are different, so their idea of a safe (calm) place will be unique. Some examples of safe places may be unsafe for someone in the group. Help them to find another image. Anything or anyone can be included as long as no danger is introduced.

In a warm and soothing voice, ask the group to close their eyes (or direct their gaze downward).

> Imagine a place that represents safety and calm for you. Whatever comes to mind, real or imagined. Paint the image, noticing the colors, the scents, the sounds, and the textures in as much detail as possible. Can you see yourself there? What do you see? Hear? Smell? How does your body feel? Is anyone there with you? Name this place so it can come to mind quickly. Say something to yourself like "I am safe here," or" I feel calm here," or use words that are meaningful for you.

Ask the group members to practice this imagery on their own at least once a day.

EXERCISE 3.2

The Safety Bubble Exercise

(Farrell & Shaw, 2018)

This exercise can be used as an alternative to Safe Place Imagery. It is help-ful for the group members and leaders alike to increase feelings of safety and as a containment exercise for overwhelming thoughts and feelings. Farrell and Shaw (2018) describe using this as a protective cocoon when triggered by a client's intense emotions.

Lead the group through this exercise

> Imagine a bubble large enough for you to fit inside. Imagine it in any color you like, as beautiful as you want to make it. It is a magic bub-ble because you can walk in and out without breaking it. You can take anything into the soothing bubble that will help you feel strong and safe. You may let other people in or choose to be by yourself. You may not take anything harmful or unhealthy into the bubble.
>
> After you have imagined your bubble and entered it with anything you want, imagine the bubble floating away wherever you want it to go. You may want to close your eyes and listen to some peaceful music as you float in your safe bubble. No unhealthy critical voices can get through the magic bubble. You may stay in this bubble as long as you need or want to. After you come out, relax for a few minutes before you do anything else.
>
> You can also put overwhelming feelings or thoughts into the bubble and let it float away until you feel less overwhelmed. You can take the feelings or thoughts out, one at a time, to address each and your under-lying need.

References

APA (2022). *Diagnostic and Statistical Manual of Mental Disorders,* Fifth Edition, *Text Revision (DSM-5-TR®).* Washington, D.C.: American Psychiatric Association.

Baldwin, M. & Korn, D. L. (2021). *Every Memory Deserves Respect: EMDR, the Proven Trauma Therapy with the Power to Heal.* New York: Workman Publishing, Hachette Book Group.

Burback, L., Brémault-Phillips, S., Nijdam, M. J., McFarlane, A., & Vermetten, E. (2024). Treatment of posttraumatic stress disorder: a state-of-the-art review. *Current Neuropharmacology,* 22(4), 557–635. https://doi.org/10.2174/15701 59X21666230428091433

Courtois, C. & Ford, J. (2009). *Treating Complex Traumatic Stress Disorders: An Evidence-Based Guide.* New York: Guilford Press.

Farrell, J. M. & Shaw, I. A. (2018). *Experiencing Schema Therapy From The Inside Out: A Self-Practice/Self-Reflection Workbook For Therapists.* New York: The Guilford Press.

Fisher, J. (2022). *The Living Legacy of Trauma Flip Chart: A Psychoeducational In-Session Tool For Clients and Therapists.* Eau Claire, Wisconsin: Pesi Publishing, Inc.

Herman, J. L. (1992). *Trauma and Recovery: The Aftermath of Violence – From Domestic Abuse to Political Terror.* New York: Basic Books.

International Classification of Diseases, Eleventh Revision (ICD-11), World Health Organization (WHO) 2019/2021 https://icd.who.int/browse11.

Javanbakht, A. (2019). Mental health of refugees and torture survivors: a critical review of prevalence, predictors, and integrated care. *International Journal of Environmental Research and Public Health,* 16(13), 2309. https://doi.org/10.3390/ ijerph16132309

Lanius, R. A., Vermetten, E., & Pain, C., (Eds.) (2010). *The Impact of Early Life Trauma on Health and Disease: The Hidden Epidemic.* Cambridge: Cambridge University Press.

Marshall, G. N., Schell, T. L. & Miles, J. N. (2009). Ethnic differences in posttraumatic distress. *Journal of Consulting and Clinical Psychology,* 77(6), 1169–1178.

Maté, G. (2018). *In the realm of hungry ghosts: Close encounters with addiction.* Chicago: Vermilion. 17th ed.

Rumball, F., Brook, L., Happé, F., & Karl, A. (2021). Heightened risk of posttraumatic stress disorder in adults with autism spectrum disorder: the role of cumulative trauma and memory deficits. *Research in Developmental Disabilities,* 110, 103848. https://doi.org/10.1016/j.ridd.2020.103848

Siegel, D. J. (2023). *Healing Trauma: IPNB Clinical Strategies for Applying the 9 Domains of Integration Toward Deep Therapeutic Growth.* Los Angeles, CA: Mindsight Institute.

van der Kolk, B. A. (2014). *The Body Keeps Score: Brain, Mind and Body in the Healing of Trauma.* New York: Viking Press.

van der Kolk, B. A., & d'Andrea, W. (2010). Towards a developmental trauma disorder diagnosis for childhood interpersonal trauma. In R. A. Lanius, E. Vermetten, & C. Pain (Eds.), *The Impact of Early Life Trauma on Health and Disease: The Hidden Epidemic.* Cambridge: Cambridge University Press, 57–68.

The Window of Tolerance

Allie recently came into my office, sat down, let out a big sigh, and bewailed, 'I cannot do this anymore – I try so hard, but once I become overwhelmed, I feel so alone. I cannot control how I react'. Allie moves between lashing out angrily or melting down in tears. Either episode is draining and exhausting, takes time to recover from, and strains her relationships. At these times, she finds herself well outside her Window of Tolerance. She feels like her emotions take over, she forgets the strategies she has learned to calm herself, and she cannot act with a more measured response. Allie laments that this pattern has been going on since she was a child when her parents were either unavailable or unable to comfort her or were the source of her upset. The feeling of being helpless and alone has pervaded much of her life.

The Window of Tolerance is a foundational concept in trauma treatment, illustrating how trauma affects the ability to regulate emotions. The legacy of trauma is to see danger all around. It shocks the system and narrows this window. When someone is within their Window of Tolerance, however, the sense of pervasive threat becomes more manageable, and the person can better regulate the intensity of their emotions. Understanding this concept can bring a profound sense of relief, as it provides a roadmap for managing overwhelming emotions. A primary goal of trauma treatment is to help clients increase their ability to regulate their intense and destabilizing emotions, offering a beacon of hope and empowerment in the process.

Goals

1 Recognize the importance of the Window of Tolerance and arousal levels in emotion regulation.
2 Understand how trauma disrupts emotion regulation.
3 Explain the metaphor of the River of Integration and its relationship to emotional well-being.

DOI: 10.4324/9781003462958-15

4 Identify the interrelationship between maladaptive schema activation, mode flipping, and arousal.
5 Develop resources to widen the Window of Tolerance.

Procedure

1 Mindfulness Exercise: **Exercise 4.1 Breath Awareness**.
2 Check-In.
3 Discuss the key points about the Window of Tolerance, differentiating the optimal zone of arousal from the zones of hyperarousal and hypoarousal. Review **The Window of Tolerance and Zones of Arousal** graphic. It may be necessary to review the material in this section repeatedly, as it is a core concept of emotion regulation.
4 Explore the group's experiences of being in or out of their window. Questions to guide discussion in the group might include: Which zone best describes the way you respond when reminders of your trauma intrude? What are you thinking and feeling at those times? What do you want to do at those moments? Can you remember past times you could stay in your Window of Tolerance? This will provide real-life examples of the concepts being explored. The **Handout 4.1 Managing Your Window of Tolerance and Level of Arousal** can help them identify their arousal levels and ways to widen their Window of Tolerance.
5 Help clients tailor strategies to widen their Window of Tolerance depending on their specific needs, preferences, and level of vulnerability or dysregulation. Review **Handout 4.2 Strategies to Help Identify and Monitor the State of Arousal**.
6 Summarize the main takeaways from the group discussion, highlighting the themes of dysregulation, disruption, distortion, disconnection, denial, and defense.
7 Check-out.
8 Grounding: **Exercise 4.2 Mountain Meditation**

Main Themes

The **Window of Tolerance** is the state in which it is possible to experience and tolerate a wide range of emotions without becoming overwhelmed and dysregulated, maintaining a flexible, adaptive, coherent, energized, and stable manner (FACES) (Daniel Siegel, 2010a,b). It is the optimal arousal zone (Siegel, 1991; Ogden et al., 2006). When an individual's Window of Tolerance narrows due to stress or trauma, they become more susceptible to the activation of schema resulting from their adverse experiences. Even minor stressors can trigger maladaptive schemas, pushing the person outside their optimal zone of functioning into the zones of hyperarousal and hypoarousal (Figure 4.1).

The **River of Integration** (Siegel, 2010a,b) is a metaphor that conceptualizes the relationship between optimal functioning and emotional regulation. A flowing river represents the state of well-being, integration, and emotional balance embodied in the acronym FACES - flexible, adaptive, coherent, energized, and stable. It is bounded on two sides by different riverbanks, each illustrating threats to well-being. The Chaos Bank symbolizes unpredictability, instability, disorganization, and lack of control. The Rigid Bank represents excessive control, inflexibility, and resistance to change.

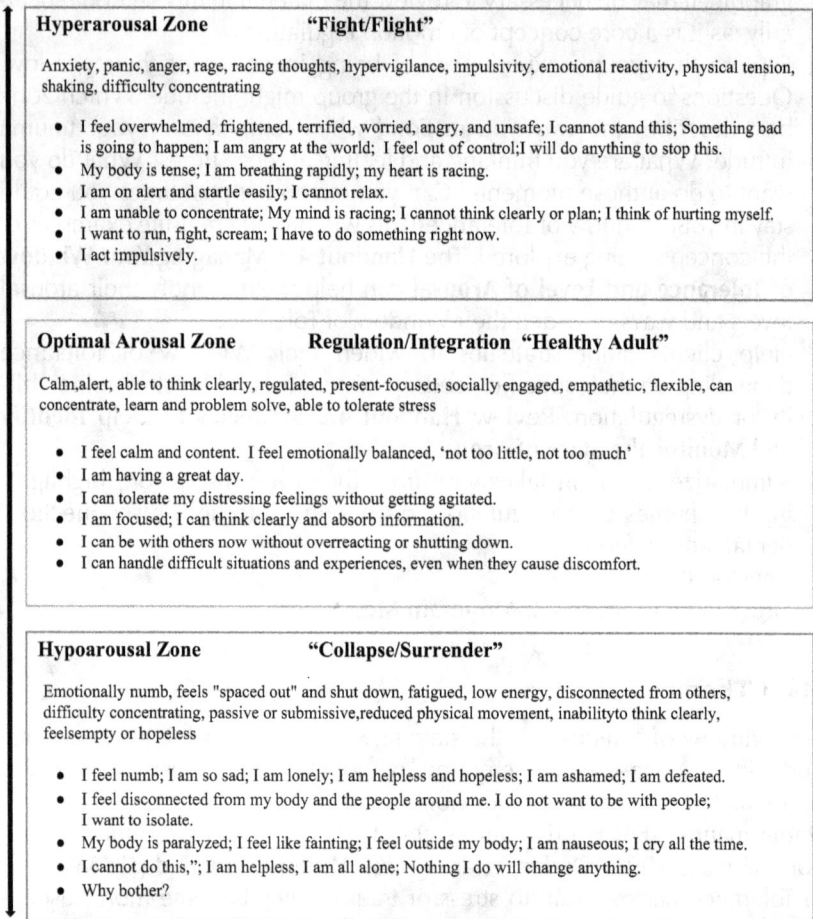

Hyperarousal Zone   **"Fight/Flight"**

Anxiety, panic, anger, rage, racing thoughts, hypervigilance, impulsivity, emotional reactivity, physical tension, shaking, difficulty concentrating

- I feel overwhelmed, frightened, terrified, worried, angry, and unsafe; I cannot stand this; Something bad is going to happen; I am angry at the world; I feel out of control;I will do anything to stop this.
- My body is tense; I am breathing rapidly; my heart is racing.
- I am on alert and startle easily; I cannot relax.
- I am unable to concentrate; My mind is racing; I cannot think clearly or plan; I think of hurting myself.
- I want to run, fight, scream; I have to do something right now.
- I act impulsively.

Optimal Arousal Zone   Regulation/Integration "Healthy Adult"

Calm,alert, able to think clearly, regulated, present-focused, socially engaged, empathetic, flexible, can concentrate, learn and problem solve, able to tolerate stress

- I feel calm and content. I feel emotionally balanced, 'not too little, not too much'
- I am having a great day.
- I can tolerate my distressing feelings without getting agitated.
- I am focused; I can think clearly and absorb information.
- I can be with others now without overreacting or shutting down.
- I can handle difficult situations and experiences, even when they cause discomfort.

Hypoarousal Zone   "Collapse/Surrender"

Emotionally numb, feels "spaced out" and shut down, fatigued, low energy, disconnected from others, difficulty concentrating, passive or submissive,reduced physical movement, inabilityto think clearly, feelsempty or hopeless

- I feel numb; I am so sad; I am lonely; I am helpless and hopeless; I am ashamed; I am defeated.
- I feel disconnected from my body and the people around me. I do not want to be with people; I want to isolate.
- My body is paralyzed; I feel like fainting; I feel outside my body; I am nauseous; I cry all the time.
- I cannot do this,"; I am helpless, I am all alone; Nothing I do will change anything.
- Why bother?

Figure 4.1 The Window of Tolerance and Zones of Arousal (Adapted from Siegel, 1999; Ogden, et.al., 2006)

The Healthy Adult mode's self-awareness, mindfulness, flexibility, emotion regulation, and integration help maintain the flow down the center of the river, balancing stability and flexibility as the "boat" veers off to the side.

Trauma survivors often experience extremes in the intensity of their emotions when even regular changes in the level of emotional arousal may become unmanageable and dysregulating. When arousal levels are too high or too low, the capacity for processing and learning is compromised. The individual may move, for example, between chaos and rigidity, hyperarousal to hypoarousal, flipping between different schema modes, depending on the situation. For instance, a sudden loud noise might trigger hyperarousal and a protector mode, while isolation might trigger hypoarousal, surrender, or a vulnerable child mode.

Hyperarousal is a state with "too much" emotion. It is often associated with a fight/flight/freeze defensive response. When pushed beyond the upper limit of the Window of Tolerance into hyperarousal, individuals may experience intense activation of schemas related to danger, abandonment, or vulnerability. "Too much" arousal increases the intrusion of trauma memories, which leads to a flood of often dysregulating feelings that can manifest as anxiety, anger, or hypervigilance. It can feel like past trauma is being reexperienced in the present, with innocuous stimuli perceived as dangerous and threatening. The present reality becomes disrupted by the intensity of what is experienced.

Hypoarousal is a state with "too little" activation. Falling below the lower limit of the Window of Tolerance into hypoarousal can reinforce schemas related to helplessness, emotional deprivation, or social isolation. Associated with the feigned death or surrender response, "too little" arousal can result in emotional numbness, feelings of helplessness, dissociation, and a disconnection from the world around them or their own body. Individuals may have difficulty thinking clearly or experiencing positive emotions.

When outside the Window of Tolerance, the ability to respond flexibly or adaptively is severely diminished, and individuals may flip into different modes. For instance, the Vulnerable Child mode might emerge during hypoarousal, while the Angry Child mode could appear during hyperarousal. Dysfunctional Coping Modes represent attempts to stay within or return to the Window of Tolerance. For example, the Detached Protector mode might activate during hypoarousal to manage overwhelming emotions. Inner Critic Modes can push individuals outside their Window of Tolerance as the harsh criticism of a punitive mode creates a state of guardedness and hyperarousal. These dysregulated emotions interfere with smooth sailing down the "river of integration" into the zone of optimal arousal and the closely aligned Healthy Adult Mode. When in the Healthy Adult mode, individuals can regulate their emotions effectively, staying within their optimal arousal zone.

The wider the Window of Tolerance, the greater the ability to tolerate a broader range of emotions. Expanding the Window of Tolerance can help heal schema by reducing the frequency and intensity of maladaptive schema activations. As individuals learn to stay within their Window of Tolerance more consistently, they create opportunities to heal maladaptive schemas and develop more adaptive responses to stress. The window widens when feeling safe and secure, which can be achieved by spending time with loved ones or engaging in activities that bring comfort and joy. Conversely, the window narrows when vulnerability is high, such as when one is not sleeping at night,

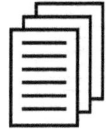

Managing Your Window of Tolerance and Level of Arousal

1 What is your current level of arousal? Are you inside or outside your Window of Tolerance? What cues help you notice whether you are inside or outside your window? (e.g., I know I am hyperaroused because my body is tense, and I feel angry and want to scream).

Hyperarousal Zone   Zone of Optimal Arousal(WOT)   Hypoarousal Zone

_____
_____
_____

2 What events contributed to your current state? Why do you think this state was activated?

_____
_____
_____

3 What do you think when you are in this zone? (e.g., I cannot trust anyone.)

_____
_____
_____

4 What are you feeling when in this zone? (e.g., I am uneasy and suspicious; I am restless and agitated)

_____
_____
_____

5 What sensations are you noticing in your body? (e.g., My body is tense. My shoulders are tight. I have knots in my stomach).

_____
_____
_____

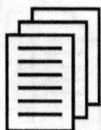

6 What is your action urge—what do you want to do in this zone? (fight, flight, freeze, submit, and attach) (I do not want to continue talking to this person; I want to run away).

_____

_____

_____

_____

_____

7 What resources help YOU return to your WOT? Jot down some helpful tips if you feel you need more or more. Refer to the STRATEGIES TO HELP IDENTIFY AND MONITOR YOUR STATE OF AROUSAL sheet for ideas or use what is helpful.

When I feel too much, I can:

_____

_____

_____

_____

_____

When I feel too little, I can:

_____

_____

_____

_____

_____

_____

_____

_____

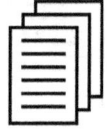

Strategies to Help Identify and Monitor the State of Arousal

Staying in and widening your Window of Tolerance increases the ability to feel emotions and make sense of experiences. You can develop the skills to soothe and regulate your feelings, thoughts, physical reactions, and behaviors as you increase awareness and understanding of how your mind and body are connected. You can manage arousal levels by utilizing the power to PAUSE before responding and not react impulsively. You can engage in activities that help you feel better and function more effectively moment-to-moment. As your Window of Tolerance widens, you find more moments that *float down the river toward well-being without being battered by the banks of chaos and rigidity.* Here are some techniques that can help you get into your **Window of Tolerance:**

1 **Downregulating Hyperarousal** (When you feel 'too much'): Use techniques that slow down physiological reactivity. Distressing feelings may be more easily tolerated when calm, decreasing the need to engage in avoidance behaviors such as using substances, overeating, or self-harming.

- **Deep Breathing:** Practice slow, deep breaths. Inhale for a count of four, hold for four, and exhale for four. Repeat until a sense of calm is achieved.
- **Breath Awareness**: One of the most effective mindfulness exercises for staying within the Window of Tolerance is breath awareness. This practice helps you stay present and can be used to regulate arousal levels. Find a comfortable seated position, close your eyes or soften your gaze, and take a few deep breaths to settle in. Begin to notice your natural breath without changing it. Observe the sensations of breathing in your body. If your mind wanders, gently bring your attention back to your breath. Continue for 5–10 minutes.
- **Body Scan and Progressive Muscle Relaxation (PMR):** Scan to identify body areas with tension. Systematically tense and then release each muscle group in the body. This helps release physical tension and promotes relaxation.
- **Distraction** can be helpful when it provides a *temporary* break from distressing emotions. This is different from intentionally avoiding

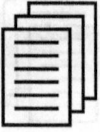

reminders of the trauma. Distraction can help you slow down, reset, breathe- and take that PAUSE.

- Match your activity to how you are feeling. Angry? Try physical activity. Sad? Try watching a funny movie.
- Art can also be helpful, as it focuses on your present experience, helping you identify, name, and express the feelings instead of holding them in your head.
- **Grounding and Reorienting** techniques engage the senses to help you reconnect with the present moment.
- Using your five senses, describe what you see, feel, hear, smell, and taste in the present moment. The 5-4-3-2-1 technique is one way to accomplish this. Name five things you can see, four things you can touch, three things you can hear, two things you can smell, and one thing you can taste.
- Listening to music, biting a sour lemon, or squatting against a supportive wall are additional techniques to help you reorient to the present.
- **Containment** can help limit access to stressful thoughts, feelings, and trauma memories *for the moment*. You choose to *temporarily* contain or put away overwhelming thoughts, feelings, and trauma memories with the understanding that you will return to address them when you are less distressed. Containment helps you remain present rather than being hijacked by your emotions. It is a technique that engages the imagination.

  Imagine your overwhelming thoughts or memories locked in a bank vault, floating in a balloon up into the air; lock them in a file cabinet or your therapist's office, or imagine putting them into your safety bubble.
- **The Diving Reflex**: This is a calming reflex and survival instinct that slows your heart rate and causes your body to conserve oxygen. It is a series of physiological responses while breathing under cold water. *Apply icy water to your face (especially the area beneath your eyes) while holding your breath, either by submerging your face or applying a cold compress. Ensure the area beneath your eyes is submerged or covered, and hold your breath for 30 seconds.*
- **Mindfulness**: Mindfulness helps you focus on the present moment *without judgment*. Focus on the facts. It can help reduce anxiety and stress at the moment and avoid being pulled back into trauma-based reactions.
- **Physical Exercise**: Engage in physical activity to release built-up tension. Exercise can also trigger the release of endorphins, which are natural mood elevators.

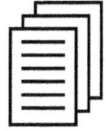

- **Guided Imagery:** Visualize a calm and peaceful place, and imagine a more effective outcome to your actions. Guided imagery can transport your mind away from stressors.
- **Limit Stimulants:** Reduce intake of caffeine, nicotine, and other stimulants, as they can contribute to increased arousal.

2 **Upregulating Hypoarousal** (when you feel "too little"): Use activating techniques to stay in your body and reengage in the present moment.

- **Physical Activity:** Engage in physical activities that increase heart rate and circulation, such as brisk walking, jumping jacks, or dancing. If you feel frozen, try moving even a tiny part of your body, such as your little finger.
- **Cold Water Splash:** Splash cold water on your face or take a cold shower. Cold stimuli can help activate the nervous system.
- **Deep Pressure:** Apply deep pressure to the body through deep tissue massage, a weighted blanket, or hugging a pillow.
- **Sensory Stimulation:** Introduce sensory stimuli like bright lights, strong scents, or invigorating music to increase alertness.
- **Change your posture:** Assume a power pose: open and confident postures help to boost feelings of empowerment. This can influence hormone levels and increase confidence.
- **Breath of Fire (Yogic Breathing):** This rapid, rhythmic breathing technique involves passive inhales and active exhales that are quick and powerful. As a form of breath control, it can be invigorating, help increase alertness, and relieve stress.
- **Aromatherapy:** Use stimulating scents or essential oils like peppermint or citrus to activate the senses.
- **Reach out for social support.** *Seek support from trusted friends, family, and therapists who can help you rebalance if you move outside your window.*

EXERCISE 4.1

Breath Awareness

This is one of the most effective mindfulness exercises to help stay present and within the Window of Tolerance. It can be used to regulate arousal levels.

1. Find a comfortable seated position.
2 Close your eyes or soften your gaze.
3 Take a few deep, cleansing breaths to settle in.
4 Begin to notice your natural breath without changing it.
5 Observe the sensations of the breath in your body.
6 If your mind wanders, as our minds do, gently bring your attention back to your breath.
7 Continue for 5–10 minutes.

EXERCISE 4.2

Mountain Meditation

This exercise is a grounding and empowering meditation that builds the Healthy Adult self by boosting self-confidence, strength, and feelings of stability. Like a mountain in a winter squall, this meditation reminds us that we can remain calm and stand tall and strong as the vagaries of life swirl around.

Imagine a majestic mountain, any mountain that you can envision. As you visualize the mountain, paint the picture with as much detail as wpossible. Notice the tall mountain, firmly rooted in the ground for thousands of years. See how the weather changes all around the mountain, from sunny skies to hurricane-force winds to snow and ice. The mountain remains unaffected, staying strong as the weather swirls around it.

Sit quietly and focus on each inhale and exhale of your breath. Relax and breathe. Sit up or stand with your shoulders back, your chest open, and your feet firmly planted on the ground as thoughts swirl through your mind. Imagine yourself as the tall, strong mountain, steadfastly grounded to the earth. Let your thoughts, stress, and worries whirl around you without letting them affect you. The thoughts that are pressuring you are just thoughts. You stand firm and grounded like the mountain. You remain who you have always been, regardless of the 'weather' around you. Breathe in and out slowly and deeply. Savor this feeling of power, strength, and majesty.

References

Ogden, P., Minton, K., & Pain, C. (2006). *Trauma and the Body: A Sensorimotor Approach to Psychotherapy*. New York: W. W. Norton & Co.

Siegel, D. J. (1999). *The Developing Mind: How Relationships and the Brain Interact to Shape Who We Are*. New York: Guilford Press.

Siegel, D. J. (2010a). *The Mindful Therapist: A Clinician's Guide to Mindsight and Neural Integration*. New York: W.W. Norton & Co.

Siegel, D. J. (2010b). *Mindsight: The New Science of Personal Transformation*. New York: Bantam Books.

Emotion Regulation

Emotion regulation is the ability to experience, manage, and tolerate a wide range of emotions to maintain a balanced emotional state. It entails creating a comfort zone where one can respond flexibly and spontaneously, inhibiting instinctive reactions that disrupt healthy functioning. Early childhood trauma often interrupts normal emotional development and the acquisition of these capabilities. The child learns to avoid painful emotions that complicate connecting with feelings and managing complex emotions. Emotional instability results when the individual uses external strategies such as substance abuse, disordered eating, or self-harm to avoid the pain.

Helping group members develop and strengthen skills to modulate their emotions and increase their tolerance of stressful experiences is a core goal of treatment. Processing traumatic material within a window that allows the individual to tolerate and reduce avoidance of distressing emotions will ultimately enable more significant healing from the traumatic experiences. Individuals gain greater control over their emotional experience as they move from reactive, impulsive coping with emotional triggers to the Healthy Adult's more mindful and reflective stance. Negative emotions such as shame or self-blame can be challenged as participants learn that their emotional responses are normal reactions to abnormal circumstances. Regulating negative emotional states opens access to positive emotions, builds healthier strategies for self-soothing, and causes emotional overwhelm and distress.

Goals

1 Increase emotional awareness and labeling of emotions.
2 Understand how trauma disrupts the ability to self-regulate.
3 Strengthen the Healthy Adult mode: Teach strategies for emotion regulation, distress tolerance, impulse control, and self-reflection.

DOI: 10.4324/9781003462958-16

4 Practice using emotion regulation skills to increase tolerance of emotions triggered within the group and in other situations.
5 Cultivate positive emotional experiences, fostering a sense of accomplishment and well-being.

Procedure

1 Mindfulness Exercise: **Aromatherapy Treasure Hunt**. Create a sensory experience by placing different scented items in front of the group and ask each member to explore them individually. Items might include soap bars, fresh herbs or flowers from outside, scented candles, and essential oils. Discuss the group's observations.
2 Check-In. Have clients pay special attention to their current emotional state. The use of a **Feelings Wheel** can assist in identifying and naming feelings. Different examples of Feelings Wheels are available on the internet.
3 Define emotional awareness and emotional regulation. Explore the functions of emotions.
4 Discuss the interrelationship between trauma and emotion regulation. How might past trauma have affected the ability to recognize and regulate emotions? How has it interfered with the ability to self-soothe? Has it affected relationships with others? Discuss **Handout 5.1 Understanding Emotions**.
5 Discuss the interconnection between a strong, Healthy Adult self and emotion regulation. Ask group members to complete **Handout 5.2 Developing the Healthy Adult** to identify and strengthen their understanding of their HA.
6 Introduce and practice emotion regulation strategies (**Handout 5.3 Emotion Regulation Activities**)
7 Summarize the main themes about emotion regulation.
8 Check-out
9 Grounding: **Exercise 5.1 Emotion Labeling and Breath Awareness**. This exercise combines mindful breathing, emotion labeling, and self-compassion to help increase emotional awareness and regulation.

Main Themes

Emotions

Emotions are normal, adaptive, and complex experiences that provide essential information, communicate feelings, guide decision-making, facilitate social interactions, energize, connect thoughts and memories, and increase self-awareness of what we think, want, or need. *Emotions* differ from feelings and moods. They are momentary reactions to specific stimuli accompanied by physiological changes, often triggered by internal or external experiences (e.g., fear during a scary movie). *Feelings* are prolonged, subjective experiences arising from emotions and influenced by personal perceptions and interpretations (e.g., feelings of love for a child). *Moods* are sustained, less intense emotional states that persist over a more extended period, may have no apparent trigger, and inform our view of the world and our behaviors (e.g., waking up with optimism and enthusiasm opens us up to positive experiences during the day, in contrast to a pessimistic attitude that shuts us off from those same experiences).

Primary Core Emotions are universal, instinctual, hard-wired reactions to stimuli, our emotional "first responders." They are easily recognizable in our facial expressions, are universal, and occur automatically (e.g., happiness, sadness, fear, anger, surprise, and disgust). **Secondary Complex Emotions** emerge from primary emotions but may not be as easily identified. They are subjective and involve self-awareness and appraisal (e.g., love, guilt, shame, jealousy, pride, envy, regret, and admiration). It is essential to identify the primary emotion behind the secondary emotion.

Emotional Awareness is recognizing, identifying, and naming experienced emotions and noticing any associated thoughts, body sensations, and urges to act. **Emotion Regulation** uses healthy strategies to decide how and when to respond to an emotion, managing its intensity and duration without spiraling out of control. **Emotional Integration** is making sense of the full range of one's emotional experiences by connecting them to one's thoughts, beliefs, and behaviors.

Emotion Regulation and Trauma

People who have experienced trauma often struggle with overwhelming emotions and labile, intense mood swings that make it difficult to manage emotions. Avoiding these intense emotions through the use of unhelpful coping modes can lead to feelings of disconnection, confusion, dissociation, and emotional numbness. People might surrender to their overwhelming distress without understanding or regulating their emotions. They may use self-harm, substances, or food to dull and avoid the pain or get angry and lash out at others and end up damaging relationships.

Emotion regulation is different from distress tolerance: Emotion regulation is like being a chef, knowing what you are cooking with (emotions are your ingredients), being prepared, following a recipe, finding a balance, and turning down the heat as necessary (Healthy Adult mode). Distress Tolerance is being the captain of a ship that guides you through the storm of emotional crises using tools to avoid sinking the ship or making the situation worse (coping modes) (Linehan, M., 2014).

The Healthy Adult mode serves as a framework for effective emotion regulation. It provides the cognitive, emotional, and behavioral tools necessary for managing emotions in adaptive ways while promoting a compassionate and balanced approach to one's emotional life. A unique aspect of this mode is its ability to balance and integrate different emotional needs: nurturing vulnerable parts, setting limits to regulate intense negative emotions, and encouraging the experience and expression of all feelings. This is particularly beneficial when experiencing distressing emotions, as it promotes self-compassion, modulates emotional experiences, and enhances the ability to reframe situations and emotional experiences in more balanced and adaptive ways.

Understanding emotions, decreasing emotional vulnerability, reducing emotional suffering, and building skills to manage emotions more effectively are fundamental skills in **Dialectical Behavior Therapy** (DBT; Linehan, 2015). The essential elements include:

1 Understanding and labeling emotions (Identify and name emotions accurately; distinguish between primary and secondary emotions; recognize the function and purpose of emotions).
2 Reducing vulnerability to negative emotions (The PLEASE skill: Treat Physical illness, Eat balanced meals, Avoid mood-altering drugs, Sleep well, Exercise)
3 Increasing positive emotional experiences (engaging in activities that bring joy or satisfaction and building mastery through accomplishments).
4 Practicing mindfulness skills (being present at the moment without judgment and observing thoughts, feelings, and sensations).
5 Changing thoughts about a situation alters emotional responses and challenges negative thought patterns.
6 Acting opposite to the urge of an unhelpful emotion (e.g., opposite action—getting up in the morning when depression makes you want to stay in bed).
7 Examining the evidence for emotional reactions and considering if the response is proportionate to the situation (Check the Facts). (When an emotion is more intense than the situation warrants, it may signal schema activation).
8 Problem-solving ways to address the causes of distressing emotions.
9 Acknowledging and accepting emotions as valid.
10 Using skills like distraction and self-soothing to manage intense emotions in the short term (e.g., use the five senses to calm and comfort).
11 Improving communication and assertiveness in relationships.

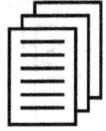

Understanding Emotions

In the past, you may have learned that it was not okay to feel or express your emotions, making it challenging to identify and express them today. This exercise is designed to help you understand what you are feeling.

1 How do you respond when you feel…how is this action helpful?
   Angry? _____
   Sad? _____
   Fear? _____
   Shame? _____
   Joy? _____

2 What are two emotions you feel comfortable expressing? How do you act when you experience these emotions?

   _____

   _____

3 What are two emotions you may try to avoid feeling? Are you afraid of them? Ashamed? How do you act when these feelings arise?

   _____

   _____

4 What do you believe would happen if you let yourself feel those emotions?

   _____

   _____

5 What do you do when difficult emotions arise? Do you engage in behaviors that help in the short term but are ineffective in the long term? (e.g., drinking, self-harm, and binging).

   _____

   _____

6 Name two other ways you might cope more effectively with these difficult emotions:

   _____

   _____

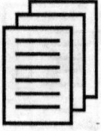

7 Do you feel uncomfortable when you experience pleasant emotions such as joy, happiness, and pride? Why do you think these feelings cause discomfort for you?

_____

_____

Adapted from pre-group reflections, S.A.F.E.T.Y.
Curriculum, Penn Medicine
Women's Program)

EXERCISE 5.1

Emotion Labeling and Breath Awareness

This exercise helps identify and regulate emotions through mindful awareness and breathing techniques.

1 Find a comfortable seated position, close your eyes, or direct your gaze toward the floor.
2 Begin with box breathing to center: Inhale for four counts, hold your breath for four counts, and exhale for four counts. Repeat this cycle 3-4 times.
3 Shift your attention to your natural breath, noticing the sensations of breathing without trying to change them.
4 As you continue mindful breathing, start to notice what emotions begin to surface. Ask yourself: "What am I feeling right now?"
5 Identify the most prominent emotion. Label the emotion by repeating its name three times in a gentle, kind voice (e.g., "worry, worry, worry" or "joy, joy, joy").
6 Return your focus to your breath for a few moments.
7 Continue alternating between breath awareness and emotion labeling: When you notice an emotion, label it, then return to your breath.
8 If an emotion feels overwhelming, stay with your breath until you feel more stable.
9 Place a hand over your heart, feeling its warmth. Cultivate a sense of loving-kindness towards yourself as you breathe through your heart.
10 If your mind wanders, gently bring your attention back to your breath without judgment.
11 Slowly open your eyes.

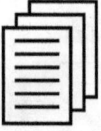

HANDOUT 5.2

Developing your Healthy Adult Mode

(Adapted from Hayes & Brockman 2022)

The Healthy Adult mode identifies and takes care of the feelings of the vulnerable child mode, offers hope and a different perspective, and deals with the reality of the present situation. This exercise will help you move through these steps as you strengthen your Healthy Adult (HA) resources and increase your ability to tolerate difficult emotions.

1 Identify an event or current/future life challenge that triggers your Vulnerable Child mode.

_____

_____

_____

2 When do you think this mode is most activated? (e.g., when you consider visiting your family for a holiday, is there a specific feeling, thought, or idea overwhelming your VC mode?

_____

_____

_____

3 Envision a Healthy Adult or other resource and identify the needed resource: "What would you need to believe about yourself to manage this situation? What quality would your HA need so you would not feel overwhelmed or inadequate (strength, empowerment, compassion, kindness, etc.)?"

_____

_____

_____

4 Envision the resource and link to times you have felt empowered. "Remember a time you have felt strong and powerful." What did that feel like? Where do you feel it in your body? Can you label that feeling (sunshine, strength, power, confidence, etc.)?

_____

_____

_____

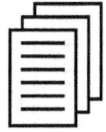

5 Identify resources that can meet the needs of your VC. Describe someone or something you know (real or imagined) who embodies the needed element of your HA.

_____

_____

_____

_____

6 Imagine this resource within you. What would it be like to have your strong HA by the side of your VC when you face a triggering situation? Try imagery to help: "Can you get a sense of me being there with you, supporting you as you…?" What does that feel like? When have you felt that in the past?

_____

_____

_____

_____

7 Expand the resource: Can you notice that your HA self is there with you, taking care of the challenge? Notice the sense of empowerment, courage, determination, and strength (HA resource) as your HA says, "You've got this; I've got your back." What does that feel like? What do you feel in your body?

_____

_____

_____

_____

8 Installs the resource: Restate the most salient elements of the HA and the sense of needs being met. "So I notice the sense of empowerment, determination, strength, and courage (HA resource) when my HA says, 'I've got this.' My HA is with me, feeling at ease and confident."

_____

_____

_____

_____

9 (Sometimes, it may be challenging to connect with your HA resources when a coping mode sets up blocks. Explore where you feel the negative beliefs in your body. What would your HA mode say to your coping mode (to your fears, anxiety, denial, avoidance, or your vulnerable mode)?

_____

_____

_____

_____

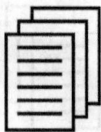

Emotion Regulation Strategies

The Healthy Adult mode aligns closely with many effective emotion regulation strategies. These strategies focus on mindful awareness, cognitive flexibility, self-compassion, adaptive coping, emotional intelligence, and balanced behavioral approaches. By strengthening these skills, you can enhance your ability to operate from the Healthy Adult mode and effectively regulate your emotions (Hayes and Dominquez, 2023).

1 **The Feelings Wheel:** Recognizing and naming emotions accurately helps the Healthy Adult mode regulate emotions. Learning to express emotions in healthy ways; neither suppressing them nor allowing them to overwhelm is a key skill of the Healthy Adult mode. (Examples of a Feeling Wheel are available online).

   a Identifying and labeling feelings is the first step in managing emotions effectively.
   b Provide participants with a feelings wheel handout and explain that this tool helps expand the emotional vocabulary and pinpoint feelings more accurately.
   c Have participants identify and share an emotion they experienced recently, the situation that triggered it, associated thoughts, physical sensations, and action urges.
   d The Feelings Wheel diagram is a helpful tool available during group check-ins.

2 **Self-Care Activities:** Engaging in activities that promote overall well-being, such as exercise, proper sleep, and healthy eating, supports the Healthy Adult mode and emotion regulation.

   a **Building Mastery** (DBT ABC-Skills, Linehan, 2015): Doing pleasant things now builds the long-term goal of a purposeful life worth living (**A**ccumulation of Positive Emotions). Doing things that make you feel competent and effective combats feelings of helplessness, hopelessness, and inadequacy (Building **M**astery). Developing and rehearsing ways to cope with emotional situations ahead of time increases their effective management (**C**ope Ahead).
   b **Reducing Vulnerability** (DBT PLEASE Skills, Linehan, 2015): Treat Physica**L** Illness, Balanced **E**ating, **A**void Mood Altering Substances, Balanced **S**leep, Get **E**xercise.

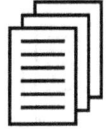

c **Adaptive Coping Strategies** include problem-solving and redirecting attention away from intense emotions when appropriate, without suppressing them entirely.

d **Opposite Action** (Linehan, 2015): The core principle of opposite action is to do the opposite of what your impulses are telling you to do. Typically, we avoid, withdraw, or escape from situations that make us uncomfortable. Sometimes, acting opposite to our emotional urge can help shift the emotion. For example, if you are feeling anxious and want to avoid a situation, purposefully approaching it can reduce anxiety over time. If a person feels judged at work, they actively engage instead of avoiding work colleagues; if they fear public speaking, they volunteer to present at a conference instead of declining speaking opportunities.

  i Explain the concept of opposite action. Have participants brainstorm examples of what they can do to change their emotions.

3 **Mindfulness-based strategies** lead to increased emotional tolerance and reduced reactivity (Present moment awareness, observing emotions as they arise, and acceptance of emotions). **Mindful Breathing**: Focusing on the breath helps regulate intense emotions by anchoring us in the present moment and activating our body's relaxation response. Guide the group through a brief mindful breathing exercise.

4 **Acceptance:** Radical acceptance means fully accepting and not trying to change reality, even as we wish it were different. This does not mean we have to agree with, approve of, or condone the situation, but that we stop fighting against what we cannot control. Paradoxically, acceptance often reduces emotional suffering. Introduce the concept of radical acceptance. This is a difficult concept for some to grasp. Acknowledge that it may take many efforts to keep "turning the mind" back to reality as it is and not how we wish it were.

5 **Reframing Situations:** Our thoughts greatly influence our emotions. We can often change our feelings about a situation by consciously shifting our perspective, developing the ability to view situations more objectively, and considering alternative viewpoints and interpretations.

  a Have participants identify a recent situation that triggered a problematic emotion, examine the evidence that supports or negates this thought, consider alternative explanations, and restructure a more balanced perspective. Guide them in reframing their thoughts about the problem.

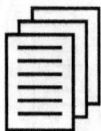

b The initial thought might be, "Everyone at work judges me and thinks I'm stupid." **The restructured thought might be, "**Even if some people might judge me, it does not define my worth. Most people focus more on themselves anyway and are not judging others."

6 **Self-Compassion:** Engaging in positive self-talk, encouraging oneself during difficult emotional experiences, and recognizing that emotional challenges are part of the human experience.

a **Gratitude Practice**: Guide the group through a brief gratitude exercise, having each person share one thing they are grateful for and how it makes them feel. Other exercises include keeping a journal of things they are thankful for, writing a letter to someone they are grateful for, and incorporating gratitude into mindfulness or meditation practice by focusing on things to be thankful for.

b **Cultivating Positive Emotion**: While working with difficult emotions is important, actively fostering positive emotions is equally crucial for emotional well-being.

i. Discuss the importance of intentionally cultivating positive emotions. Explore what this means to the group.

References

Brockman, R. N., Simpson, S., Hayes, C., van der Wijngaart, R., & Smout, M. (2023). In *Cambridge Guide to Schema* Therapy (pp. i–ii). half-title-page, Cambridge: Cambridge University Press.

Hayes, C. & Brockman, R. (2022). Healthy Adult Development. https://www.schematherapytrainingonline.com

Hayes, C. & Dominguez, S. (2023 personal communication). Modified Schema Healthy Adult/EMDR Resource Development and Installation Protocol. https://www.SchemaTherapyTraining.com

Linehan, M. (2014) personal communication. *DBT Skills Training Manual, Second Edition*. New York: Guilford Press.

Linehan, M. M. (2015). *DBT Skills Training Handouts and Worksheets, Second Edition*. New York: Guilford Press. https://www.dialecticalbehaviortherapy.com/emotion-regulation/

The Neurobiology of Trauma

Early childhood trauma has a profound impact on the brain's structure and function, nervous system regulation and integration, information processing, and memory. It leads to dysregulated emotions, stress responses, and compromised mental and physical health. This is the neurobiological basis for the diverse range of reactions observed in trauma survivors.

Goals

1 Recognize how brain structure and function changes after prolonged trauma disrupt nervous system regulation and integration.
2 Understand the three levels of nervous system development, information processing, and integration as conceptualized in the Triune Brain model.
3 Explain the concept of bottom-up hijacking and its relation to the nervous system's threat response (the Threat Detection System).
4 Understand how trauma disrupts memory, executive functioning, stress regulation, and social engagement.
5 Identify the role of the **Autonomic Nervous System (ANS)** (Sympathetic NS, Parasympathetic NS, and the Vagus Nerve [VN]) in regulating the unconscious neuroception of safety.

Procedure

1 Mindfulness Exercise: **Box Breathing**: Inhale for four seconds, hold the breath for seven seconds, and exhale for eight seconds. This rhythmic breathing pattern helps activate the VN and calm the autonomic nervous system.
2 Check-In.
3 Review the effects of trauma on nervous system regulation and functional integration *(Figure 6.1)*.
4 Discuss the **Threat Detection System** and **the Stress Response System**. These models provide a framework for understanding how the brain

DOI: 10.4324/9781003462958-17

disconnects and dysregulates in threatening situations. Review **Handout 6.1 Understanding Your Brain's Response to Trauma**, *Figure 6.2*.

5   Understanding the differences between implicit and explicit memory is crucial for trauma recovery. It is important to explore how implicit memory is stored in the body after trauma and why this is significant for trauma recovery.

6   Discuss the Polyvagal Theory and its pivotal role in the neuroception of safety and social engagement. Neuroception is the process by which the nervous system subconsciously detects and evaluates safety and danger. Use the Polyvagal Ladder graphic to illustrate the body's response to threat.

7   Discuss the relationship between Schema Modes and the three neural circuits described in the Polyvagal Theory *(Figure 6.3)*.

8   Discuss the role of neuroplasticity in healing from trauma.

9   Summarize the group's discussion about dysregulation of the nervous system, the role of innate defenses and coping modes, and the disruption and disconnection in social engagement due to trauma.

10   Check-out.

11   Grounding: **5-4-3-2-1**. Have the group engage their senses by identifying five things you can see, four things you can touch, three things you can hear, two things you can smell, and one thing you can taste. Engaging multiple senses anchors in the present moment and signals safety to the nervous system. It can help interrupt traumatic flashbacks or panic attacks by engaging the logical, "rational" side of your brain and reconnecting the mind and body to the present.

Main Themes

The Nervous System's Response to Threat

The Brain is an interconnected and adaptive system with a complex interplay between its neural networks. When detecting a threat, the brain activates protective mechanisms to defend against the imminent danger. The chronic activation of this threat response directly impacts the nervous system's structures and functions. Regulating emotions in response to stress and recalling specific memories is impaired as the medial prefrontal cortex (MPFC) (the thinking brain) and the hippocampus (explicit memory) are "hijacked." Trauma is remembered implicitly through body sensations stored in the instinctual and emotional parts of the brain. This affects the ability to regulate emotions in response to stress and to recall and consolidate memories. Social engagement and access to the safety of social support become disrupted.

Information Processing

In the 1960s, neuroscientist Paul D. MacLean introduced the model of the **Triune Brain** as a way to explain brain development, information processing, and nervous system integration (MacLean, 1990; Reiner, 1990). Although it has been criticized for its oversimplified and hierarchical approach, the model has helped explain how complex trauma can affect the flow of communication in the brain, defensive stress responses, the role of the amygdala in detecting threat (e.g., fight-flight-freeze), and the role of the prefrontal cortex in emotional regulation. The caution is to remember that current research emphasizes the brain's interconnected and adaptive nature and the complex interplay between different neural networks in trauma responses.

The **Triune Brain** Model differentiates three areas of information processing (sensorimotor, emotional, and cognitive). Brain development is organized from bottom to top, with the lower brainstem and midbrain regions developing first and then increasing in complexity as the midbrain limbic system and outer cortex develop. When we perceive a threat, the information flows from the bottom up.

- The **Instinctual Brain** is the oldest and most essential part of the brain, often called the "survival brain." Situated in the brainstem and basal ganglia, it manages vital functions like respiration, heart rate, digestion, and instinctual reactions to threats. It is concerned with sensory awareness and processing **sensorimotor information.** "Am I physically safe?"
- The **Emotional Brain** and the limbic system evolved in mammals to process emotions, memory, and stress regulation. It is essential for social behaviors, pleasure, and alerting to danger (the "smoke alarm"). This system is involved with the processing of **emotional information**. "Am I loved? Am I emotionally safe?"
- The **Thinking Brain,** or neocortex, is highly developed in humans. The cortex manages executive functions, abstract thinking, language, problem-solving, conscious awareness, and **cognitive processing of information**. It is vulnerable to going "offline" during trauma, challenging the integration of incoming data. "What can I learn from this?"

The brain has two hemispheres, right and left, connected by the corpus callosum, each with different functions. It operates as a connected and intricate system; both hemispheres must function well.

- The **Left Hemisphere** dominates language, logic, speech, and problem-solving and is critical for conscious functions and explicit tasks. Trauma may impair the capacity to think and speak, partly due to the shutdown of the area in the brain responsible for speech (Broca's Area).

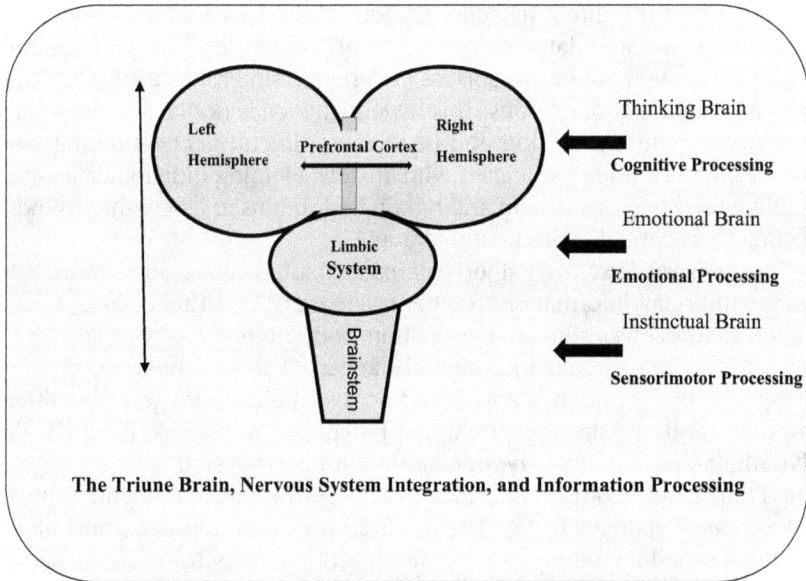

The Triune Brain, Nervous System Integration, and Information Processing

Figure 6.1 The Triune Brain, Nervous System Integration, and Information Processing (McClean, 1990)

- The **Right Hemisphere** is associated with spatial abilities, holistic thinking, creativity, emotional processing, nonverbal communication, emotions, recognizing facial expressions, and interpreting language tone. This hemisphere processes information unconsciously and implicitly.
- Information flows between the left and right cerebral hemispheres through the **Corpus Callosum**, a collection of nerve fibers that facilitate communication, coordination of functions, and sharing of sensory, motor, and cognitive information. Thinning of the corpus callosum after complex trauma disrupts the interconnection and communication between the two hemispheres.

The Threat Detection System

The "Threat Detection System" (Parasuraman & Galster, 2013; van der Kolk, 2014; Levy & Schiller, 2021) refers to a rapid alert system in the brain that identifies potential threats in the environment and instantly triggers the body's "fight or flight" response, even when no threat exists. The brain is constantly in a heightened state of vigilance as it scans for cues of past trauma. The thalamus, amygdala, hypothalamus, hippocampus, and MPFC are fundamental brain structures that activate the protective mechanisms involved in threat detection (Figure 6.2). The amygdala is the central component of the threat detection system, the "smoke alarm" alerting to danger. An overstimulated threat detection system leads to exaggerated responses to even minor stressors, as the brain misinterprets everyday situations as potentially dangerous. This hypervigilance is noticeable physically in increased muscle tension and heart rate, difficulty concentrating, and other symptoms often associated with anxiety. Helping individuals learn to regulate their nervous system and retrain their brains to assess threats more accurately is central when treating trauma.

The **Sensory Systems** gather external stimuli (e.g., sight, sound, and touch) and relay information to other brain areas. The **Thalamus** is a relay station that receives sensory information from the environment and alerts the different brain areas to potential danger ("I smell smoke now"). The **Amygdala** (the "smoke alarm") broadcasts THREAT, triggers the threat response, and initiates emotional and behavioral responses. It signals the **Hypothalamus** and the **Hypothalamic-Pituitary-Adrenal axis** to release stress hormones (Cortisol and Adrenaline). Cortisol and Adrenaline initiate a cascade of changes in heart rate, blood pressure, alertness, and blood flow that mobilize the organs and muscles of the body to respond quickly to stress. Prolonged trauma may cause heightened sensitivity of the Amygdala, intensified fear and anxiety, and chronic dysregulation of the body's stress response system (Thomas et al., 2023).

The **Hippocampus**, responsible for memory formation, storage, retrieval, and consolidation, also provides contextual information that helps the brain differentiate between safe and threatening stimuli. The MPFC is the "watchtower" that mediates abstract thought, planning, organization, and decision-making, regulates emotional responses and modulates activity that allows for the regulation of threat responses based on context and learning. Activation of the threat detection system results in bottom-up, emotional "hijacking" when instinctual reactions to perceived threats cause the Hippocampus and the MPFC to go "offline." The shutdown of these structures leaves unintegrated sensory elements set off by the amygdala to remain implicitly stored in the body without witnessing or processing what happened (van der Kolk, 2014; Teicher & Samson, 2016; Teicher et al., 2016).

Under normal circumstances, the **Parasympathetic** branch of the **ANS** helps the body return to a calm, resting state. Terrifying experiences and perceived threats change the brain by prolonging and disrupting the normal functioning of the stress response. The state of chronic hypervigilance interferes with a return to baseline and recovery. The failure to return to a baseline resting state can contribute to the development of psychosomatic disorders, sometimes without a clear medical cause. Coined "MUPS" or multiple unexplained physical symptoms, they are often manifested as chronic pain, headaches, gastrointestinal or autoimmune impairments, and chronic stress and anxiety.

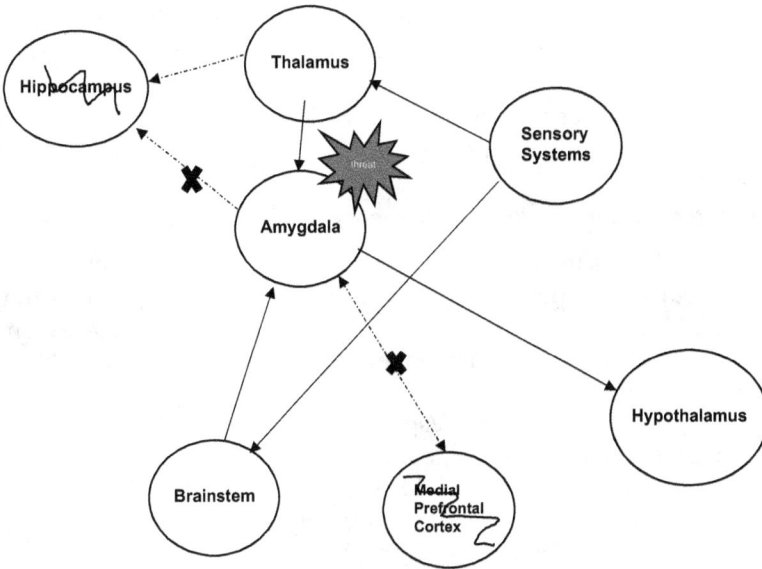

Figure 6.2 Brain Structures and Pathways Involved in Threat Detection (adapted from Parasuraman & Galster, 2013, van der Kolk, 2014; Levy & Schiller, 2021)

The Polyvagal Connection

The Polyvagal Theory describes how the different components of the **ANS, the Sympathetic Nervous System (SNS), the Parasympathetic Nervous System (PSNS), and the Vagal Nerve (VN)** are differentially involved in regulating the unconscious physiological and emotional responses that promote social engagement, restoration, and recovery (Porges, 2011; Porges & Dana, 2018). *Neuroception* is the process by which the nervous system subconsciously detects and evaluates environmental threats, safety, and danger. It is a primitive process that occurs in parts of the brain that evolved before conscious thought. The chronic neuroception of threat in unresolved trauma has a significant influence on shaping the responses of the ANS.

The VN is at the center of the Polyvagal Theory. The dorsal vagal branch of the VN mediates "rest and digest" bodily functions (breathing, digestion, and heart rate) as well as immobilization in the face of extreme life threats (a shutdown that conserves energy). In contrast, the ventral vagal branch promotes connection in social relationships when it neurocepts safety. Prolonged trauma and neurocepted threat create chronic disconnection by creating distance from the relationships and social connections that keep us safe.

A three-tiered model is captured in the image of the Polyvagal Ladder *(Figure 6.3)*. This model describes the movement away from safety and social engagement in the face of threat. We feel calm, relaxed, and socially connected when the ventral vagal branch of PSNS neurocepts safety.

Moving down the ladder, the SNS mobilizes the fight/flight/freeze survival defenses, increasing hyperarousal and hypervigilance when danger is neurocepted. If neither of those responses avails in the face of extreme life threats, the dorsal vagal branch of the PSNS leads to immobilization, dissociation, shutdown, and numbness.

Schema Modes and the Polyvagal Theory

Schema modes are the nervous system's attempt to cope with overwhelming experiences and perceived safety or threat. This corresponds with the Polyvagal Theory's emphasis on the ANS's role in regulating our responses to environmental cues. Schema modes can be conceptualized as different autonomic states that parallel the three neural circuits described in the theory *(Figure 6.3)*. The Ventral Vagal Complex or Social Engagement System is seen in interested, social, curious, connected, playful, compassionate, and happy modes (Happy Child/Healthy Adult modes). Schema modes involving mobilization, fight, or flight (Angry Protector or Overcompensator modes) correspond to the SNS. This may be seen as fighting to destroy or repel the threat (contemptuous, tactless, rageful, and explosive) or fleeing to

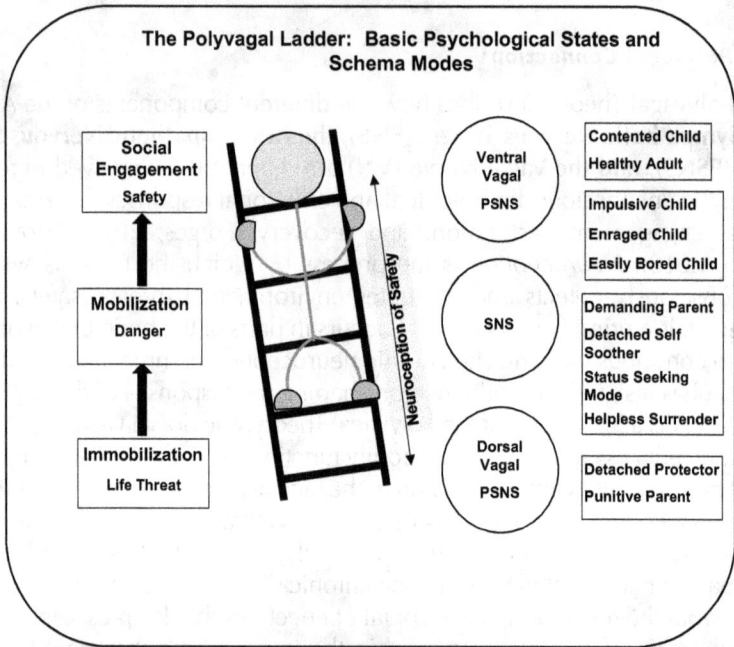

Figure 6.3 The Polyvagal Ladder: Basic Psychological States and Schema Modes (adapted from Dana, 2018; Karaosmanoğlu, et al., 2023)

stay entirely out of its way (reluctance, independence, and substance use). Other overcompensating modes (status-seeking, self-soothing, demanding, rude) are more socialized forms of attacking responses (staying beyond the threat's reach or intimidating and discouraging the danger). SNS frozen immobility and fawn may be compared to the Helpless Surrender and Compliant Surrender modes. Other Schema modes related to immobilization or disconnection (Detached Protector (dissociation), and Inner Critic modes) are associated with the shutdown of the Dorsal Vagal Complex that reflects surrender as a way to immobilize the individual without provoking the attacker (Karaosmanoğlu & Kose Karaca, 2020; Karaosmanoğlu et al., 2023). The philosophy of treatment for both Schema Therapy and Polyvagal Therapy is to help the individual move up the ladder from immobility (dorsal vagal activation/Surrender Modes) through mobility (sympathetic activation/SNS Helpless Surrender and Compliant Surrender modes, Angry Protector/Overcompensator Modes) to achieve a sustained social engagement state (ventral vagal activation/Healthy Adult/Happy Child modes).

Trauma's Impact

As noted, the thinking brain, executive functioning (MPFC), and explicit memory (Hippocampus) may be "hijacked" during trauma, leading to a shutdown of conscious functions or memory consolidation. Trauma is remembered implicitly through the body sensations stored in the instinctual and emotional parts of the brain (e.g., right, nonverbal hemisphere). Explicit memory of events is disrupted, impairing the integration of the experience. Communication across hemispheres is disrupted due to a thinning of the corpus callosum. The ability to consolidate memory, make meaning of the event, and develop a straightforward, coherent narrative—"this happened to me, and it happened in the past" is impaired.

Neuroplasticity—Rewiring the Brain

The brain's intricate, interconnected system can remarkably influence mental and physical health through communication between its two hemispheres, structures, and systems. The brain's resilience is the foundation for healing and recovery from trauma. Calming the dysregulated body, strengthening the ability to monitor sensations, resetting the stress response (bottom-up processing), and re-engaging the cortex and hippocampus (top-down processing) help the individual make meaning of their experience. While trauma can negatively impact brain development, the brain's ability to reorganize itself (neuroplasticity) is a central aspect of healing from trauma. Our neurons do not know "right" from "wrong." They follow the most frequented path, whether it is helpful or not, which can entrench anxious, obsessive, or depressive patterns and thoughts. Suppose adults frequently tell a child that they are stupid and will not amount to anything in life. In that case, a well-worn neural pathway develops, leading to persistent feelings of unworthiness and incompetence (e.g., defectiveness schema). Neuroplasticity explains how a trauma response becomes habitual and also provides a road map for bypassing a neural pathway that no longer serves us. When the child receives messages of support and encouragement, new neural pathways replace the old, outdated pathways in the brain (Hossain, 2022).

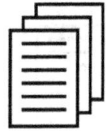

HANDOUT 6.1

Understanding Your Brain's Response to Trauma

1 Your Brain's Alarm System and Response to Stress

    a How does your body respond to stress? Mark which responses you commonly experience.

        ___ Heart racing
        ___ Difficulty breathing
        ___ Muscle tension
        ___ Sleep disruption
        ___ Digestive issues
        ___ Other: _____

    b Rate your physical responses: 1–5 (no noticeable change—extreme change in physical response).

        ___ Heart rate changes
        ___ Breathing changes
        ___ Muscle tension
        ___ Digestive issues

2 Understanding Your Nervous System States—Which state do you most commonly experience?

    a When I feel safe, I notice: (Social Engagement—e.g., able to connect with others, calm breathing, and feeling present).

        _____

    b When I feel threatened, I notice (Fight/flight—e.g., racing thoughts, fight/flight urges, and on guard).

        _____

    c When I feel overwhelmed, I notice: (Shutdown and immobilization—e.g., numbness, disconnected, and foggy).

        _____

3 Your Recovery Tools

    Body Scan

- Areas of tension: _____
- Areas that feel calm: _____
- Physical sensations: _____

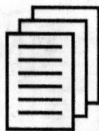

4 Building Safety

   a Identify your safety anchors. Why do they feel safe?

- Safeplaces: _____
- Safe people: _____
- Safe activities: _____

   b Identify activities that help you feel:

- Grounded: _____
- Connected: _____
- Safe: _____

References

Hossain, Y. (2022). *Trauma-Informed Toolkit: A Resource for Educators*. Oregon: Oregon State University.

Karaosmanoğlu, H. A., Ateş, N., & Köse Karaca, B., (2023). A new viewpoint to schema modes and mode domains through polyvagal theory: could schema modes be just a way of coping? *Current Psychology, 42*, 21119–21132. https://doi-org.proxy.libraries.rutgers.edu/10.1007/s12144-022-03176-x

Karaosmanoğlu, A., & Kose Karaca, B. (2020). Reviewing schema therapy concepts through the frame of polyvagal theory. *The Schema Therapy Bulletin*. Bad Vilbel, Germany: International Society of Schema Therapy, 21–29.

Levy, I. & Schiller, D. (2021). Neural computations of threat. *Trends in Cognitive Sciences, 2*(2), 151–171. https://doi.org/10.1016/j.tics.2020.11.007

MacLean, P. (1990). *The Triune Brain in Evolution: Role in Paleocerebral Functions*. New York, Plenum Press.

Parasuraman, R., & Galster, S. (2013). Sensing, assessing, and augmenting threat detection: behavioral, neuroimaging, and brain stimulation evidence for the critical role of attention. *Frontiers in Human Neuroscience, 7*, 273. https://doi.org/10.3389/fnhum.2013.00273

Porges, S. W. (2011). *The Polyvagal Theory: Neurophysiological Foundations of Emotions, Attachment, Communication, and Self-Regulation*. New York: W.W. Norton & Co.

Porges, S. W., & Dana, D. (Eds.). (2018). *Clinical Applications of the Polyvagal Theory: The Emergence of Polyvagal-Informed Therapies*. New York: W.W. Norton & Company.

Reiner, A. (1990). The Triune Brain in Evolution. Role in Paleocerebral Functions. Paul D. MacLean. Plenum. *Science, 250*(4978), 303–305.

Teicher, M. H., & Samson, J. A. (2016). Annual research review: enduring neurobiological effects of childhood abuse and neglect. *Journal of Child Psychology and Psychiatry, 57*(3), 241–266.

Teicher, M. H., Samson, J. A., Anderson, C. M., & Ohashi, K. (2016). The effects of childhood maltreatment on brain structure, function, and connectivity. *Nature Reviews Neuroscience, 17*, 652.

Thomas, M., Rakesh, D., Whittle, S., Sheridan, M., Upthegrove, R., & Cropley, V. (2023). The neural, stress hormone and inflammatory correlates of childhood deprivation and threat in psychosis: a systematic review. *Psychoneuroendocrinology, 157*, 106371 https://doi.org/10.1016/j.psyneuen.2023.106371

van der Kolk, B. A. (2014). *The Body Keeps the Score: Brain, Mind and Body in the Healing of Trauma*. New York: Viking Press.

Session 7

Trauma and the Body

When the "fight/flight/freeze/collapse/submit/attach" responses are activated, chronic emotional distress and nervous system dysregulation become embedded in the cellular memory and muscles of the body. When trauma is stored in the body, it is no longer safe. The unresolved trauma expressed somatically as persistent physical symptoms or sensations disrupts the ability to differentiate internal and external bodily states. Individuals become numb to and avoid their bodily sensations to control these experiences (van der Kolk, 2014). Health problems such as chronic pain or fatigue, headaches, and autoimmune, gastrointestinal, or cardiovascular issues frequently develop. Ogden and Fisher (2015) remind us that simply talking about trauma may not address the somatic sequelae of trauma. Our physical body holds the emotional pain resulting from past pain. To heal, the body must learn to live in the present (van der Kolk, 2014). Increasing awareness of the internal physical experiences and the unconscious, implicit memories stored in the body is the foundation for working through physical and emotional pain caused by trauma (Payne et al., 2015).

Goals

1 Increased understanding of the mind-body connection as reflected in the statement "the body keeps score" (van der Kolk, 2014).
2 Understand that physical responses to trauma are not abnormal but rather a natural part of the healing process. The body's reactions, such as chronic pain or fatigue, are its way of processing and coping with the trauma it has experienced.
3 Recognize that traumatic experiences held in the body are deeply embedded in the body's cellular memory, often manifesting as persistent physical symptoms or sensations.
4 Recognize the link between health problems such as chronic pain or fatigue, headaches, autoimmune gastrointestinal or cardiovascular

DOI: 10.4324/9781003462958-18

disorders, and persistent physical symptoms resulting from unresolved trauma.

5 Understand the importance of both top-down and bottom-up approaches in trauma treatment.
6 Understand the importance of embodiment and mindfulness to nervous system regulation and recovery from trauma.
7 Introduce body-focused approaches to help members develop a more integrated sense of self and improve emotional regulation as they process traumatic experiences somatically.

Procedure

1 Mindfulness Exercise: Mindful Awareness of Bodily Sensations or Body Scan. Examples and scripts abound on the internet (e.g. Jon Kabat Zinn mindfulness of other body sensations (Bodyscape) https://jonkabat-zinn.com/downloads/
2 Check-In.
3 Discuss how the statement "the body keeps score" relates to remembering trauma.
4 Explore how the defensive survival responses in the body contribute to dysregulated arousal, disruption of normal somatic functions, and disconnection from the body.
5 Discuss the differences between top-down vs. bottom-up approaches to treatment. How do body-focused interventions and mindfulness practices help regulate the nervous system and heal from trauma? Discuss potential triggers related to body awareness or touch.
6 Review **Handout 7.1 How Can I Learn to Live in My Body?** Ask clients to consider how they experience schema activation and traumatic memory in their bodies.
7 Practice **Exercise 7.1 Felt Sense Focusing**
8 Check-out.
9 Grounding Exercise: **Mountain Meditation** (use this exercise to counterbalance the Felt Sense Focusing Exercise if necessary. This exercise can be found in Chapter 6 Trauma, Mindfulness and the Health Adult).

Main Themes

Trauma Is Stored in the Body

"The body keeps score" (van der Kolk, 2014) is a concept that underscores how traumatic experiences are stored in the body when the nervous system's defensive responses (fight/flight/freeze or feigned death/collapse/

submit) are activated. The body's natural response to imminent threat is to enter an alert, hyperaroused state, ready to fight back or run away, or shut down into a hypoaroused state of immobilization, collapse, or surrender when it is impossible to escape. Freeze is an active defense state that combines a high level of distress with immobility (watchful alertness), while feigned death is a state of physical or mental collapse. These defenses allow assessment of the immediacy of the threat and prevent detection until an escape is possible. (Think of the deer in the headlights or a mouse that plays dead while caught in a cat's mouth). While these actions are natural survival mechanisms in the face of imminent threat, they become maladaptive as the body becomes stuck in chronic states of hyperarousal (e.g., anxiety, intrusive memories, anger, and irritability) and hypoarousal (e.g., dissociation, despair, hopelessness, and numbing) as it remembers past trauma even in the absence of immediate threat.

Body Memories

Traumatic memory manifests as physical symptoms or somatic sensations when survival actions get stuck in chronic dysregulation. These memories are encoded and stored in implicit memory as fragments of disconnected sensory and bodily experiences. These memories are not consciously recalled, like explicit memories of last night's dinner or your favorite teacher's name. Sensory experiences, smells, sounds, or physical sensations linked to traumatic experiences (e.g., the time of day or the smell of a particular aftershave) can trigger implicit memories held in the body. Sensitivity to body sensations is heightened, and tolerance for physical discomfort decreases.

Emotional distress and chronic dysregulation become ingrained in the body's visceral responses, posture, movement, emotions, and sensations. For example, a person's muscle patterns may become habitually contracted or tightened when they are chronically tense and ready to fight, leading to entrenched postural inflexibility and constriction of movement. They may unconsciously avoid physical contact and touch if reaching out has resulted in unpleasant consequences in the past (e.g., rejection, punishment, and abuse). They may unconsciously slump their shoulders forward and draw inward into a diminished, unassertive posture if standing tall drew unwanted attention, abuse, or shame.

Chronically elevated stress hormones (adrenaline and cortisol) contribute to the development of physical illness and health problems across core physiological systems (chronic pain, fatigue, headaches, and autoimmune, gastrointestinal, or cardiovascular illnesses). Multiple unexplained physical symptoms can persist for years, serving as a somatic expression of unresolved trauma.

In addition, trauma (especially that involving physical or sexual abuse or bodily harm) may lead to feelings of shame, disgust, or distrust toward one's own body. Some may feel that their body "betrayed" them, that it is unworthy or damaged. Body image issues, disordered eating, or self-harm behaviors may develop from distorted beliefs about the body ("I should not have experienced pleasure. I was not strong enough to resist"; "I was not pretty enough (or I was too pretty); I do not like to look nice; I feel uncomfortable when attention is paid to how I look"; "Being fat will make me feel less vulnerable," or "If I don't look like a woman, I will be safer"). Excessive focus on the body and health may lead to obsessions about germs and illness and fears of vulnerability to harm. Substance abuse, overeating, restriction, or excessive exercise may become coping modes that help avoid feelings of discomfort in the body.

Bottom-Up Approaches

Talking about and reflecting on the different aspects of one's trauma during traditional "top-down" talk therapy engages the "thinking brain" and provides meaning and context to the person's trauma narrative. Though necessary, talking about trauma alone does not sufficiently address the nonverbal, emotional, and body-based sequelae that result when the body's alarm system is chronically activated. It does not quiet the unconscious physiological responses that occur involuntarily when flooded with emotions. Bottom-up approaches (e.g., Somatosensory Psychotherapy, Somatic Experiencing, and Hakomi) make meaning of the implicit sensations or feelings in the body that are linked to memories of the trauma. Mindfulness and somatic approaches serve to widen the Window of Tolerance. Connection with the moment-to-moment bodily experience helps clients regulate their fluctuating emotions and tolerate discomfort better. (Ogden & Minton, 2000; Fisher & Ogden, 2009; Levine, 2010; Siegel, 2010; Winblad, et. al. 2018; Fisher, 2019);

Schema Therapy and Bottom-Up Interventions

Schema Therapy incorporates bottom-up strategies to address maladaptive schemas' physiological and emotional aspects. The strong emphasis on accessing and processing emotions aligns with the bottom-up approach of targeting the brain's limbic system and emotional centers. By focusing on emotional experiences, therapists help clients connect with their bodily sensations and feelings before engaging in cognitive restructuring. Limited reparenting taps into the client's nervous system responses and attachment-related issues. Imagery rescripting rewires physiologically based trauma responses by having clients vividly imagine and physically feel alternative, more nurturing scenarios. Body awareness exercises help clients notice their physical reactions associated with maladaptive schema activation (Young et al., 2003). For example, someone about to give a presentation in front of a large audience might notice butterflies in the stomach, a dry mouth and difficulty swallowing, a rapid heartbeat, shallow breathing, feeling flushed and sweating, or shaking. A schema such as approval seeking, defectiveness, or unrelenting standards may have triggered the body's stress response, leading to the physical reactions described above. Once the person is aware of this connection, they can use somatic resources to calm their body and regulate their threat detection system.

Mindfulness and Embodiment Interventions

Using body-focused and mindfulness resources in groups develops a sense of safety, stability, and a greater capacity for emotional regulation. The group space helps the members observe symptoms, tolerate their discomfort without becoming overwhelmed, and challenge the experiential avoidance that is a hallmark of Post Traumatic Stress Disorder (PTSD).

- **Embodiment** interventions are bottom-up approaches to treating trauma that orient the individual to spontaneous changes and shifts in moment-to-moment bodily responses, thoughts, and feelings. Connecting the conscious mind with bodily sensations helps integrate the body's communications (gestures, posture, facial expressions, eye gaze, affect, intrusive images, pain, smells, constriction, and numbing) with the meaning of the traumatic experience. (Fraleigh, 2015; Tempone-Wiltshire, 2024). Bodily and emotional shifts also occur when feelings of danger and helplessness are counteracted by the therapist's modulation of the sound of their voice, eye contact, rhythm and pace of their speech, and proximity to the client (Treleaven, 2018; Baldwin & Korn, 2021).
- **Grounding and Centering exercises** increase the ability to feel grounded in the body and anchored in the present moment. "Plant feet firmly on the ground." **Deep breathing exercises** connect breath patterns to emotional states and help regulate the nervous system. For example, group members can explore the relationship between their quickening breath and heart rate and the presence of a perceived threat. **Gentle, deliberate movements** such as stretching, yoga, mindful walking, shaking, or rocking motions incorporated into group activities can facilitate emotional release and reduce physical tension. **Guided rocking** is a vestibular, proprioceptive movement that involves swaying the body from side to side. This movement increases body awareness and fosters a sense of safety that can be helpful even during talk therapy. What does the client notice when rocking her

body? **Humming** for about five seconds in a low, deep tone, breathing, and humming again creates vibrations at the back of the throat. This type of movement and sound stimulates the ventral vagus nerve and helps calm the threat response.

- **Mindfulness** is considered a top-down and bottom-up intervention. Mindfulness of changes in body movements, sensations, feelings, and thoughts brings awareness to what is still held by the body. It is described as a present-centered and non-evaluative mode of awareness that interrupts ruminative thoughts that give rise to suffering (Chiesa et al., 2013). As awareness grows and the mind consciously regulates affective and sensory responses, clients gain an understanding of the relationship between their trauma and behavioral patterns, such as the need to sit near the door, face the room, experience anxiety when going home for a visit, or when good things happen.

  - **Mindful awareness of bodily sensations** can be integrated into the group process as group members are taught to track changes in heart rate, breathing, or muscle tension as they notice and describe the related physical sensations. **Mindful body scans, somatic journaling, and sound healing** encompass mindful attention, awareness of thoughts, and bodily attunement. They involve mapping body sensations in the present moment to understand their responses to specific environments and emotions. A prompt for journaling might be "When you think about the event, what do you feel in your body? Where do you feel it?" **Sound healing** (sound bowls and "sound baths") increases awareness of body-centered clues that indicate when trauma memories take over. They may help lessen tension, anxiety, fatigue, anger, and depressed mood. A sound bath is a full-body meditative experience where people lie down and listen to resonant sounds. Sound bowls 'bathe' people in their echoing sound. A prompt might be "How does it feel to be immersed in the sound bath? Where do you feel it most? How is sound impacting you in your body?" **Tracking felt bodily sensations, emotions, and thoughts** and completing "stuck" physiological responses can increase awareness and integration of the impact of unresolved trauma (Levine, 2008, 2010). Tracking felt sensations can help group members slow down as they become aware of how their nervous system reacts to interactions in the group ("Am I in 'survival brain' or 'ready-to-explore brain'?"). This can increase their capacity to tolerate increasingly intense experiences without dissociating, overriding, or relying on habitual patterns (Taylor & Saint-Laurent, 2017).

Monitoring Arousal with Titration and Pendulation

As trauma survivors begin to reconnect with their bodies within the group setting, safety, and choice are always prioritized. Before introducing body-focused interventions, clear guidelines should be discussed to ensure everyone feels secure and respected. Members can manage the pace of their healing by opting out of the exercises if necessary as they learn to respect their body's limits and boundaries. At the same time, they should be gently encouraged to tolerate some discomfort to widen their Window of Tolerance.

Somatic experiencing and body-based trauma processing can be gradually introduced to the group. Describing objects in the room using all five senses, mindful eating of a small snack, or texture-based grounding (e.g., holding smooth stones) are exercises that promote present-moment sensory awareness. **Titration,** limiting exposure to traumatic distress, can help participants process their experiences gradually and safely. In this way, the group can slowly build tolerance for distressing material when trauma-related content is introduced in small "doses" rather than all at once. The goal is to help the group maintain the "therapeutic window" – the zone between inadequate and overwhelming activation of trauma-related emotion during treatment. Frequent check-ins and gradual increases in sharing can help manage the group's intensity level. **Pendulation** alternates arousal triggered by recalled traumatic content with non-stressful topics, resource states, or activities that build coping skills, identify strengths, and promote resilience (Siegel, 2010). "Going in for a short time, then coming out" reduces emotional intensity over time and avoids overpowering the nervous system. For example, as the group tracks the physical sensations that arise during the group discussions, they can then be directed toward personal and shared resources (e.g., breathing, pacing, the supportive presence of others, and the safety of the room) to pendulate between states of arousal and calm. The group might practice a calming visualization (e.g., imagining a peaceful place) or group grounding exercise (e.g., feeling feet on the floor) before they are asked to recall a mildly activating situation or notice any areas of tension in their body. Their attention is then redirected to a neutral topic or pleasant body sensation (the breath, a safe space, or talking about the weather or plans for the day) until members can return to their therapeutic window. The group can be encouraged to notice how others' experiences might resonate in their bodies. The group's collective energy can become a resource as they learn to pendulate together like the ebb and flow of ocean waves.

EXERCISE 7.1

Felt Sense Focusing

(Adapted from Gendlin, 1996)

Focusing is a psychotherapeutic and self-help technique designed to help individuals access and work with their "felt sense" (the subtle, bodily awareness of an issue or situation that is not yet fully articulated) (Gendlin,1996). Simpson (2020) has adapted this Felt Sense Focusing practice to increase bodily awareness of the felt sense of the Vulnerable Child mode. The practice can foster a deeper connection between the bodily sensations and the conscious understanding of the mode.

The practice includes six steps

1 **Clearing a Space**, relaxing and paying attention to the body at the moment, and connecting with the Vulnerable child ("How am I feeling right now?"). Sensing whatever arises (the felt sense), noticing feelings and concerns that might arise without becoming attached to them.
2 **Getting a Felt Sense** means noting and accepting whatever felt sensations arise in the body. Different modes, thoughts, or perhaps particular bodily sensations compete for attention, and the felt sense may still be unclear. Many different sensations and implicit knowledge about unresolved issues can all be experienced together as they emerge naturally.
3 **Finding a Handle** acknowledges the felt sensation, even as its quality may remain unclear. The sensation is labeled, and the label becomes the handle. Finding the handle may mean playing with words (e.g., tight, sticky, scary, stuck, heavy, and jumpy), phrases, or images that emerge from the felt sense until something fits and feels 'just right' (e.g., "on edge" or "tightness").
4 **Resonance** entails moving back and forth between the "handle" and the felt sense until the handle accurately reflects the felt sense. For example, feeling 'jumpy' might mean "crawling out of my skin," or another feeling in the body might signal a better fit. This felt sense is one part of the whole, the Vulnerable Child (feeling) part.
5 **Asking questions** about the felt sense of the Vulnerable Child helps identify any obstacles or needs (What makes it challenging to stay with the sensation, or what is needed?). This can bring more awareness to any shifts, "give," or releases (e.g., less heaviness, tension-relaxing feeling, or a more general sense of lightness) in the body, the Vulnerable Child mode, and the felt sense.
6 **Receiving and experiencing** whatever comes up during the session with curiosity and nonjudgment allows a befriending of the sense of the Vulnerable Child felt in the body. The goal is to engage in experiencing the felt sense even if there is no immediate resolution to the issues or whether you believe or agree with what the felt sense is communicating (Simpson, 2020).

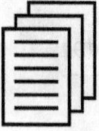

HANDOUT 7.1

How Can I Learn to Live in My Body?

Quietening the body will quiet the mind

Many people who have experienced early childhood trauma have an aversion to thinking about or experiencing their bodies as part of who they are. The body may have become their enemy, leading to disgust, shame, numbness, detachment, and disconnection. Pain, fatigue, and other somatic ailments may increase their awareness of how the body has "let them down." Nevertheless, the body is communicating something about how the trauma is remembered. Recognizing the mind/body connection can lead to more significant healing of the effects of trauma.

1 How does your body react when you experience intense emotions? Check off the ways you have noticed your body reacting.

__ Tensing muscles   __ Hot flashes

__ Racing heart   __ Rapid breathing

__ Difficulty catching your breath   __ Collapsed posture (slumping)

__ Increased pain   __ Uncomfortable feeling in your stomach

__ More frequent illness, reduced immunity   __ Increased energy

__ Calming   __ Warmth

__ Constriction in your throat   __ Sick feeling in your stomach

__ Nausea   __ Feeling frozen, unable to move.

__ Unable to talk   __ Feeling like you want to hide.

__ Butterflies in your stomach   __ Digestive ailments

__ Migraines   __ Inflammation

2 What experiences trigger these reactions in your body?

_____

_____

_____

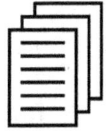

3 What is your body telling you? What are its messages?

_____

_____

_____

4 What calms your body?

_____

_____

_____

5 What helps you feel more connected to your body?

_____

_____

_____

6 Describe your bodily sensations and emotions when you sit slumped over, shoulders collapsed, and head hung. Compare this to sitting upright, shoulders back, head erect, and chest open. What do you notice? What is your body communicating in each position? Do you feel differently in the different postures?

_____

_____

_____

7 Hum for about five seconds in a low, deep tone from the back of your throat, breathe deeply, and repeat. What do you notice happening in your body?

_____

_____

_____

8 Sway back and forth, rocking your body gently. Combine this with breathing. Track the changes you notice in your body. What do you notice?

_____

_____

_____

9 Identify three strategies you can use to calm your body

a _____

b _____

c _____

References

Baldwin, M. & Korn, D. L. (2021). *Every Memory Deserves Respect: EMDR, the Proven Trauma Therapy with the Power to Heal*. New York: Workman Publishing, Hachette Book Group.

Chiesa, A., Serretti, A., & Jakobsen, J. C. (2013). Mindfulness: top-down or bottom-up emotion regulation strategy? *Clinical Psychology Review*, 33(1), 82–96. https://doi.org/10.1016/j.cpr.2012.10.006

Fisher, J. (2019). Sensorimotor psychotherapy in the treatment of trauma. *Practice Innovations*, 4(3), 156–165. https://doi.org/10.1037/pri0000096

Fisher, J., & Ogden, P. (2009). Sensorimotor psychotherapy. In C. A. Courtois & J. D. Ford (Eds.), *Treating Complex Traumatic Stress Disorders: An Evidence-Based Guide*. New York: Guilford Press, 312–328.

Fraleigh, S. (Ed.). (2015). *Moving Consciously: Somatic Transformations Through Dance, Yoga, And Touch*. Champaign, Illinois: University of Illinois Press. https://doi.org/10.5406/illinois/9780252039409.001.0001

Gendlin, E. T. (1996). *Focusing-Oriented Psychotherapy: A Manual of the Experiential Method*. New York: Guilford Publications.

Levine, P. A. (2010). *In An Unspoken Voice: How the Body Releases Trauma and Restores Goodness*. Berkley, CA: North Atlantic Books.

Levine, P. A. (2008). *Healing Trauma: A Pioneering Program for Restoring the Wisdom of Your Body*. Louisville, CO: Sounds True.

Ogden, P., & Fisher, J. (2015). *Sensorimotor psychotherapy: Interventions for trauma and attachment*. New York: W. W. Norton & Company.

Ogden, P., & Minton, K. (2000). Sensorimotor psychotherapy: one method for processing traumatic memory. *Traumatology*, 6(3), 149–173. https://doi.org/10.1177/153476560000600302

Payne, P., Levine, P. A., & Crane-Godreau, M. A. (2015). Somatic experiencing: using interoception and proprioception as core elements of trauma therapy. *Frontiers in Psychology*, 6, 93. https://doi.org/10.3389/fpsyg.2015.00093

Siegel, D. J. (2010). *The Mindful Therapist: A Clinician's Guide to Mindsight and Neural Integration*. New York: W. W. Norton & Company.

Simpson, S. (2020). Manual of group schema therapy for eating disorders. In Simpson, S. & Smith, E. (Eds.) *Schema Therapy for Eating Disorders: Theory and Practice for Individual and Group Settings*. P. 136–184. London: Routledge.

Taylor, P. J., & Saint-Laurent, R. (2017). Group psychotherapy informed by the principles of somatic experiencing: moving beyond trauma to embodied relationship. *International Journal of Group Psychotherapy*, 67(Suppl. 1), 171–181. https://doi.org/10.1080/00207284.2016.1218282

Tempone-Wiltshire, J. (2024). The role of mindfulness and embodiment in group-based trauma treatment. *Psychotherapy and Counselling Journal of Australia*, 12(1), 1–27. https://doi.org/10.59158/001c.94979

Treleaven, D. A. (2018). *Trauma-Sensitive Mindfulness: Practices for Safe and Transformative Healing*. New York: W. W. Norton & Company.

van der Kolk, B.A. (2014). *The Body Keeps Score: Brain, Mind, and Body in the Healing of Trauma*. New York: Viking Press.

Winblad, N. E., Changaris, M., & Stein, P. K. (2018). Effect of somatic experiencing resiliency-based trauma treatment training on quality of life and psychological health as potential markers of resilience in treating professionals. *Frontiers in Neuroscience*, 12, 70. https://doi.org/10.3389/fnins.2018.00070

Young, J. E., Klosko, J. S., & Weishaar, M. E. (2003). *Schema Therapy: A Practitioner's Guide*. New York: Guilford Press.

Session 8

Traumatic Memory

Overwhelming experiences profoundly shape the development of the brain, the mind, and body awareness, as well as how we remember these events. Our understanding of this process has been significantly advanced by research showing that traumatic memories are processed differently in the brain than regular memories. These studies have revealed that brain regions involved in memory do not activate in the same way when recalling traumatic experiences, indicating that traumatic memories may not be treated as typical memories by the brain (Barry et al., 2018).

> Albert described an inexplicable feeling of dread whenever he took a shower. Samantha experienced a sense of panic when she was near a swimming pool. Evie repeatedly became involved with partners who were not available to her. Anna experienced a great sense of calm when experiencing the smell of baking bread. These are all examples of implicit memories of abuse occurring in the shower or the swimming pool, unavailable partners reflecting the memory of an absent parent, or a sense of safety reminiscent of times spent with a beloved grandparent.

Goals

1 Understand how traumatic memory is encoded, stored, and retrieved differently than other memories.
2 Understand the impact of traumatic memories on current functioning.
3 Enhance control over and management of trauma-related memories.

Procedure

1 Mindfulness Exercise: **Exercise 8.1 Exploring a Raisin Mindfully**
2 Check-In.
3 Review the main points about traumatic memory. Discuss the differences between explicit and implicit memory. Explore how traumatic

DOI: 10.4324/9781003462958-19

memories show up as "body memories" or triggers. Discuss the state-ment: "Trauma memory is remembering by reliving."
4 Review the group's responses to **Handout 8.1, The Trauma Memory Questionnaire.**
5 Summarize group discussion.
6 Check-out.
7 Grounding Exercise: **Exercise 8.2 Stretching**

Main Themes

Memory is a complex process that involves encoding, storing, and retriev-ing past feelings, images, beliefs, and sensations. Memories are laid down in the brain implicitly and explicitly as the individual develops. **Implicit Memory** is the dominant form of memory in the early years of life. It is information that is remembered automatically and is resistant to forget-ting. It is encoded, stored, and retrieved through body sensations, move-ments, emotions, and perceptions. It involves skills, habits, and associative learning rather than verbal content (riding a bike, salivating when smell-ing food). **Explicit Memory** is information you must consciously work to remember (such as recalling items on your to-do list). The conscious recall of past events, facts, and experiences becomes available after 1½ years as the hippocampus develops. It is the basis for the verbal narrative that helps us develop a coherent sense of who we are across time. It is the memory of facts and general knowledge (semantic) and the memory of our his-tory and personal experiences (episodic). We know we are remembering something, such as when we recall the morning's breakfast or the name of a favorite childhood teacher.

Traumatic Memory—Remembering by Reliving

Trauma impacts both implicit and explicit memory systems. Some people may have detailed recollections of their trauma, while others may experi-ence fragmented memories, amnesia, or even complete repression of the event due to the mind's protective mechanisms.

> *Explicit memory is like looking into a room in daylight: you can look around confidently and see how one object or piece of furniture is arranged next to another. You can see how big the room is and what color the walls are and describe it to someone else. Implicit memory is like looking into a room through a keyhole or with a flashlight in the dark: you cannot see the whole room, just one disconnected part at a time, and it is hard to describe the room to anyone else*
>
> (Stern, in Hershler, et al., 2021, p. 45).

This analogy helps to illustrate the difference between explicit and implicit memory, with explicit memory providing a full, detailed view of the "room" and implicit memory offering only a fragmented, partial view.

Traumatized people remember both too much and too little. High arousal disconnects the memories from areas of the brain necessary for storing and integrating incoming information: the thalamus, the hippocampus, and the cortex. While narrative memory (the stories one tells about oneself) is adaptive, social, and purposefully integrated into the account of the person's experiences, traumatic experiences appear in fragmented sensory and emotional traces (images, sounds, and physical sensations) precipitated by specific triggers. The memories are held in the body without the words to explain them and appear as "body memories" or triggers—the urge to avoid distressing memories conflicts with the need to make sense of and remember what happened. To know, but not to know. While the urge to avoid distress is understandable and self-protective, it aggravates feelings of fear and anxiety (van der Kolk, 2014).

> Arlene, Jim, Michelle, and Barbara each shared their unique experiences with trauma triggers. Arlene described the days leading up to the anniversary of her abuse as filled with a sense of foreboding and doom. Jim reported feeling paralyzed by anxiety at dusk and during the early evening hours. Panic would engulf him, and he would turn to alcohol to quell his distress. Michelle's "skin would crawl," and her heart would start racing whenever she smelled a particular scent of aftershave. Barbara could not swallow gelatinous foods because they caused sudden nausea and disgust. These personal accounts shed light on the diverse ways trauma triggers can manifest, often below a level of conscious awareness or understanding.

Triggers are reminders of past traumatic experiences that are encoded by implicit memory and make it feel as if the trauma is being relived all over again. They can be anything that activates the memory of the event and results in intense, dysregulating, and disruptive emotional and physical reactions (people, places, sounds, smells, anniversaries, or even the time of day). Flashbacks, intrusive bodily sensations, and images of traumatic events that "seem to come out of the blue" are all elements of blocked explicit/enhanced implicit processing (Siegel, 2012).

When these memories are activated, a person often feels helpless, out of control, and retraumatized; those who experienced the traumatic event want to forget it, but the memories keep being forced into consciousness in the reliving of the experience. The reenactments of the trauma become frozen in time and are experienced as immediate life threats, as if they were happening *now*, in the present moment (van der Kolk, 2014, p. 180; Ogden et al., 2006). Disruptions in consolidating and retrieving traumatic memories can lead to emotional dysregulation, the persistence of fear-based traumatic memories, dissociation, and fragmentation of the self (Siegel, 2012).

Situations that lack context and do not seem to be connected to the trauma (birthdays, anniversaries, developmental milestones, or experiences) become linked to past events when they contain similarities to stimuli present during the earlier trauma (similar color, shape, smell, or body sensations) (Ehlers & Clark, 2000; Ehlers et al., 2010). Physical reactions are an expected part of the body's survival responses. These responses, often called "fight, flight, freeze, fawn," are automatic reactions the body initiates in response to a perceived threat. Symptoms such as increased heart rate, nausea, upset stomach, dizziness, trouble concentrating, or sweaty palms can be warning signs of a trigger. As in the earlier examples, a person may become anxious and hypervigilant after smelling a particular brand of aftershave without realizing that the smell triggered memories of the aftershave worn by an abuser, or they may become distressed as the anniversary of an event occurs.

The area of the brain supporting language capacities (Broca's area) impacts the inability to put the traumatic experience into words, "I can feel it in my gut but cannot find the words to describe it.". Frequently unable to speak about their experiences or construct a narrative, those who have experienced trauma are compelled to *(relive, reexperience and)* re-enact them, often remaining unaware of what their behavior is saying (Howell, 2006, pp. 56-57; van der Kolk, 2014; Levine, 2015).

Working with Traumatic Memory

Working with traumatic memory can often be quite activating and distressing as it triggers the implicit memories without a clear understanding of what is happening. The goal of memory work is not to reexperience the events or remember every detail of everything that happened but to identify and integrate the effects of these memories, understanding their impact on the person's well-being and current life (Ogden et al., 2006; Eftekhari, et al.,2006). Curiosity, patience, and a non-judgmental attitude can help reduce their impact. *The goal is not to eliminate all triggers but to react to them less.* (The next session will focus on identifying and managing triggers and intrusive phenomena).

Memory Reconsolidation

To heal, the split-off or dissociated elements of the implicit memories need to be integrated into the person's personal story, differentiating memories of the past from present-day experiences. Once the story is told, it changes;

when the memories are retrieved, they are stored with modifications—the act of telling changes the tale. As the mind makes sense of what it knows, it changes how and what is remembered. The meaning changes to what happened then is not happening now (van der Kolk, 2014). Traumatic memory is modified and reconsolidated through a memory reconsolidation process that alters its narrative. Reconsolidation includes recalling parts of a memory, identifying the associated negative beliefs and the current desired beliefs, creating new meaning that reflects the desired beliefs, and integrating the new meaning into the memory. Sue describes the transformation that occurred when she was able to visualize her younger self (neglected child) differently:

> When I looked back on myself as a child, all I saw was a disgusting, dirty, pitiful child. During therapy, I was able to visualize my younger self differently. I saw a child who had been neglected by those who were supposed to care for her. She was dirty and unkempt through no fault of her own. I imagined her being cared for how she needed (bathing her, combing her hair, and dressing her in clean clothes). I could see how delightful she was when she was taken care of. I never again envisioned my vulnerable child as a dirty, pitiful part of myself.

The negative image of the child as disgusting, defective, or unlovable was reconsolidated into a new memory.

Memory reconsolidation is a promising technique for processing traumatic memory (Armstrong, 2019), but its use in group settings is still developing. This intervention is not suggested for use in the group and is included here for informational purposes only.

Traumatic Memory and the Group

The impact of traumatic memory can be addressed in a group without directly processing individual memories that may overwhelm or re-traumatize its members (Clifford, et. al., 2018). Other components of PTSD, including loss, grief, sadness, inability to experience pleasure, anger and rage, and feelings of shame, can be addressed. Group members can learn to recognize specific situations that trigger intrusive memories. Mindful awareness of the present-day reactions indicating implicit memories helps develop resources to create a different experience (Stedman, et al., 2007). The **Trauma Memory Questionnaire** (TMQ) can help group members identify the various ways trauma has impacted them (re-experiencing, avoidance, mood changes, and hyperarousal) while maintaining the focus on coping with current symptoms rather than recalling details of past events.

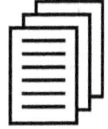

Trauma Memory Questionnaire

This questionnaire explores the current impact of early childhood trauma. It has been designed to help you understand various aspects of your traumatic memories, including re-experiencing symptoms, memory clarity issues, emotional impacts, integration difficulties, and coping mechanisms. It is not a diagnostic tool. It can serve as a starting point for discussions about managing traumatic memories. Please answer each question as honestly as possible. You may skip any questions you do not wish to answer.

Instructions: Please answer the following questions about your traumatic memories. For each item, indicate how much you agree or disagree using the scale: 0 (Not at all), 1 (A little), 2 (Moderately), 3 (Quite a bit), and 4 (Extremely).

1 Re-experiencing

___ I have unwanted memories or thoughts related to my past trauma
___ I experience flashbacks, feeling as if the traumatic event is happening again in the present.
___ My traumatic memories feel more intense than other memories.
___ I recognize when specific triggers (e.g., sounds and smells) suddenly bring back traumatic memories.

2 Memory Clarity

___ My memories of the traumatic event are fragmented or incomplete.
___ My memories of the traumatic event are vivid and clear.
___ I have difficulty recalling important aspects of the traumatic event.
___ The timeline of the traumatic event is unclear in my memory.
___ My traumatic memories sometimes feel disconnected from reality.

3 Emotional Impact

___ Remembering the traumatic event causes me significant emotional distress.
___ I experience physical reactions (e.g., sweating and heart racing) when I am triggered and remember the trauma.
___ I avoid thinking about or remembering the traumatic event.

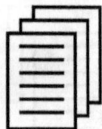

___ I avoid certain places, people, or activities to prevent these memories.

___ My traumatic memories interfere with my daily life and functioning.

4 Memory Integration

___ I have difficulty integrating my traumatic memories with my other life experiences.

___ My traumatic memories feel separate from my everyday autobiographical memories.

___ I struggle to make sense of my traumatic memories in the context of my life story.

___ My traumatic memories have changed how I view myself and the world.

5 Coping and Resilience

___ I have found ways to cope with intrusive traumatic memories.

___ I use different resources to manage difficult memories or emotions (e.g., tracking thoughts, feelings, and sensations to limit automatic reactions, mindfulness, grounding/reorienting exercises, imagery, and somatic resources).

___ I can talk about my traumatic memories without becoming overwhelmed.

___ I understand that my traumatic memories are a normal response to an abnormal event.

___ I believe I can heal and grow despite my traumatic memories.

Scoring: Calculate the sum for each section (Re-experiencing, Memory Clarity, Emotional Impact, Memory Integration, Coping, and Resilience) separately. Higher scores in the first four sections indicate more significant issues with traumatic memories, while higher scores in the Coping and Resilience section suggest better adaptation.

EXERCISE 8.1

Exploring a Raisin Mindfully

This exercise can help improve overall cognitive function, including attention, working memory, and long-term memory formation. It helps enhance episodic memory by promoting focused attention. Strong, detailed memories can be better encoded by paying close attention to sensory details and focusing on a single object, which helps calm the mind and improve recall.

1 Distribute a few raisins (or any small food item with an interesting texture) to each group member.
2 Ask them to imagine that they've never seen a raisin before.
3 Before eating the raisin, ask them to focus on it as they observe what it looks like, how it feels in their hand, how it feels to touch it, and what it smells like.
4 Next, ask them to observe what happens when they place the raisin in their mouth. What does the mouth do to receive the raisin? Do they salivate more? What does it feel/taste like when they chew it? What does it feel like to swallow the raisin?
5 Debrief.

EXERCISE 8.2

Stretching

Simple stretching exercises help group members reconnect with their bodies and the present moment. Physical grounding promotes body awareness and reduces physical tension. The body's relaxation response activates as attention moves from anxious thoughts to physical sensations. Encourage the members to move slowly and mindfully, focusing on their breath and physical sensations as they notice how their body feels before and after each stretch. Emphasize that they should avoid any pain while stretching. Stretches can also be "passed" as each member models one stretch for the group to practice.

1 **Seated Neck and Shoulder Stretch**: Guide the group members gently tilt their head to one side, bringing the ear toward the shoulder and holding the stretch for 10–15 seconds before switching to the other side. Finish by rolling their shoulders forward and backward in slow, deliberate circles.
2 **Standing Forward Bend:** Members stand with feet hip-width apart and slowly bend forward from the hips, letting arms hang down. They hold the stretch for 15–30 seconds while focusing on the stretch in the back of the legs before slowly rolling up vertebra by vertebra to standing.
3 **Gentle Spinal Twist:** Members sit sideways with both hands on the back of the chair as they gently twist toward the back of the chair. After 10–15 seconds, they switch to the other side.
4 **Mountain Pose with Arm Raises:** Standing with feet together, members slowly raise their arms overhead while inhaling, then lower them back down while exhaling. This can be repeated 5–10 times while focusing on the breath and the movements.

References

Armstrong, C. (2019). *Rethinking Trauma Treatment: Attachment, Memory Reconsolidation and Resilience*. New York: W.W. Norton & Co.

Barry, T. J., Lenaert, B., Hermans, D., Raes, F., & Griffith, J. W. (2018). Meta-analysis of the association between autobiographical memory specificity and exposure to trauma. *Journal of Traumatic Stress*, 31(1), 35–46. Https://Blueknot.Org. Au/Resources/Blue-Knot-Publications/The-Truth-of-Memory-and-the-Memory of-Truth-Different-Types-of-Memory-and Significance-of-Trauma.

Clifford, G., Meiser-Stedman, R., Johnson, R. D., Hitchcock, C., & Dalgleish, T. (2018). Developing an emotion- and memory-processing group intervention for PTSD with complex features: a group case series with survivors of repeated interpersonal trauma. *European Journal of Psychotraumatology*, 9(1), 1495980. https://doi.org/10.1080/20008198.2018.1495980

Eftekhari, A., Stines, L. R., Zoellner, L. A. (2006). Do you need to talk about it? Prolonged exposure for the treatment of chronic PTSD. *The Behavior Analyst Today*, 7(1), 70–83.

Ehlers, A., & Clark, D. M. (2000). A cognitive model of posttraumatic stress disorder. *Behavior Research and Therapy*, 38(4), 319–345.

Ehlers, A., Clark, D. M., Grey, N., Liness, S., Wild, J., Manley, J., Waddington, L., & Mcmanus, F. (2010). Intensive cognitive therapy for PTSD: a feasibility study. *Behavioral and Cognitive Psychotherapy*, 38, 383–398. https://doi.org/10.1017/S1352465810000214

Hershler, A., Huges, L., Nguyen, P., & Wall, S. (2021). *Looking at Trauma: A Tool Kit for Clinicians*. Pittsburgh, PA: Penn State University Press.

Howell, E. (2006). *The Dissociative Mind*. London: Routledge.

Levine, P. (2015). *Trauma & Memory*. Berkley, CA: North Atlantic Books. Penguin Random House.

Meiser-Stedman, R., Smith, P., Yule, W. & Dalgleish, T. (2007). The trauma memory quality questionnaire: preliminary development and validation of a measure of trauma memory characteristics for children and adolescents. *Memory*, 15(3), 271279.

Ogden, P., Minton, K., Pain, C. (2006). *Trauma and the Body: A Sensorimotor Approach to Psychotherapy (Norton Series on Interpersonal Neurobiology)*. United Kingdom: W. W. Norton.

Siegel, D. J. (2012). Pocket Guide to Interpersonal Neurobiology: An Integrative Handbook of the Mind. United Kingdom: W. W. Norton.

Stern, E. (2021). How trauma impacts memory. In Hershler, A., Hughes, L., Nguyen, P., Wall, S., (Eds.) *Looking at Trauma*. University Park, PA: University of Pittsburgh Press, 44-48.

van der Kolk, B. A. (2014). *The Body Keeps Score: Brain, Mind, and Body in Healing Trauma*. New York: Viking Press.

Session 9

Intrusive Symptoms of PTSD

Flashbacks, Nightmares, and Intrusive Memories

Intrusive memories are when I remember a small part of my trauma and then am unable to think of anything else while it loops over and over. They do not stop without much long, focused effort or worsen into flashbacks. They are different from flashbacks because there are no sensory symptoms and are always obviously just memories, not something that seems to be happening right now.

A flashback is when a part or all of me thinks and feels like my trauma is happening for the first time. I cannot remember. It is just a memory. I see it. I can turn around, look, and move; it appears, sounds, tastes, smells, and feels like that memory is happening. I can feel the pain, numbness, terror, or whatever of that memory as if it were happening right now. It is so intensely real that afterward, I still impulsively check to see if my body is intact and if nothing has been broken. Lately, I might know that what my senses are experiencing is not accurate. I might be able to move away from the experience, so it is almost an opaque overlay. However, that is a good day.

Nightmares are so bad. It is like a flashback; it feels like it is happening for the first time but a hundred times worse. The experiences in the nightmares are much more terrifying and painful than they even seemed in real life the first time. The memory track tends to last longer than in a flashback, too. Eventually, I wake up, but it is almost always a transition into flashbacks. By the time I am aware of where and when I am for real and that what just happened did not happen, I still cannot move, breathe, or think clearly. The fear and pain remain for a while, taking minutes to hours to fade. Nightmares are intense. And they are a humiliating mess to recover from. Nightmares are traumatizing in their own right. They are often the same half dozen memories over and over and over.

(Abby, 2023)

Flashbacks, nightmares, and intrusive memories are intense and disruptive emotional and physical reactions that are a normal part of the trauma

DOI: 10.4324/9781003462958-20

recovery process but also can leave people feeling helpless and out of control. Intrusive memories are characterized as looping recollections without active sensory components, while flashbacks involve complete sensory immersion that feels like reliving the trauma. Nightmares are intensified versions of flashbacks that often transition into waking ones. Avoiding reminders of the trauma is a defense against the emotional upset, but it also limits and constricts living life fully. Individuals can regain control over their reactions and engage more thoroughly when facing situations that might otherwise be avoided. The frequency and intensity of the distressing experiences decrease as a person differentiates the traumatic past from the present experiences. With its understanding and supportive environment, the group plays a crucial role in normalizing these reactions and helping members learn to cope with these dysregulating phenomena.

Goals

1 Increase awareness of triggers and intrusive phenomena.
2 Reduce the impact of and reactivity to triggering stimuli, as well as the frequency and intensity of flashbacks, nightmares, and intrusive memories.
3 Improve participants' ability to manage and cope with the short and long-term effects of intrusive symptoms by developing skills in the short and long term when faced with triggering situations and difficult emotions. These coping strategies can significantly reduce intrusive symptoms' impact when practiced consistently.

Procedure

1 Mindfulness: Suggested Meditation: **A Guided Meditation to Label Difficult Emotions** (Germer, 2019). (https://www.mindful. org/a-guided-meditation-to-label-difficult-emotions/; Neff & Germer, 2018). This practice is a proactive approach to help group members stay present and manage intrusive trauma-related experiences. By learning to label and acknowledge difficult emotions, they can begin to take control of their reactions and reduce the impact of intrusive symptoms.
2 Check-In.
3 Discuss critical points about identifying triggers and differentiating flashbacks, nightmares, and intrusive memories.
4 Explore how these intrusive phenomena represent activated schema and associated coping modes.

5 Have group members complete part 1 of **Handout 9.1, Take Charge of Your Triggers: Identifying Triggers**. How do triggers and intrusive symptoms disrupt their normal functioning and disrupt the ability to regulate emotions?

6 Review short-term and long-term strategies for managing triggers and intrusive symptoms **(Handout 9.1 Take Charge of your Triggers: Managing Triggers; Handout 9.2 Managing Intrusive Symptoms)**. How can mindfulness change the experience of the intrusive phenomena? How can engaging the Healthy Adult mode (HA) help manage these symptoms?

7 Practice a rescripting exercise with the group. This exercise involves revisiting mildly traumatic material and 'rescripting' it by imagining a different, more positive outcome. By doing so, participants can change how their brain stores and recalls the memory, reducing its intrusive impact on their daily lives.

8 Summarize the main takeaways from the group discussion and debrief the group exercise.

9 Check-out

10 Grounding **Exercise 9.1 Sensory Awareness.**

Main Themes

Intrusive symptoms are continuous reminders of the past that may stem from the brain's difficulty processing and storing unresolved traumatic memories. They can be triggered by external cues (e.g., sounds, smells, sights, time of day), internal sensations, or body memories (e.g., rapid heartbeat, feelings of foreboding, 'gut' feelings, and body postures that remind the individual of the trauma). Identifying, anticipating, and managing triggers helps reduce their destabilizing impact (Iyadurai, et al., 2018). (Triggers can also elicit pleasant emotions that help reorient and ground in present-day positive experiences. The smell of baking brownies, the surf at the beach, or snuggling in a blanket knitted by a beloved grandparent are all enjoyable experiences that can bring feelings of warmth, calm, and contentment).

Flashbacks

Flashbacks are sudden and vivid re-experiences of past trauma that overwhelms the individual's ability to differentiate past from present as they feel like they are happening now. Avoidance might be a temporary safety solution, but it is necessary to face the flashbacks to heal from trauma. *When a group member is experiencing a flashback, the therapist's role is to help manage the moment and help ground the person in the present. The trauma is not explored during a flashback.

Nightmares

Nightmares are disturbing and vivid dreams laced with fear, panic, and physiological arousal that cause emotional dysregulation and disrupt sleep and daytime functioning. Considered a learned sleep disorder, nightmares may help individuals remember essential details for survival or processing trauma. When nightmares become chronic, they can take on a life of their own, however, maintaining dysfunctional beliefs underlying schema activation.

Schemas, Schema Modes, and Intrusive Symptoms

Schema Therapy offers several practical techniques for treating intrusive symptoms, triggers, nightmares, and flashbacks associated with trauma and PTSD. This approach addresses the underlying schemas and emotional patterns contributing to these distressing experiences.

Intrusive trauma symptoms can be understood as activations of trauma-related schemas that often correspond to specific schema modes (the moment-to-moment emotional states) triggered by situations that remind the individual of past trauma. The emotionally charged intrusions evoke fear and cause extreme distress, with symptoms ranging from hyperarousal (e.g., agitation, anxiety, and panic) to hypoarousal (e.g., dissociation and numbing of affect). This can lead to flashbacks, nightmares, intrusive memories, and further avoidance that constrict and disrupt daily life by interfering with sleep, concentration, and relationships.

Nightmares and flashbacks often represent the activation of child modes or vulnerable emotional states related to unmet core emotional needs. For instance, a 'Vulnerable Child' mode might be associated with feelings of helplessness during a flashback. These symptoms link to maladaptive coping styles: avoidant coping strategies may manage intrusive symptoms in the short term. However, they can also reinforce the schemas and maintain the symptoms in the long term. Immediate and long-term strategies can help manage acute reactions and long-term patterns. Identifying and working with the different schema modes activated during flashbacks or nightmares helps patients manage these experiences more effectively. Some individuals might overcompensate by becoming hypervigilant or engaging in risk-taking behaviors as a way to cope with intrusive memories, while others may avoid them through dissociation.

Immediate responses utilize resources to calm the nervous system (controlled breathing), distance from the triggering experience (moving away, distraction, mindfulness), and reduce the intensity of the response (grounding/reorienting exercises). Long-term strategies help anticipate personal triggers, link them to past trauma, and reconstruct their meaning as they increase control over automatic reactions and buffer against the effects of triggers. Maladaptive thoughts and beliefs associated with intrusive symptoms are challenged and reframed: What negative schemas fuel the intrusive thoughts and flashbacks? Experiential exercises help change the power of the distressing experience. Imagery rescripting reduces the emotional impact of flashbacks and nightmares as the person revisits and modifies the distressing material. Chairwork helps confront and process different aspects of the trauma. Identifying and challenging the "schema modes" or emotional states activated during intrusive experiences can help the client develop more adaptive responses. Making sense of the intrusive symptoms within the context of the client's life experiences can help them process traumatic material in a way that reduces their intrusive nature. Strengthening the HA mode is a central focus of treatment to improve the management and integration of these experiences. Gradual exposure in a controlled environment and using grounding to manage the dysregulated responses reduce the impact of triggers.

Imagery Rehearsal Therapy

Imagery Rehearsal Therapy (IRT) (imagery rescripting) is a strategy for changing the repetitive nightmare script and challenging the maladaptive beliefs. Imagery is used to reduce nightmare distress and frequency. IRT allows patients to revisit and modify the distressing material, reducing the emotional impact of flashbacks and nightmares.

The person experiencing the intrusive symptoms can gain control over their experience as they create, imagine, and rehearse a new ending for the nightmare multiple times throughout the day (Krakow & Zadra, 2010). IRT helps bridge daytime and nighttime imagery, with patients practicing pleasant imagery to counter disturbing images. In the rescripting phase, patients select an alarming dream, change it as they wish, and rehearse the new dream daily. This process is repeated, with patients choosing new dreams to rescript every few days to a week. The focus is on promoting positive practice and using imagery to master harmful dream elements (Ellis, 2023). Practicing rescripting, especially during non-triggering times, improves the management of nightmares. Rescripting reduces fear by providing distance from the frightening dream and increasing a sense of control.

The group plays a crucial role in helping identify and address triggering situations as they arise during the group session. Their guidance and support ensure that individuals feel supported in managing their distress as they learn to anticipate triggering situations. Rescripting can be taught to the group and practiced at home. Homework assignments involving daily mental rehearsal of rescripted nightmares help reduce their frequency and intensity. Group members can also practice within the group. Participants select a recurring nightmare or flashback to work on and write down the details of their chosen nightmare or flashback. Using imagery techniques, each person mentally transforms the distressing elements into less threatening or positive images. The group members then take turns sharing their rescripted scenarios and brainstorming alternative scripts. Each participant can reflect on how they might adapt this script to the intrusive phenomena they experience. Participants are instructed to mentally rehearse their rescripted nightmare or flashback for 10–20 minutes daily, preferably before sleep. They keep a log of nightmare frequency and intensity to track progress.

Coping modes can be challenged with mindfulness exercises that encourage engagement with present-moment experiences rather than avoiding trauma-related thoughts and feelings. Promoting a balanced awareness of one's surroundings and internal states can help counteract modes that might manifest as excessive daydreaming or hypervigilance. Grounding techniques (see attached exercise) can help individuals who might surrender to feelings of helplessness in the face of intrusive memories or flashbacks. Regular mindfulness practices can strengthen the HA by developing skills in emotional regulation, present-moment awareness, and self-soothing that help interrupt patterns of repetitive, intrusive thoughts that often accompany PTSD symptoms (Edwards, 2022).

Janey became quite distressed, agitated, anxious, and tearful when the group spoke about their relationships with their parents. She became confused, not understanding the source of her distress. The group helped Janey identify the situation as a memory of past neglect and feelings of abandonment linked to her early childhood experiences. They emphasized that her reactions were related to past experiences and not what was happening in the present. They empathically acknowledged Janey's feelings and reminded her she was no longer alone. The group's understanding and support allowed Janey to explore how memories of abandonment, isolation, and helplessness were triggered during the discussion, reminding her of her absent and neglectful mother. The group leaders simultaneously monitored other members' reactions (e.g., overt agitation or dissociation) to this common and distressing theme. They encouraged the group to join an activity that helped them refocus on the present (e.g., deep breathing, awareness of bodily reactions, grounding in the body, and reorienting to the therapy room). Exploring ways to manage triggers during difficult group discussions distanced Janey from the intrusive in-the-moment experiences. The group returned to the discussion of family dynamics in a titrated, paced manner that allowed all the participants to engage within their Window of Tolerance.

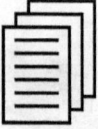

HANDOUT 9.1

Take Charge of Your Triggers

Identifying Triggers

Can you think of a time when you experienced a strong reaction or trauma-related symptom, such as feeling disconnected from your body, anxiety or panic, sudden nausea, or intrusive thoughts or feelings?

1 Where were you when you experienced this reaction? _____
_____
_____

2 When did it happen (time of day, year)? _____
_____
_____

3 Were you alone or with someone else? _____
_____

4 What did you hear? See? Smell? How were you feeling emotionally? What physical sensations did you experience? _____
_____
_____

5 Were your survival actions activated (fight/flight/freeze/submit/attach)? What happened? _____
_____
_____

6 Was it difficult to control or step back from your reactions? _____
_____
_____

7 Was your reaction "bigger" or more intense than warranted by the situation? Explain. _____
_____

8 Can you link these reactions to any past experiences? _____
_____
_____

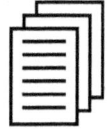

Managing Your Triggers

Managing triggers can feel overwhelming at times. Curiosity, patience, and a non-judgmental attitude can help reduce their impact. *The goal is not to eliminate all triggers but to react to them less.*

1 Anticipate triggering situations. Notice and observe any sudden shifts in your mood, increase in the intensity of emotions, or intrusive symptoms (thoughts, feelings, body sensations, and actions). Is your response more intense than is warranted by the situation? Are your survival actions activated (fight/flight/freeze/submit/attach)?
2 Patterns may emerge that help you identify specific triggers. Write down your thoughts, feelings, and physical reactions when you experience an intense emotional reaction. Pay attention to your surroundings, including sights, sounds, and smells, noting the date, time, and location.
3 Understand the origin of these triggers. Can you link these reactions to any past experiences? Differentiate the past experiences from the present situation.
4 Distance from the triggering situation to reduce the intensity of the emotional response. Give yourself time to reframe negative thoughts into more balanced perspectives.
5 Develop a coping plan to counterbalance the destabilizing reactions— list the skills you can use to challenge intense reactivity and buffer against long-term effects.
6 Practice skills to decrease reactivity, avoid being pulled back into memories, and calm an aroused nervous system. These include distancing and defusing triggering situations, controlled breathing, grounding, mindfulness, safe place imagery, developing supportive relationships, and regular self-care.

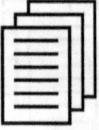

HANDOUT 9.2

Managing Intrusive Symptoms

Avoiding or pushing away a flashback or a nightmare might seem helpful initially, but it leads to more problems over time, increasing the intensity and frequency of the intrusive material. It is like putting unpaid bills in a drawer – it might seem helpful at first, but it leads to more problems over time. Imagine getting a credit card bill, saying, "I cannot afford this," and then putting it away without dealing with it. More bills come, and the situation worsens (Lloyd, 2023).

1 Create a feeling of safety in the present moment to counteract being pulled into the past.
2 Use imagery rescripting, mindfulness, and grounding to help quiet the body when overwhelming circumstances leave you feeling helpless and out of control.
3 *Orient to the present moment.* Mindfulness helps us refocus on the present, reminding us that intrusion is a memory that is not happening now. A grounding phrase or mantra helps make these intrusive experiences more manageable (e.g., "I know what I am experiencing is not accurate. I can feel my feet on the ground. I know this is not happening to me now"). Note that the date, time, and location can anchor the present.
4 Create a sense of safety in the mind and body to reduce the activation of negative thoughts and emotional stress.
5 *Practice grounding and calming activities* such as safe place imagery, safety bubble, relaxation, deep breathing, distancing, or distraction to shift these sensations. These techniques help maintain a here-and-now, reality-based orientation when intrusive symptoms occur. Engaging all five senses is an effective grounding technique. Other examples include sipping a warm or cold drink, smelling a strong scent such as lavender, unwrapping and sucking on a peppermint candy.
6 *Identify and label the emotions associated with the intrusive symptoms.* Notice the sensory cues and physical sensations accompanying the intrusive experiences (e.g., rapid heartbeats, shallow breathing, and body tension). What mode are you in when these intrusions occur? What does it feel like in your body?
7 Engage the Healthy Adult to soothe and nurture the vulnerable parts of you. Challenge the inner critic modes' critical messages of guilt, self-blame, and shame.

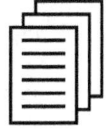

8 *Imagine* a safe place with as much sensory detail as possible (light, color, texture, scents, and images), helpful when internal or external experiences are overwhelming. Visualization of successful navigation out of a distressing situation restores a feeling of control and creates distance from the intrusive experience.

9 *Practice Imagery Rescripting* when confronting nightmares. It changes the repetitive nightmare script, challenges maladaptive beliefs, and reduces nightmare distress and frequency. Create, imagine, and rehearse a new ending for the nightmare multiple times throughout the day (Krakow & Zadra, 2010). Pleasant imagery and visualization help master harmful dream elements and counter the disturbing images from the nightmare. (Ellis, 2023). In the rescripting phase, select a frequent nightmare, replace it with a neutral or positive image, and rehearse it daily. If helpful, include supportive others, a power animal, or a suit of armor (anything that increases the sense of safety and control). This process is repeated, with new dreams chosen to rescript every few days to a week.

EXERCISE 9.1

Sensory Awareness

1 Find a comfortable seated position in a safe space.
2 Begin with deep, slow breaths to center yourself:

- Inhale for four counts through your nose
- Hold for four counts
- Exhale for four counts through your mouth
- Repeat this cycle 3–4 times

3 Engage your senses using the 5-4-3-2-1 technique:

- Name five things you can see
- Touch four different textures around you
- Listen for three distinct sounds
- Identify two scents in your environment
- Notice one taste in your mouth

4 As you breathe steadily, mentally repeat this affirmation: "I am safe in the present moment. What I am experiencing is a memory, not current reality."
5 If an intrusive memory or flashback occurs:

- Acknowledge its presence without judgment
- Gently redirect your focus to your breath or one of your senses
- Remind yourself: "This is a flashback. I am remembering what happened before. It is not happening now."

6 Practice body awareness by tensing and relaxing different muscle groups, starting from your toes and moving to your head.
7 If emotions become overwhelming, place a hand over your heart, feeling its warmth and steady beat.
8 Conclude the exercise by taking three deep breaths and slowly opening your eyes.

References

Edwards, D. J. A. (2022). Using schema modes for case conceptualization in schema therapy: an applied clinical approach. *Frontiers in Psychology*, 12, 763670. https://doi.org/10.3389/fpsyg.2021.763670

Ellis, L. A. (2023). Solving the nightmare mystery: the autonomic nervous system as missing link in the aetiology and treatment of nightmares. *American Psychological Association*, 33(1), 45–74.

Germer, C. (2019). A guided meditation to label difficult emotions. Mindful Magazine, January.

Iyadurai, L., Visser, R. M, Lau-Zhu, A., Porcheret, K., Horsch, A., Holmes, E. A., & James, E. L. (2018). Intrusive memories of trauma: A target for research bridging cognitive science and its clinical application. *Clinical Psychology Review*, 69, 67–82. https://doi.org/10.1016/j.cpr.2018.08.005

Krakow, B., & Zadra, A. (2010). Imagery rehearsal therapy: principles and practice. *Sleep Medicine Clinics*, 5(2), 289–298. https://doi.org/10.1016/j.jsmc.2010.01.004

Lloyd, M. (2023). The surprising thing about flashbacks (part one). *CTAD Clinic* https://www.youtube.com/watch?v=RFu3eDp7kEE

Neff, K. & Germer, C. (2018). *The Mindful Self-Compassion Workbook*. New York: Guilford Press.

Trauma and Dissociation

Trauma and Dissociation

Jane's parents were both neglectful and abusive. She remained with her father and older brothers after her parents divorced when she was ten. She felt abandoned when her mother left her behind with her father and violent siblings while taking an older sister to live with her. She did not understand why her mother left her behind, why there were no pictures of her as a child, or why her mother never showed interest in her activities (abandoned child mode). Jane was left to fend for herself, in the care of her aggressive father and siblings or with an abusive uncle. She yearned for love and acceptance but was frightened by the anger, violence, and abuse surrounding her (frightened, vulnerable child). The internal push and pull for connection, while simultaneously being frightened of it, created a state of conflict resolved when Jane's mind split into dissociated parts, resulting in internal fragmentation and disorganization. Jane's "going on with life" part detached from the memories of her traumatic experiences, which allowed her to excel at school and become an accomplished athlete (detached protector). This way, she adapted to a dangerous, dismissive environment that ignored her basic needs and feelings. The parts that endangered day-to-day functioning were walled off, allowing the parts interacting with her environment to become identified as 'me'.

(Fisher, 2017)

Dissociation is strongly linked to early childhood trauma, particularly abuse and neglect. Many experts believe that long-term trauma is the root cause of dissociation, as dissociative disorders occur more often in those with a history of childhood abuse or neglect than in other mental health disorders. At least 90% of people with dissociative disorders have experienced adverse childhood experiences (Stein et al., 2013). Dissociation is a considered defensive survival strategy, or coping mode, developed to help deal with overwhelming stress or trauma.

DOI: 10.4324/9781003462958-21

As individuals begin to make sense of their experiences, they recognize the importance of integration and coherence to their well-being. A primary goal of trauma-informed therapy is to help integrate dissociated aspects of past experiences within a stable identity, moving from avoidance to an acceptance and tolerance of the past. This does not mean erasing memories or blending self-states into one single self. Instead, it means integrating the notion that "it happened, it happened to me, and it happened in the past" into a consistent sense of self within a coherent life narrative.

The cornerstone of this work is the therapeutic relationship, a crucial element that provides the empathic support and validation needed for healing. The effect of dissociation on interpersonal relationships and emotion regulation, as it is addressed here and now, facilitates the integration of the dissociated aspects of self and experience.

Goals

1 Understand dissociation and innate action tendencies as adaptive defensive responses that help survive trauma.
2 Identify symptoms of dissociation that impair the ability to be connected to the present.
3 Review how the Structural Dissociation of the Personality (SDP) model explains brain disconnection and dysregulation in threatening situations.
4 Understand how Schema Therapy (ST) informs the treatment of dissociation.

Procedure

1 **Mindfulness Exercise: Passing Stretches**. Each member demonstrates their favorite stretch and passes it to the group to imitate. Ask them to pay attention to their muscles' sensations as they practice the different stretches.
2 Check-In.
3 Review key points about dissociation. How does dissociation manifest?
4 Discuss how the themes of dysregulation, disruption, distortion, disconnection, denial, and defense relate to dissociation. Discuss the need to recognize signs of dissociation, as early detection and intervention can significantly improve outcomes for individuals experiencing dissociation.
5 Explore the group's experiences of dissociation as reflected in **Handout 10.1, Your Dissociative Experience**. Discuss how the group, through its collective understanding and support, can address these behaviors when noticed in the group. This will provide real-life examples of the concepts being explored.

6 Compare and contrast the Structural Dissociation and ST conceptualizations of dissociation. Discuss the framework for understanding how the brain disconnects and dysregulates in threatening situations. Identify the different functions and needs underlying the different schema modes.

7 Discuss how modes relate to innate survival defenses. Refer to the NICABM idiographic **"The Structural Dissociation Model"** https://www.nicabm.com/working-with-structural-dissociation/.Review **Handout 10.2 Structural Dissociation, Action Tendencies and Modes, Handout 10.3. Recognizing the Presence of the Action Heroes and Modes and/or Handout 10.4 The Structural Dissociation Model.**

8 Summarize the main takeaways from the group discussion.

9 Check-out.

10 Grounding: Introduce **Sensory Anchoring** during dissociative episodes (*Touch*: Hold an ice cube, place your hands in water, or stroke a pet; *Smell*: Inhale a strong scent like an essential oil or your favorite lotion; *Taste*: Bite into a lemon or another fruit with a strong flavor; *Sight*: Look around the room and focus on specific objects, noticing their details *Sound*: Listen carefully to ambient noises or play soothing music).

Main Themes

Dissociation is a mental process where a person disconnects from their thoughts, feelings, memories, or sense of self. It exists on a spectrum, with symptoms ranging from mild and transient emotional detachment (highway hypnosis or daydreaming) to severe and chronic dissociation [dissociative identity disorder (DID)]. When the traumatic experience is so intense that it overwhelms the ability to tolerate the painful emotions it provokes, it splits off from the rest of our lives. Non-realized experiences (inner experiences, thoughts, physical actions, sensations, memories, emotions) fail to integrate into the person's current reality and sense of self (van der Hart & Horst, 1989; Lyons-Ruth, K. 2003; van der Hart et al., 2005; Harricharan, et al. 2021). Dissociation is viewed as an innate defensive strategy developed to survive the emotional and psychological impact of overwhelming trauma so that the individual can continue to function in their daily life. "The essence of dissociation is splitting off from the experience and the parts or modes that hold those experiences to survive otherwise unendurable trauma" (Spring, 2010). ST normalizes dissociation as a coping mode that helps individuals through experiences that might otherwise be too disturbing or unbearable and also recognizes that these coping modes become dysfunctional when the environment is no longer traumatic, but the person continues to respond as if it is.

Diagnoses and Symptom Presentation

Diagnostic types of dissociation include **Otherwise Specified Dissociative Disorder**, a partial disruption in identity, memory, or consciousness through dissociative experiences such as identity confusion or identity alteration or **DID** where the primary symptoms include sudden discontinuities in sense of self (reflected in separate identities, alters, modes that are created to cope with and compartmentalize the prolonged traumatic experiences) and sense of agency (when different aspects of self or modes take executive control of the person's conscious functioning).

These discontinuities result in the person experiencing "too little." Loss of memory or time that is more than usual forgetting (*dissociative amnesia*), a distortion in time (*time distortion, age regression*), feeling alienated or disconnected from your body (*depersonalization*) or your surroundings (*derealization*), or a loss of coordinated functioning that causes uncertainty about self-identity (*identity confusion*) are common sequelae of dissociation. Experiencing "too much" may include *intrusive dissociative symptoms* such as flashbacks, unexplained feelings, thoughts, behaviors, impulses, and body sensations that inexplicably come "out of the blue, feeling as if your thoughts, feelings, behaviors, and memories do not belong to you" ("not me" hearing voices, switching).

The individual's experience is characterized by emotional *dysregulation*, a *disruption* in daily functioning and psychological processes, *distorted* beliefs about self, others, and the world, *disconnection* from others, avoidance or *denial* of the experience, and *defensive* reactivity. Some parts of the individual may remain stuck in the unresolved aspects of the trauma. In contrast, other parts deny or avoid any associations with the overwhelming stressors to be able to "go on with life as normal" (Boon et al., 2011; Fisher, 2017). This becomes complicated when unresolved experiences intrude into daily life (nightmares, flashbacks, intrusive memories, and dysregulated emotions).

Structural Dissociation

The Structural Dissociation of the Personality Model (SDP) (van der Hart et al., 2005; Fisher, 2017) proposes that humans have two motivational systems: attachment and defense. We are motivated to connect and attach to the primary caregivers we depend on. However, we also need to defend ourselves when the source of attachment is also the source of danger. This theory proposes that in trauma, dissociation of personality is maintained over time by chronic breaking points that overwhelm integrative capacity, the need to depend on caregivers who are dangerous and frightening, a lack of regulating attachment figures, and conditioned phobic avoidance of inner experiences (van der Hart et al., 2005) (see Figure 10.1).

The systems in our mind and body are like large plates that make up the earth. In complex trauma, a "fault line" is created when the innate defense system instinctively seeks to shield from harm while the attachment system seeks connection, love, and caring. Disorganized attachment results when parts of the child's mind and body disconnect from the frightening stimulus (e.g., an abusive parent) to survive in a relationship they are dependent on. When systems have differing goals, two incompatible systems engage in a tug-of-war, not unlike an earthquake (Steele, 2024). A person's personality divides these subsystems, each with its first-person perspective, rigid in their functions, and often unavailable to each other. The child develops divided and compartmentalized trauma responses (Fight, flight, freeze, attach/cry for help, collapse/submit, and appease/please) as dissociation develops along these fault lines.

The model of hemispheric specialization of function is a helpful way to illustrate the disruption caused by structural dissociation (even while remembering that this is an oversimplification of the intricately interconnected and involved nervous system) (Fisher, 2017). According to the SDP model, the brain's left hemisphere represents the rational, present-oriented, and grounded "Going on with Normal Life" parts of the self that manage the responsibilities of present-day life. In contrast, the right hemisphere represents the "traumatized child" or "Emotional Parts" stuck in the survival defensiveness when activated by reminders of the trauma.

Crying out for help, giving in, collapsing or submitting, pleasing or appeasing, fighting back, fleeing or freezing are innate survival responses and trauma-based coping modes that defend against trauma. The SDP model posits that these survival responses become embodied as different trauma-related parts or alters.

ST describes these survival responses as coping modes, although the DID modes may be three-dimensional and more multifaceted than traditional Schema Modes. The most common modes observed in dissociation and DID patients include inner critic, angry protector, angry overcontrolling modes (fight/vigilant), detached, avoidant protectors or detached self-soother coping modes (flight/escape), avoidant dissociative, hidden coping modes (freeze/immobilization), vulnerable child modes (cry for help, and attach), and compliant surrenderer, self-sacrificing, pleasing or appeasing modes (submit/shame). These modes represent extreme expressions of dysfunctional states in dissociation. They differ from those in other disorders primarily in the degree of experienced dissociation from other modes. They may have different levels of knowledge about their experience, with varying degrees of co-consciousness that contribute to dissociative amnesia. Modes may hold unique memories, assume executive control over the system, and function as usual while avoiding inner experiences and traumatic memories held by the "trauma parts" (vulnerable child parts).

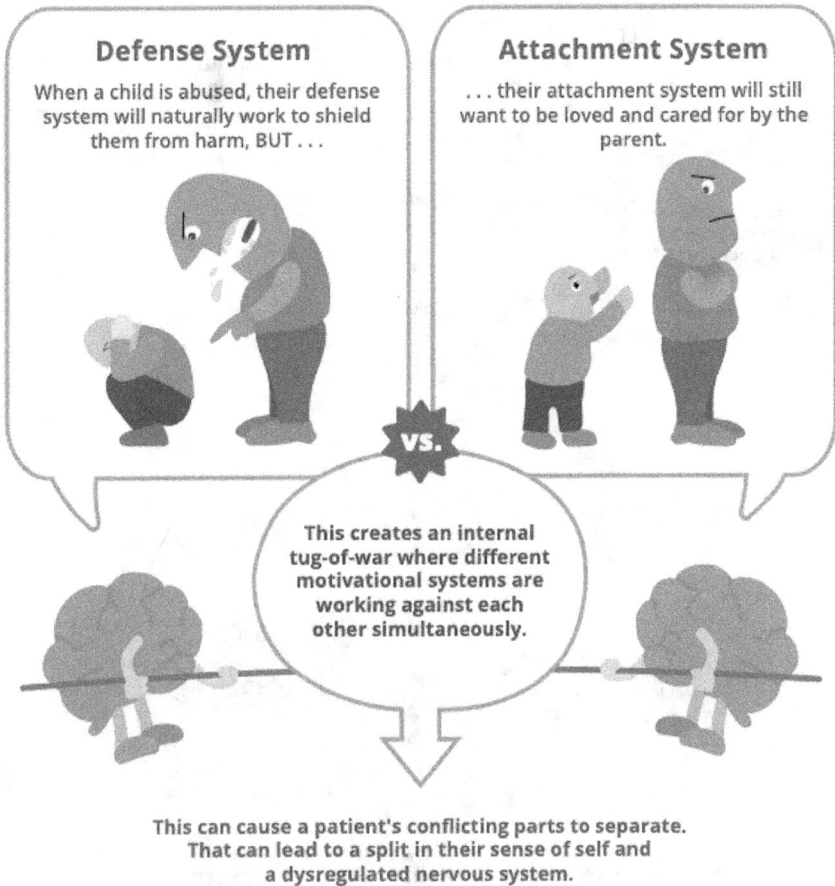

Figure 10.1 The Structural Dissociation Model

STRUCTURAL DISSOCIATION MODEL

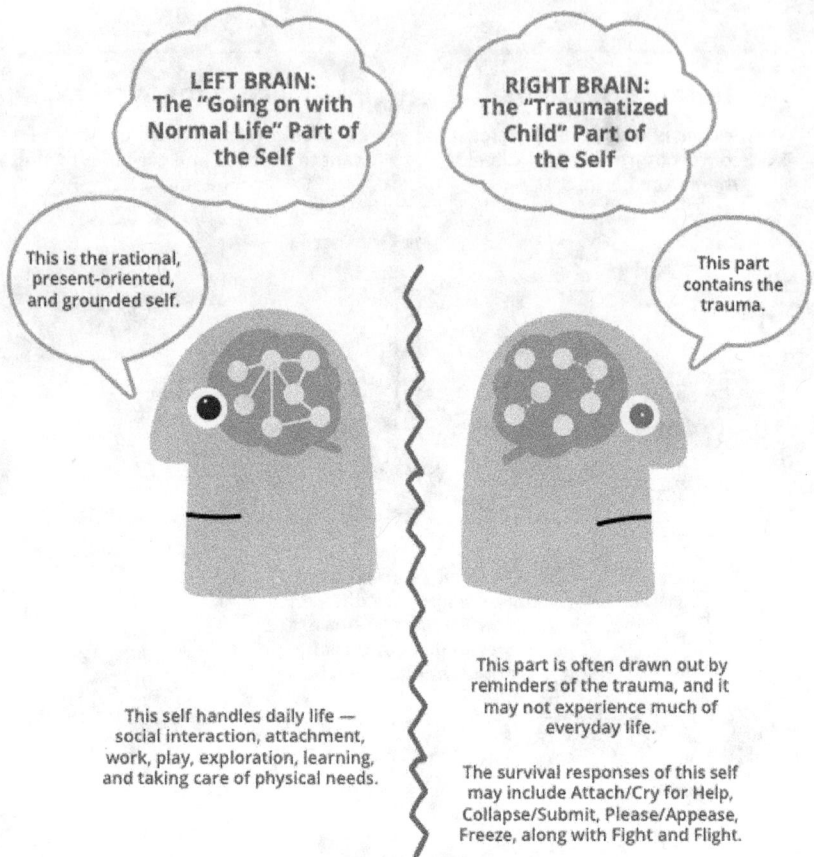

LEFT BRAIN:
The "Going on with
Normal Life" Part of
the Self

RIGHT BRAIN:
The "Traumatized
Child" Part of
the Self

This is the rational,
present-oriented,
and grounded self.

This part
contains the
trauma.

This self handles daily life —
social interaction, attachment,
work, play, exploration, learning,
and taking care of physical needs.

This part is often drawn out by
reminders of the trauma, and it
may not experience much of
everyday life.

The survival responses of this self
may include Attach/Cry for Help,
Collapse/Submit, Please/Appease,
Freeze, along with Fight and Flight.

The key to recovery is helping a patient have full awareness of
all their parts without feeling overwhelmed.

nicabm
www.nicabm.com

Figure 10.1 (Continued)

In the SDP model, **"going on with normal life"** parts disown the survival-oriented parts. From an ST perspective, the modes that experience the painful feelings and PTSD symptoms (vulnerable, frightened child) become hidden behind the avoidant coping modes that actively avoid triggering situations, disconnect emotionally, and defend against perceived threats (Detached Protector, Avoidant Protector, Self-Soother, and Angry Protector), or behind the critical and demanding modes that reflect self-hatred, self-punishment, unrealistic standards and push for perfection (Inner Critic modes). These modes allow the person to function in their daily lives. Disowning them or detaching from them distances from the painful, destabilizing, and harmful effects of the trauma and allows a focus on the tasks of everyday life. Separation and disconnection develop between these parts of the self, or modes as the vulnerable (sad, lonely, needy, angry, distrusting) parts become "not me" while the "going on with everyday life" parts are seen as "me." As healing occurs, the healthy adult mode facilitates, manages, negotiates with, and nurtures all the other modes.

Unlike the SDP model, which may inadvertently reinforce the idea of separate identities, ST Treatment focuses on integrating the modes activated during dissociative episodes by grouping them by their function and underlying needs. ST does not consider the extreme expressions of the dysfunctional coping modes as separate, compartmentalized identities (Shaw et al., 2014; Huntjens, et al., 2014; Huntjens et al., 2019). Treatment involves engaging with the modes that interact with the external world, connecting with those modes that remain hidden, and attuning to the different roles and functions of the behaviors exhibited by each. Addressing the needs and functions of the dissociated modes in DID can be compared to addressing the unmet needs of the child modes (Edwards, 2022; Margolin, 2022).

Strategies for Working with Dissociation

Dissociative patients are often exceptionally vulnerable and highly avoidant. Their vulnerable, hurt, threatened, and often dissociated parts can emerge in these different ways that make group treatment challenging. Group discussions or activities may inadvertently trigger traumatic memories or flashbacks, exacerbating dissociative symptoms. A person who is dissociating may have difficulty engaging in the group, become disoriented and confused, and lose contact with reality. They may experience intense emotional distress and withdraw or isolate from the group during these episodes. Dissociative episodes involving self-harm, impulsivity, or aggressive behavior may pose safety risks to the individual or others in the group.

Identifying these behaviors as defensive action tendencies in the face of some perceived threat can help reduce the associated shame and stigma.

As the individual reassesses their reactions, they can be redirected toward more effective present-oriented responses. Reminding them that slower is faster, less is more validates their experience without pressuring them to participate. Providing trigger warnings when discussing potentially sensitive topics, identifying needs, and reviewing coping strategies for managing triggers can redirect them toward more effective present-oriented responses.

Group members can be taught to recognize notable changes that occur with dissociation (spacing out, blank stare, physical stilling, switching of self-state with changes in style, behavior, eye contact, voice tone, etc.) to support the dissociated member. Attending to the person's different postures or movements may help identify different modes or parts of the self that are reflected in the body. A collapsed posture or shutdown may represent a hopeless mode, while speaking out and standing erect may be an assertive or healthy adult mode.

Mindfulness and grounding techniques for dissociation help reconnect with the senses and redirect attention from dissociative states. Dissociation is an automatic reaction, while mindfulness is intentional. Dissociation stems from difficulty holding in awareness present experience; mindfulness purposefully cultivates that awareness. It targets stabilizing attention and emotional regulation through acceptance (Bishop et al., 2004; Shapiro et al., 2006; Zerubavel & Messman-Moore, 2015; Vancappel et al., 2021).

Mindful awareness can help bring the client's attention back to what they are experiencing. For example, increasing early awareness of "mode flipping," switching between different parts, or signs of spacing out (quick eye movements, vacant stare, changes in (shallow, more rapid?), lack of responsiveness) may decrease the intensity of dissociative episodes. "I'm noticing your 'spacing out' mode (part) is here. Do you sense that?" "Let's be curious – what mode are you in? What are you thinking/feeling/doing when in that mode? What happens when you have that thought/feeling/action? What do you need?").

While mindfulness is beneficial for many people, it may be contraindicated for pathological dissociative patterns or dissociative disorders like DID. Asking individuals to pay attention to internal body sensations may trigger dissociative episodes, exacerbate symptoms such as depersonalization or derealization or lead to emotional blunting. For some individuals with trauma, focusing on the breath can be triggering.

Mindfulness practices can be introduced gradually, in brief segments that allow the participants to choose the focus of their attention. External anchors may reduce the triggering effect of some mindfulness activities. Techniques that are considered "safer" for dissociation include physical grounding (focus on the sensation of the feet on the ground or the feeling of sitting in a chair); gentle movement (yoga, mindful walking, especially in nature or barefoot on grass or sand, stretching or postural changes); the 5-4-3-2-1 technique (naming five things you can see, four things you can touch, three things you can hear, two things you can smell, and one thing you can taste) and engaging the senses (scented oils, different textures).

Farrell et al. (2014) suggest a fleece strip to connect the dissociated member and the therapist symbolically (and literally). The strip is long enough to keep the patient and therapist at a comfortable distance but still connected. Whenever the patient is "zoning out" or starts to dissociate, the therapist gives the fleece a slight tug. The member feels the connection and becomes more aware of what is happening at that moment.

In addition to the fleece strips, the group can create colorful bead bracelets as a grounding exercise that strengthens the cohesiveness of the group and functions as a transitional object to symbolize the care of the vulnerable child. Balloons and bubble-blowing devices are ways to reengage a dissociated member, decrease the hold of the detached protector or the inner critic when feeling stuck, work with anger, or have fun in the group (Farrell et al., 2014).

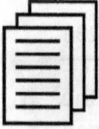

HANDOUT 10.1

Your Dissociative Experience

While dissociative experiences such as highway hypnosis are everyday experiences, people with a history of trauma may have more prolonged or chronic episodes of dissociation. Noticing the signs of dissociation can help you better understand and manage your reactions to specific trauma triggers.

1 Check the dissociative symptoms you have experienced in the past week:

___ Losing time.
___ Disconnected from, outside your body.
___ Feeling numb.
___ Difficulty concentrating and focusing.
___ Feeling like things around you are unreal.
___ Experiencing flashbacks, nightmares, intrusive memories.
___ Feeling little, small.
___ Feeling spacey or "checked out."
___ Hearing internal "chatter" or voices in your head.
___ Unexplained sensations or feelings that seem to come out of nowhere.
___ Feeling like you do not have control over your body or behavior.
___ Watching your actions as if from a distance.
___ Other: _____

2 How did your experience of these symptoms affect your functioning at the time?

_____
_____
_____
_____
_____

3 Which symptoms are most disruptive for you?

_____
_____
_____
_____
_____

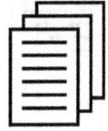

4 What has helped you cope with these symptoms in the past? What helps you currently?

_____

_____

_____

_____

5 Are you aware of any distinct and differentiated parts of self? Describe what you notice and what you know about this part. What function does it serve?

_____

_____

_____

_____

_____

6 Can you identify which modes are activated when you dissociate? Please describe what you notice and what it feels like in this mode. What function does it serve?

Child Modes: _____

_____

_____

_____

Avoidant Modes (Detached Protector, Detached Self-Soother, Angry Protector, etc.)

_____

_____

_____

Critic Modes: _____

_____

_____

_____

Healthy Adult Mode: _____

_____

_____

_____

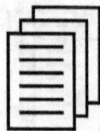

Structural Dissociation, Action Tendencies and Modes

The mind's ability to dissociate is an adaptive response to trauma and has often been described as a heroic response (Fisher, 2019). How does each action tendency hero or schema mode help survive trauma? Consider how this shows up in your life.

Fight: This part tries to rescue by controlling and defending against danger. Negative self-talk and defensive/controlling behaviors can disconnect us from people or situations perceived as dangerous and from parts of our internal self that threaten our ability to function. (ST: **Angry child or angry adult, a demanding or punitive inner critic, or an overcompensating mode**).

Flight: This part tries to rescue us by fleeing to safety. Flight can be seen in thoughts or actions that remove us from situations sensed as threats. (ST: **Detached Protector, Self-Soother, Avoidant modes**). Disordered eating, substance abuse, or self-harm serve this function.

Freeze: Freezing is an active response that helps immobilize us in the face of a perceived threat. The message might be, "Do not move – or else you will die!" (tonic immobility). We can hide in plain sight from a predator to survive. Freezing also helps orient as we try to detect or identify the threat, e.g., hearing brakes squeal or a siren blaring, "Where is this sound coming from, and am I in its path?" (ST: **Detached Protector, Compliant Surrenderer modes**).

Fawn (Submit/Please/Appease): Complying with, pleasing, appeasing, or surrendering to those with power is safer when fighting back or running away is impossible. (ST: **Compliant Surrenderer mode**).

Collapse/Shutdown: This part resembles the submit and freeze parts. In the collapsed state, however, the person is shut down and hypoaroused. Endorphins serve to numb the pain. (ST: **Detached Protector mode, Helpless Surrender**).

Attach: The attach part cries out for help and engages others to provide safety. (ST: **Compliant Surrenderer, Vulnerable Child modes**).

Going on with everyday life: This part shuts out the other trauma responses and tries to maintain normalcy in the present everyday world. (ST: It may appear as a **Healthy Adult mode** or wise mind, but it may also be a **Detached Protector mode** as seen in intellectualizing behaviors).

If a burglar broke into your home, the fight part would threaten with a gun; the flight part would run out of the house, freeze would be quiet

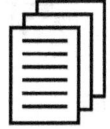

and unmoving; submit would turn over all the valuables to appease the burglar, and attach would call 911 or run to someone for help. Collapse would disconnect or dissociate to avoid the danger.

Adapted by McDonald, L. (2010). **S.A.F.E.T.Y Curriculum**, Penn Medicine Princeton House Behavioral Health Women's Program, Penn Medicine Princeton Health.

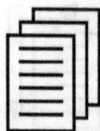

Recognizing the Presence of the Action Heroes and Modes

1 The alarm clock goes off. Sharon does not feel like facing the day. She hits the snooze button even though she knows this will make her late. Who is trying to be the hero? What mode is she in?

Fight Flight Freeze Fawn Submit Attach Going on with Life
Child Mode Detached/Soother Surrenderer Overcompensator Critic Healthy Adult

2 Sharon finally gets up. She is rushed. As she hurriedly showers and dresses, she finds herself out of her window of tolerance. She can't find her cell phone. She can't find her keys. She can't concentrate. She stops in the middle of the room. She feels like she is going to panic. Who is trying to be the hero? What mode is she in?

Fight Flight Freeze Fawn Submit Attach Going on with Life
Child Mode Detached/Soother Surrenderer Overcompensator Critic Healthy Adult

3 Sharon hears her thoughts. "I am so stupid. I can't believe I am late again. They are going to fire me. I know it". As these thoughts scare and shame her more and more, she runs out the door. Who is trying to be the hero? What mode is she in?

Fight Flight Freeze Fawn Submit Attach Going on with Life
Child Mode Detached/Soother Surrenderer Overcompensator Critic Healthy Adult

4 Sharon drives and gets stuck behind a school bus. She bangs the steering wheel and swears out loud. She thinks. "If I left earlier, I wouldn't be stuck behind this bus. I am such an idiot." Who is trying to be the hero? What mode is she in?

Fight Flight Freeze Fawn Submit Attach Going on with Life
Child Mode Detached/Soother Surrenderer Overcompensator Critic Healthy Adult

5 She pulls out her cell phone and calls her friend. She knows her friend always makes her laugh and feel better about herself. Who is trying to be the hero? What mode is she in?

Fight Flight Freeze Fawn Submit Attach Going on with Life
Child Mode Detached/Soother Surrenderer Overcompensator Critic Healthy Adult

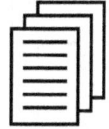

6 Sharon remembers that she didn't eat breakfast. She thinks, "F... it! I am late already; I'm stopping at Wawa." Who is trying to be the hero? What mode is she in?

Fight Flight Freeze Fawn Submit Attach Going on with Life
Child Mode Detached/Soother Surrenderer Overcompensator Critic Healthy Adult

7 When in Wawa, she gets her favorite large mocha cappuccino even though she started a diet yesterday. "The day is blown already." she thinks. "I am getting that doughnut." Who is trying to be the hero? What mode is she in?

Fight Flight Freeze Fawn Submit Attach Going on with Life
Child Mode Detached/Soother Surrenderer Overcompensator Critic Healthy Adult

8 Sharon gets to work. She is only a few minutes late. She breathes a sigh of relief and forgets about the frantic start to her day. She concentrates on work. Who is trying to be the hero? What mode is she in?

Fight Flight Freeze Fawn Submit Attach Going on with Life
Child Mode Detached/Soother Surrenderer Overcompensator Critic Healthy Adult

Adapted by McDonald, L. (2010). **S.A.F.E.T.Y Curriculum**, Penn Medicine Princeton House Behavioral Health Women's Program, Penn Medicine Princeton Health.

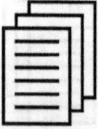

HANDOUT 10.4

Structural Dissociation Model

Emotional Parts that Defend and Protect

	Behaviors	Emotions	Thoughts	Relationships
Fight Takes control of danger	yells, verbally and physically abusive of others, takes action to commit suicide, self-harms, road rage	Irritability, anger, rage	Judgmental, critical of self and others, preoccupations with control	Must have her own way, excessive emotional intensity when setting limits, challenges others' boundaries and sees them as threats, distrustful of others
Flight Runs to Safety	avoidance, procrastination, disappearing through addictions, eating disorders (that create numbing or high), depersonalization	Trapped then relief, emotional numbing, cravings	Fantasies of escape including suicide and self-harm, preoccupations with addictions	Creates boundaries by distancing from others and fears being trapped. Avoids commitment
Freeze	Hides by not moving, physically or emotionally, unable to talk, paralysis	Fear, anxiety, panic attacks, waiting	Confusion, can't think, Ruminations, OCD	Doesn't trust herself to set limits with others, may appear calm on the outside Doesn't initiate

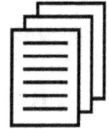

	Behaviors	Emotions	Thoughts	Relationships
Fawn	Seeks safety by pleasing others in power, poor eye contact, collapsed posture	Shame, waiting, hopelessness, hypo-aroused, emotionally numb	Self-critical thoughts from Fight that keep her ashamed	More aware of others' needs than her own, tries to be "good" and please others, compares self to others and always finds himself deficient
Attach	Seeks safety through connection, repetitive bids for attention (ex. over texting), crying, seduction	Desperate, lonely, helpless, abandoned	Fantasies of safe others, preoccupied with abandonment: "Why did he leave me," "Where is she?"	Communicates less powerfully than the one she is with, presents as helpless, experiences boundaries as abandonment, difficulties in saying "good-bye" at the end of an encounter and in the loss of a relationship, seductive, flatters

The Part(s) that Functions in Peacetime

Carry on with Normal Life (HA)	Completes tasks of daily living works; plays; takes care of others; creates; maintains food, shelter, clothing	Determination, compartmentalization, access to all emotions, gut feelings	Avoids trauma triggers, thoughts about completing tasks, motivated by potential reward, wisdom	Social defenses with the goal of protecting social attachments and status and managing social impression

McDonald (2024). Adapted from Fisher (2022).

References

Bishop, S. R., Lau, M., Shapiro, S., Carlson, L., Anderson, N. D., Carmody, J., Segal, Z. V., Abbey, S., Speca, M., Velting, D., & Devins, G. (2004). Mindfulness: a proposed operational definition. *Clinical Psychology: Science and Practice*, 11(3), 230–241. https://doi.org/10.1093/clipsy.bph077

Boon, S., Steele, K., & Hart, O. v. d. (2011). *Coping with Trauma-related Dissociation: Skills Training for Patients and Therapists*. New York: W. W. Norton.

Edwards, D. (2022). Kelly's circle of safety and healing: an extended schema therapy narrative and interpretative investigation. *Pragmatic Case Studies in Psychotherapy*, 18(3), 210–261.

Farrell, J.M., Reiss, N., & Shaw, I.A. (2014).*The Schema Therapy Clinician's Guide : A Complete Resource for Building and Delivering Individual, Group and Integrated Schema Mode Treatment Programs*. New York: John Wiley & Sons.

Fisher, J. (2019). Sensorimotor psychotherapy in the treatment of trauma. *Practice Innovations*, 4(3), 156–165. https://doi.org/10.1037/pri0000096.

Fisher, J. (2017). *Healing the Fragmented Selves of Trauma Survivors: Overcoming Internal Self-Alienation*. New York: Routledge/Taylor & Francis Group.

Fisher, J. (2022). *The Living Legacy Instructional Flip Chart*. Eau Claire: PESI Publishing. Https://www.Nicabm.Com/Working-With-Structural-Dissociation/

Harricharan, S., McKinnon, M. C., & Lanius, R. A. (2021). How processing of sensory information from the internal and external worlds shape the perception and engagement with the world in the aftermath of trauma: implications for PTSD. *Frontiers in Neuroscience*, 15, 625490. https://doi.org/10.3389/fnins.2021.625490

Huntjens, R. J. C., Wessel, I., Hermans, D., & Van Minnen, A. (2014). Autobiographical memory specificity in dissociative identity disorder. *Journal of Abnormal Psychology*, 123(2), 419–428.

Huntjens, R. J. C., Rijkeboer, M. M., & Arntz, A. (2019). Schema therapy for dissociative identity disorder (DID): rationale and study protocol. *European Journal of Psychotraumatology*, 10(1), 1571377. https://doi.org/10.1080/20008198.2019.1571377

Lyons-Ruth, K. (2003). The two-person construction of defenses: disorganized attachment strategies, unintegrated mental states, and hostile/helpless relational processes. *Journal of Infant, Child, and Adolescent Psychotherapy*, 2, 105–114.

Margolin, J. (2022). Applying the schema therapy approach of Edward's case of Kelly to patients with dissociative identity disorder (DID): the cases of Susie and Anna. *Pragmatic Case Studies in Psychotherapy*, 18 (3), 272–286.

McDonald, L. (2010). Heroes. In *S.A.F.E.T.Y Curriculum*. Penn Medicine Princeton House Behavioral Health Women's Program, Penn Medicine Princeton Health, private correspondence.

Shapiro, S. L., Carlson, L. E., Astin, J. A., & Freedman, B. (2006). Mechanisms of mindfulness. *Journal of Clinical Psychology*, 62(3), 373–386. https://doi.org/10.1002/Jclp.20237

Shaw, I., Farrell, J., Rijkeboer, M. M., Huntjens, R. J. C., & Arntz, A. (2014). Schema therapy for dissociative identity disorder: a treatment protocol. Unpublished Manuscript.

Spring, C. (2010). A brief guide to working with dissociative identity disorder. Https:// Www.Carolynspring.Com/Blog/A-Brief-Guide-To-Working-With-Dissociative-Identity-Disorder/

Steele, K. (2024). *Application of Somatic Interventions in Clinical Practice: Attachment, Trauma, Neurobiology, and the Body*. Calgary, Canada: Envision Workshop.

Stein, D. J., Karestan, K. C., Friedman, M. J., Hill, E., Mclaughlin, K. A., Petukhova, M., Meron Ruscio, A., Shahly, V., Spiegel, D., Borges, G., Bunting, B., Caldas-De-Almeidaj, J. M., De Girolamo, G., Koen Demyttenaere, K., Silvia Florescu, S., Haro, J. M., Karam, E. G., Viviane Kovess-Masfety, V., Lee, S., Matschinger, H., Mladenova, M., Posada-Villa, J., Tachimori, H., Viana, M. C., & Kessler, R. C. (2013). Dissociation in posttraumatic stress disorder: evidence from the world mental health surveys. *Biological Psychiatry*, 73(4), 302–312.

Vancappel, A., Guerin, L., Reveillere, C., & El-Hage, W. (2021). Disentangling the link between mindfulness and dissociation: the mediating role of attentional and emotional acceptance. *European Journal of Trauma & Dissociation*, 5(4), 100220. https://doi.org/10.1016/J.Ejtd.2021.100220

van der Hart, O. & Horst, R. (1989). The dissociation theory of Pierre Janet. *Journal of Traumatic Stress*. 2(4), 397–412.

van der Hart, O., Nijenhuis, E. R. S., & Steele, K. (2005). Dissociation: an insufficiently recognized major feature of complex posttraumatic stress disorder. *Journal of Traumatic Stress*, 18, 413–423.

Zerubavel, N., & Messman-Moore, T. (2015). Staying Present: Incorporating Mindfulness into Therapy for Dissociation. *Mindfulness*, 6(2), 303-314. https://doi.org/10.1007/s12671-013-0261-3

Session 11

Trauma and Attachment

Attachment theory, a cornerstone in psychology, underscores the pivotal role of early relationships and attachments in molding an individual's emotional and psychological well-being. This theory, initially formulated by psychologist John Bowlby and later enriched by Mary Ainsworth and Mary Main, posits that the quality of these early attachments influences an individual's temperament, ability to form and sustain relationships with self and others, ability to regulate emotions and function in daily life (Bowlby, 1969; Main & Hesse, 1990). The quality of those early bonds becomes the model for later relationships. When a caring, dependable adult responds with understanding when they are upset, hungry, tired, or scared, the child is better able to tolerate stress and learns to regulate their emotional states. When these early interactions are characterized by repetitive, prolonged, and inconsistent caregiving, neglect, or abuse by those responsible for the child's safety, security, and protection, the child may fail to learn how to regulate their own emotions. They may see themself and others through a misshaped lens, developing the belief that they are unlovable or of little value, are not worthy of healthy relationships, or that others cannot be relied on to meet their basic needs. They may not learn what being in a safe, secure, healthy relationship means. These patterns of distorted beliefs about self and others can result in ineffective relational patterns that persist into adulthood.

Goals

1 Understand how the quality of early relationships shapes the development of attachment style, internal working models, and schema.
2 Discuss how early childhood trauma impairs the ability to feel secure and develop trust in others.
3 Identify each individual's unique attachment style and its impact on their current relationships.
4 Discuss the potential for growth and change through the development of earned secure attachment.

DOI: 10.4324/9781003462958-22

Procedure

1 Mindfulness **Exercise 11.1 Secure Base Visualization**
2 Check-In.
3 Discuss the interrelationship of early attachment, internal working models and schemas, self-regulation, and interpersonal relationships.
4 Discuss how trauma impacts attachment style (**Handout 11. 1 Attachment Styles**).
5 Explore how attachment trauma contributes to emotional dysregulation and disconnection in relationships and disrupts and distorts beliefs about oneself and others. (*The goal is not to blame but to see how trauma impacts relationships in adult life: no caregiving environment is perfect or absolute- explore what it means to be a good enough parent*).
6 Discuss how developing Earned Secure Attachment and strengthening the Healthy Adult (HA) mode can change insecure attachment styles and self-defeating behavior patterns.
7 Review **Handout 11.2 Exploring Relationship Challenges**. What did the individual notice about how their attachment style impacts current relationships? Are they able to identify any patterns? What changes can they make to develop earned secure attachment and strengthen the HA mode?
8 Summarize the main takeaways from the group discussion.
9 Check-out.
10 Grounding: Suggested activity: **The Butterfly Hug** (Artigas & Jarero, 2014; https://emdrfoundation.org/toolkit/butterfly-hug.pdf). This is a grounding technique combining mindfulness and bilateral stimulation elements. It is beneficial for individuals experiencing anxiety or overwhelming emotions. One can gain greater control over one's emotional state as the ability to self-soothe in stressful situations improves. The hug provides an immediate calming effect during moments of acute anxiety and, over time, helps improve emotional regulation.

Main Themes

Attachment lies at the core of healthy development and emotional regulation. Early attachment experiences are pivotal in shaping our behaviors and expectations of how significant others will respond to our needs. Schemas and internal working models originate from early childhood experiences and represent internalized patterns of thinking about oneself and others. Both affect how individuals perceive and interact in relationships throughout their lives. The concept of core emotional needs in Schema Therapy closely aligns with Attachment Theory. The most fundamental need identified is secure attachment, mirroring Bowlby's emphasis on the importance of a secure base for healthy development. Responsive caregiving fosters secure attachment, while inconsistent or abusive care has detrimental effects on a child's emotional development and self-worth.

The capacity to understand the mental states that underlie one's own and others' behaviors (mentalization) develops through emotionally responsive attachment relationships in childhood. This capacity is a social-cognitive function necessary for healthy interpersonal engagement. Being able to rely on others for information about the social world permits children to develop the ability to accurately and flexibly appraise social situations (Fonagy et al., 2017; Karantzas et al., 2023).

Primary caregivers become a "haven" and "secure base" when the child knows they are available and responsive when needed. Children who are consistently and responsively cared for by their primary caregivers develop a profound sense of security, safety, and emotional equilibrium. "Good enough" parenting fosters the development of **secure attachment** that allows the child to explore the world with curiosity and develop autonomy and independence. The *regulating* comfort and soothing provided by the caregiver foster secure attachment and allow the child to learn how to manage their emotions (self-regulation) (Johnson, 2019; Corry & Gladstone, 2022). Consistent care and responsiveness in childhood allow adults to confidently seek support, closeness, comfort, and protection when feeling threatened physically or emotionally.

The Effect of Early Trauma

Secure attachment is disrupted when those responsible for the child's care and security are also the source of danger. Schema Therapy recognizes that adverse early attachment experiences, attachment trauma, and unmet emotional needs in childhood influence the formation of self-defeating core patterns that are repeated throughout life (Early Maladaptive Schemas-EMS). The ability to regulate emotions, explore the environment, and navigate the challenges of daily life become severely constricted without a secure base. Negative internal working models increase the difficulty of forming secure adult relationships. A cycle of re-traumatization can occur as the person reenacts the dynamics that mimic experiences of abuse or neglect (van der Kolk, 2005).

Resulting insecure attachment styles that play out in later relationships may be expressed as a **preoccupied attachment** (insecure anxious), **dismissive attachment** (insecure avoidant), or **disorganized attachment** (fearful-avoidant). These insecure attachment styles (anxious, avoidant, fearful) were positively associated with early maladaptive schemas across all domains, while secure attachment was negatively associated. Anxious attachment showed stronger associations with schemas in the disconnection/rejection and other-directedness domains, particularly with abandonment and subjugation schemas (Karantzias et al., 2023).

Fears of abandonment, too much intimacy, or yearning for connection with a primary caretaker who is threatening and dangerous can impair the ability to trust and establish intimate connections (Fisher, 2017). *Will someone be close, present, responsive, and engaged, or will they be inconsistent, unpredictable, unavailable, and harmful?*

Earned secure attachment can develop when an insecure attachment style is changed into a secure attachment later in life. Earned secure attachment works to heal past traumas or negative experiences by developing healthier ways of thinking, feeling, and behaving that challenge the underlying attachment disruptions perpetuating unhealthy adult relationships (Olufowote et al., 2020; Siegel, 2022). This process involves intentionally making internal and interpersonal changes that strengthen the Healthy Adult's ability to meet core emotional needs in a kinder and balanced way, regulate emotions, and engage in healthier relationships.

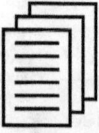

Attachment Styles

Attachment Style	Qualities of Child	Qualities of Caretaking Environment	Expression in adult relationships
Secure "It is easy for me to be close to others emotionally"	• Comfortable with intimacy, balances dependence and independence. • Healthy, trusting, and emotionally close relationships without fear of abandonment or separation or threat to autonomy. • Trusting, secure, self-confident, independent, autonomous, curious, affectionate, accepting. • Communicates openly, healthy expression of emotions and needs.	• Warm and responsive to the child's needs • Safe and secure environment. • Sensitive and attuned to the child's emotional and physical signals. • Reliable, predictable, and consistent. • Emotionally availability to offer comfort, support, positive reinforcement, and encouragement.	• Is sensitive to the needs and concerns of romantic partners • Calmly addresses areas of conflict. • Shares ideas and feelings in a flexible, appropriate manner and differentiates thoughts from feelings. • Comfortable both in relationships and alone. • Able to sustain a balanced sense of self and confidence.
Anxious (Preoccupied) "I need to be in a relationship but often worry whether my partner is available and committed"	• Attuned to small fluctuations in partner's mood and actions. • Fears abandonment or rejection • Seeks reassurance, approval, and validation. • Sensitive to criticism.	• Emotionally distant, inconsistent, insecure, unpredictable, unavailable to the child's needs. • Overprotective, enables dependency and fear of separation. May use fear or guilt to control the child's behavior.	• Preoccupation with attachment needs and potential losses, imagines things going wrong. • Often feels unappreciated by others and has difficulty receiving criticism and rejection.

(Continued)

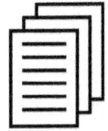

Attachment Style	Qualities of Child	Qualities of Caretaking Environment	Expression in adult relationships
		• Inappropriate boundaries, oversharing personal information or expecting the child to take on adult roles. • Excessively controlling, expects the child to conform to their expectations.	• Fears separation from loved ones, independence and autonomy. May be jealous, clingy, and overly dependent. • Self-sacrificing to maintain relationships. • Negative view of self
Avoidant (Dismissive) " I don't need to depend on others or have close relationships"	• Self-sufficient, emotionally unavailable, aloof detachment. • Rigid boundaries. • Avoids commitments, vulnerability, and intimacy to safeguard independence. • Struggles to express needs and wants.	• Emotionally distant and unresponsive to the child's needs. • May dismiss or minimize the child's emotional needs. • Values independence over emotional connection, • Little physical affection, negative or critical attitude	• Difficulty asking for help or seeking comfort from partner. • Avoids expressing feelings and emotional commitment. • Overly self-reliant and independent. Maintains distance in relationships. • Thinks highly of self, less of others. • Fantasizes about or engages in sexual encounters and affairs.

(Continued)

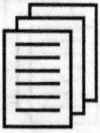

Attachment Style	Qualities of Child	Qualities of Caretaking Environment	Expression in adult relationships
Disorganized (Fearful Avoidant) "I want connection but fear connection. It is difficult to trust people"	• May have experienced early childhood trauma. Blend of both the Anxious and the Avoidant styles. • Contradictory behaviors as both yearns for and fears intimacy. Clingy and aloof. • Difficulty maintaining healthy boundaries. • Unpredictable, emotional extremes – intense hyperarousal or dissociative shut down. • Chaotic relationships.	• Traumatic and chaotic environment • Confusing, disorienting, unpredictable or contradictory behaviors. • Neglectful or abusive • Lack of appropriate boundaries, safety, or security.	• Inconsistent and unpredictable • Difficulty self-soothing and regulating emotions. • Approach-Avoidance moves between clinginess and avoidance. • Fears abandonment as well as intimacy. • Difficulty expressing needs clearly. • Emotional vulnerability • Instability in relationships.
Earned Secure Attachment "I can develop healthy relationships as I understand the impact of my early experiences"	• Adverse early attachment experiences. • Comfortable with intimacy, trusting, and emotionally open. • Positive sense of self. • Balances intimacy, dependence, and independence.	• Supportive and safe environment • Responsive, consistent and predictable adult relationships. • Present, warm, comforting	• Like secure attachment patterns after working through impact of attachment trauma.

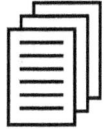

Exploring Relationship Challenges

This worksheet is designed to help you identify and explore your relationship challenges in the context of complex trauma. Take some time to reflect on the questions below and answer them as honestly and openly as possible. There are no right or wrong answers.

1 Describe what it was like growing up when you were young. What were your early attachment experiences like with your primary caregivers?

_____

_____

_____

2 Check the qualities that best describe these relationships.

__ consistent	__ stable	__ punitive	__ comforting
__ inconsistent	__ warm	__ understanding	__ encouraging
__ responsive	__ reliable	__ sensitive	__ intimidating
__ unresponsive	__ cold	__ chaotic	__ frightening
__ predictable	__ neglectful	__ unpredictable	__ overprotective
__ critical	__ supportive	__ controlling	__ affectionate
__ unaffectionate	__ detached	__ engaged	__ dismissive
__ unsafe	__ confusing	__ safe	__ unstable
__ flexibility			

3 How has the quality of your early relationships impacted your ability to regulate your emotions and deal with stress?

_____

_____

_____

4 How has your attachment to your primary caregivers influenced your adult relationships? Can you identify your attachment style?

_____

_____

_____

5 How have your early childhood experiences impacted your relationships with others?

_____

_____

_____

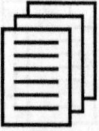

6 Did your early experiences impact your feelings about safety, security, and trust? If so, how?

_____

_____

_____

7 Do you find trusting others and forming close relationships easy or difficult?

_____

_____

_____

8 In what ways have you experienced challenges with trust, emotional regulation, and communication?

_____

_____

_____

9 Are there any specific triggers or events that make it difficult to maintain healthy relationships? How have you coped with these challenges in the past?

_____

_____

_____

10 What can you do more of to improve your relationships? What can you do less of?

_____

_____

_____

11 What steps can you take to address these challenges and build a stronger, Healthy Adult model? What skills or strategies can improve your attachment and relationship patterns and prioritize self-care and emotional regulation in your daily life?

_____

_____

_____

EXERCISE 11.1

Secure Base Visualization

This grounding exercise combines visualization, sensory grounding, and self-soothing to help reinforce a sense of secure attachment.

1 Find a comfortable seated position and close your eyes.
2 Take three deep, slow breaths to center yourself.
3 Visualize a person, place, or object that represents safety and security for you. This could be a loved one, a favorite childhood location, or a comforting item.
4 As you hold this image in your mind, engage your senses:

   - Notice what you can see in vivid detail
   - Imagine any sounds associated with this secure base
   - Feel the textures or sensations you might experience
   - If applicable, recall any scents or tastes

5 Now, focus on the feelings of comfort, safety, and calm that this secure base provides. Allow these sensations to spread throughout your body.
6 Place one hand on your heart and the other on your belly, creating a self-soothing gesture similar to the butterfly hug technique.
7 As you maintain this connection, slowly repeat to yourself: "I am safe. I am supported. I am grounded."
8 Stay with this visualization and the associated sensations for 2–3 minutes or longer if desired.
9 When ready, slowly bring your awareness back to your surroundings, opening your eyes and taking a final deep breath.

References

Artigas, L., & Jarero, I. (2014). *The Butterfly Hug Method for Bilateral Stimulation.* https://emdrfoundation.org/toolkit/butterfly-hug.pdf.

Bowlby, J. (1969). Attachment and Loss: Volume I Attachment, Second Edition. New York: Basic Books.

Corry, J. & Gladstone, G. (2022). *Schema Chemistry Analysis Workbook,* The Red Flag Project. theredflagproject.com.

Fisher, J. (2017). *Healing the Fragmented Selves of Trauma Survivors: Overcoming Internal Self-Alienation.* New York: Routledge/Taylor & Francis Group.

Fonagy, Peter & Campbell, Chloe & Bateman, Anthony. (2017). Mentalizing, Attachment, and Epistemic Trust in Group Therapy. *International Journal of Group Psychotherapy.* 67. 176-201. 10.1080/00207284.2016.1263156.

Johnson, S. (2019). Attachment in action – changing the face of 21st-century couple therapy. *Current Opinion in Psychology,* 25, 101–104.

Karantzas, G. C., Younan, R. & Pilkington, P. D. (2023). The associations between early maladaptive schemas and adult attachment styles. *Clinical Psychology: Science and Practice,* 30(1), 1–20. https://doi.org/10.1037/cps0000108

Main, M., & Hesse, E. (1990). Parents' unresolved traumatic experiences are related to infant disorganized attachment status: is frightened and/or frightening parental behavior the linking mechanism? In M. T. Greenberg, D. Cicchetti, & E. M. Cummings (Eds.), *Attachment In The Preschool Years: Theory, Research, And Intervention.* Chicago, Illinois: The University of Chicago Press, 161–182.

Olufowote, R., Fife, S., Schleiden, C., & Whiting, J. (2020). How can i become more secure? A grounded theory of earning secure attachment. *Journal of Marital and Family Therapy,* 46(3), 489–506.

Siegel, D. J. (2022). Understanding and Treating Disorganized Attachment and Dissociation (Live Course). Los Angeles, CA: Mindsight Institute.

van der Kolk, B. A. (2005). Developmental trauma disorder: toward a rational diagnosis for children with complex trauma histories. *Psychiatric Annals,* 35, 401–408. https://doi.org/10.3928/00485713-20050501-06

The Trauma Triangle

The Trauma Triangle

The Trauma Triangle is a framework for understanding how early childhood trauma can shape interpersonal dynamics. The roles of the Trauma Triangle are closely linked to early childhood experiences and attachment relationships. Introduced initially as the Drama Triangle (Karpman, 1968), this model describes how troubled individuals switch between the roles of Victim, Rescuer, and Persecutor within the same relationship, contributing to the development of maladaptive behavioral patterns and the perpetuation of dysfunctional relationships. These patterns are often reflected in the themes of responsibility, power, boundaries, and control.

> Jane has primary responsibility for her home and the family's needs. She puts her needs and wants last as she sacrifices to meet those of her family (rescuer-compliant surrenderer role). She is very demanding and self-critical through internalized messages from the past, such as "you are lazy (if you relax)" or "you are not good enough" (persecutor/inner critic). Jane eventually begins to feel resentful, unappreciated, and used (rescuer/self-pity/victim mode). When she tries to express this to her husband, he tells her that she is imagining things, that she is crazy, and that there is no problem. He becomes angry at her when she expresses these feelings (victim role). At this point, Jane blames and judges herself for asking too much (persecutor/flagellating over controller). She shuts down and feels helpless to change the situation (helpless surrenderer/self-pity/victim role).

The above example vividly demonstrates the fluidity of roles in the Trauma Triangle. As one interacts, the roles shift seamlessly from victim to persecutor to rescuer, depending on the nature of the interaction or the roles others adopt. This dynamic interplay fuels each role, eliciting coping modes and creating an illusion of protection from further trauma. However, in reality,

DOI: 10.4324/9781003462958-23

each role keeps a survivor trapped in the traumatic experience and prevents actual needs from being met.

Goals

1 Understand how trauma influences the development of different roles in relationships.
2 Recognize how the roles in the Trauma Triangle play out in current relationships.
3 Identify how the role of the Healthy Adult offers a positive alternative to those in the Trauma Triangle.
4 Develop and implement strategies to move into the Recovery/Empowerment triangle and foster healthier relationships.

Procedure

1 Mindfulness: **Exercise 12.1 Role Awareness Meditation**
2 Check-In.
3 Discuss how the roles in relationships reenact past trauma. Explain how these patterns relate to concepts of dysregulation (inability to manage emotions), disruption (interference with healthy functioning), distortion (misinterpretation of reality), disconnection (lack of emotional intimacy), and defenses (protective mechanisms).
4 Discuss how each role reflects a coping mode. How has this helped or hindered them from getting their needs met? **Handout 12. 1 Breaking the Cycle** can guide this discussion.

   (In this context, the use of the term "victim" is not intended to diminish the experiences of individuals who have been through trauma. Instead, each label recognizes the protective coping function and survival value inherent in each role due to past traumatic experiences. These terms are not intended to overlook or minimize the strength, resilience, and agency instrumental in overcoming adversity).
5 Encourage group members to share their observations about their roles in relationships. What do they notice as they flip into different modes? How do these modes show up in group interactions? Foster a non-judgmental and non-blaming atmosphere to ensure open and honest discussion.
6 Ask group members to complete **Handout 12.2 Strengthening the Healthy Adult Mode: Supporting Your Vulnerable Child Mode.** Discuss with the group.
7 Summarize the main takeaways from the group discussion.
8 Check-out.
9 Grounding: **Exercise 12.2 Strengthening the Healthy Adult Mode.**

Main Themes

The Trauma Triangle emphasizes the dynamics of trauma and abuse as it focuses on roles in relationships that reflect a lack of control, power differentials, unhealthy boundaries, and emotional instability. The triangle identifies patterns of behavior in unhealthy relationships that are reenactments of trauma-based survival behaviors and coping responses.

Attachment

The roles in the triangle are closely linked to early childhood experiences and attachment styles. Attachment style is based on the relationship formed with primary caregivers during the first few years of life. Internal working models develop primarily through early interactions with caregivers. Positive experiences with responsive caregivers lead to positive views or internal working models, while negative experiences with unreliable or neglectful caregivers result in negative representations. For example, an infant with a responsive parent will likely see themselves as worthy of comfort and others as available to support when needed. In contrast, the infant with an unresponsive parent may view themself as unworthy of care and attention without the expectation that others will reliably provide the support they need.

The internal working models formed through early attachment experiences play a crucial role in shaping how individuals perceive themselves and others in relationships. These models align with the roles in the Trauma Triangle and influence which roles are assumed in adult relationships. People with secure attachment are more comfortable with intimacy and autonomy. They have healthier relationship patterns and better emotional regulation skills that help them navigate relationships outside the triangle dynamics. Adverse experiences and insecure attachment styles (anxious, avoidant, and disorganized) can predispose individuals to adopt specific roles within the Trauma Triangle. For example, individuals with histories of early childhood trauma may feel disempowered and taken advantage of (a victim role), focus on others' needs at the expense of their own (rescuer role), or become overly judgmental, critical, and controlling (persecutor role).

Anxiously attached individuals may seek co-regulation from others and feel powerless without external support. They may overinflate their needs and what others must do to meet them, reflecting their fear of abandonment. They may unconsciously seek out situations or partners that reinforce their belief that they are powerless or mistreated (Victim role). Someone in the Rescuer role may prioritize and take responsibility for another person's needs, often neglecting their own. Those with an avoidant attachment may be critical of others, using perceived flaws to justify maintaining emotional distance, suppressing emotions, and avoiding intimacy (Perpetrator role).

Liotti (2004) proposed that disorganized attachment, often resulting from early traumatic experiences with caregivers, creates a complex working model for how individuals view themselves, others, and relationships. He suggested that children with a disorganized, fearful-avoidant attachment may view themselves and their attachment figures in all three roles of the Trauma Triangle. A central aspect of Liotti's theory is the role of dissociation in trauma and disorganized attachment. This dissociative process can help explain why individuals may unconsciously oscillate (flip) between all three roles in the trauma triangle without fully integrating their experiences, reflecting the push and pull of their yearning for and fear of closeness.

Triangle Roles and Coping Modes

Childhood trauma can significantly affect attachment and intimacy in adult relationships and lead to reenacts of these roles. Individuals may unconsciously seek out unhealthy relationships that mirror their childhood experiences, recreating familiar dynamics. Adults who engage in Trauma Triangle dynamics often find themselves stuck in repetitive, unhealthy patterns of interaction. They can unconsciously flip between roles, perpetuating negative interactions and conflicts, leading to chronic relationship problems. "The point of the trauma (drama) triangle is that none of these positions is an authentic way of relating. They are all, in the language of schema therapy, coping modes" (Edwards, 2015, p.3).

The three roles can be understood as different schema coping modes. The rescuer may be seen as a compliant surrender mode; the persecutor as a Bully and Attack mode, a Self-Aggrandizer that puts itself above others by being disdainful of them, or a self-righteous Scolding Overcontroller. The victim role lends itself to the Self-pity/Victim mode (Edwards, 2012). The 'poor me' victim role protects one from shame and self-criticism. However, these coping modes keep the person out of touch with their actual needs.

Flipping between modes may explain the fluid nature of role-switching in the trauma triangle. Movement between these roles frequently escalates conflicts rather than working toward constructive solutions. The roles often lead to feelings of shame and guilt, blaming others or denying responsibility, making it challenging to address and resolve the underlying issues. For example, someone in the rescuer role may shift into a persecutor role or victim role if they become resentful and feel mistreated (see Figure 12.1).

Persecutor

"I'll hurt you before you hurt me".

- Defensive, angry, rageful. Reactive
- Control through criticism and punishment.
- Contemptuous, judgmental, hostile, abusive.
- Rigid boundaries. Create distance to avoid pain and emotional vulnerability.
- "I feel safest when I am in control."

Bystander

"It doesn't involve me".

- Passive
- Uninvolved
- Distances self

The Trauma Triangle

Lack of control

Unhealthy Boundaries

Instability

Victim

"Poor me." "Why me?"

- Powerless, helpless, distrusting
- Vulnerable, overwhelmed.
- Limited agency for change
- Little motivation to help self.
- "I feel safest when others take care of me."
- Weak boundaries
- Dependent

Rescuer

"I will take care of you".

- Focus on needs of others.
- Loose boundaries
- Self-sacrificing, overextends themselves.
- Feels guilty when not helping.
- High expectations of others. May feel unappreciated, leading to resentment and burnout.
- "I feel safest when I care for others and avoid focusing on my own needs."

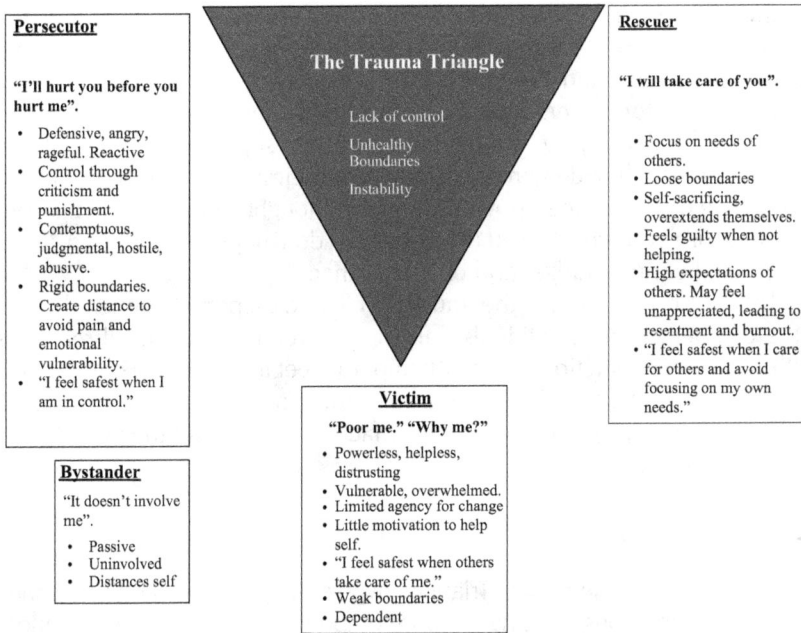

Figure 12.1 The Trauma Triangle

Victim, Rescuer and Perpetrator

The inverted triangle represents three aspects of the victim, no matter which role is assumed in the triangle (Lac & Donaldson, 2022). It places the victim (please help me) in the bottom corner, with the rescuer (you need my help) and the persecutor (you are helpless; it is all your fault) both on the top of the triangle. Sometimes, a fourth role of bystander is added, as the role, perhaps, of the parent who failed to protect from abuse. This may be reenacted when individuals do not defend themselves in present-day relationships.

The Victim (Self Pity/Victim mode) lacks agency and control and avoids acknowledging painful and frightening feelings of powerlessness, persecution, helplessness, and shame. Everyday thoughts of the victim might include: "There is nothing I can do," "I cannot cope on my own," "Poor me," "I am not ok, and everyone else is," "Nothing will ever change," "I feel safe when others take control and help me."

The Rescuer/Caretaker (Compliant Surrender mode) feels good about themselves when rescuing another, neglecting their needs and problems. Rescuers are self-sacrificing and often feel unappreciated and guilty if they do not "help" others (even when that help is not wanted). Caregiving appeases others as a way to meet their needs. Common thoughts might include: "Let me help you." "You are not OK, I will fix you," "I am the only one who can help," "I feel safe when helping others," "You will love me if I take care of you," and "You need me."

The Persecutor (Inner Critic mode) is critical, angry, resentful, dominating, bossy, rigid, bullying, self-aggrandizing, and superior. Lashing out and blaming others, they deny responsibility for their actions and discount the destructive quality of their power. Common thoughts include, "This is your fault because you are..." "You are not ok, so do what I tell you," and "I feel safe when I control, judge, and criticize others."

The three roles entrench the trauma cycle and perpetuate unhealthy patterns of interaction. Individuals can flip between any of the three roles within a given interaction as they attempt to meet their needs. For example, a victim may lash out and become a persecutor, or a rescuer may become a victim if their help is rejected or if they face backlash from the person they are trying to help.

Breaking the Cycle

Moving away from the Trauma Triangle involves taking responsibility for one's actions and emotions, leading to more empowered and balanced relationships. Awareness of one's tendencies to adopt specific roles is the first step in breaking the cycle. Strengthening the Healthy Adult mode is central to breaking the cycle of dysfunctional relational patterns reflected in the Trauma Triangle. The healthy adult mode is self-reflective and can acknowledge the impact of the past while emphasizing their resilience and strength. The healthy adult confidently embraces adult responsibility and accountability, sets clear boundaries, and trusts others to make their own choices and decisions while remaining flexible, compassionate, and supportive. As this mode strengthens, the individual can gain a balanced perspective outside the triangle roles.

Targeting dysfunctional schemas (e.g., fears of abandonment, self-sacrifice, feelings of powerlessness, or helplessness) that contribute to prioritizing others' needs over one's own helps individuals break out of Victim or Rescuer roles. They can focus on their needs and emotions and nurture and protect their vulnerable self. Edwards (2015) suggests that accessing the Healthy Adult is the only way to get off this merry-go-round. Only the Healthy Adult can disidentify from the roles of the trauma triangle, recognize them for what they are, and find healthy alternative ways to respond to the other person.

Victim (Helpless, Self Pity Mode)	Rescuer (Savior/ Compliant Surrender Mode)	Perpetrators (Bully/Overcompensating Controller/Inner Critic Modes)	The Healthy Adult Mode	Bystander Detached Protector Modes
"I can't cope on my own". "Poor me. I'm not ok and everyone else is". "I feel safe when I submissive".	" I am worthy when I help others." "You need my help. You are not OK, "I must save you". "I feel safe when I rescue/enable others".	"I know best". "I will hurt you before you hurt me". "I get to feel safe by controlling, dominating hurting others, putting them down."	"I am hopeful and capable of taking care of my needs in a healthy way". "I am physically and emotionally safe, I am connected and appropriately trusting of others".	"It does not involve me."
Overwhelmed by own vulnerability. Doesn't take responsibility for own power. Gives up control.	Neglects own needs and vulnerability; self-sacrificing. Fears being abandoned, unloved, unneeded if they stop helping. Takes control of situation.	Dominates and controls. Bully, abusive, contemptuous, critical, judgmental, hostile. Avoids personal responsibility and blames others. Self-aggrandizing. Takes control of situation	Responsible to and for self. Embraces adult responsibility. Makes choices that help decrease helplessness, shame, and defeat. Holds self and others accountable.	Passive witness, uninvolved. Detached.
Feels helpless, hopeless, powerless, ashamed.	Feels angry, resentful, guilty, anxious, unappreciated.	Feels angry, resentful, bossy, dominating, critical, unpleasant; defensive, guarded, rageful, self-righteous, also feels inadequate.	Feels strong, capable, confident, action oriented, self-compassionate.	Feels distant, detached.
Discounts own capacity to think and act for themselves.	Discounts capacity of others to think and act for themselves. Creates dependency and indispensability. May offer help even when not asked for or needed. Results in burnout, resentment, feeling unappreciated.	Discounts capacity of others to think and act for themselves. Aggressor controlling victim Retaliates, believing that it is what the victim deserves.	Trust others to make their own choices and decisions. Empowers others to ask for what they need rather than deciding for them.	
Feels let down by rescuer; increases demands	Works hard to "help" others, even when doesn't want to, even when others don't want help, and doesn't ask what they need to be supported.	"This is your fault; You are not ok, but I am so do what I tell you".	Sets clear boundaries and prioritizes their own needs. Flexible, compassionate, supportive, reflective.	
Goals are to acknowledge own vulnerability and strengths, minimizes self-pity and take personal responsibility.	Goals are to take responsibility for self, connect with their power while acknowledging own vulnerability, establish clear boundaries and provide choices.	Goals are to recognize own their power, rather than being afraid of it, or use it covertly and to establishes clear structure, boundaries and expectations.	Goals are to accept responsibility for oneself, allow clear choices and boundaries and accept vulnerability" **How can I get what I really want in a healthy way?**	

Figure 12.2 The Roles of the Trauma Triangle

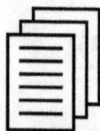

HANDOUT 12.1

Breaking the Cycle

Healing through Safety, Connection, and Coping

Taking responsibility for your actions can change the damaging trauma-based patterns that may be re-enacted in current relationships and prevent your needs from being met. How does each role of the trauma triangle play out in your relationships? What can you do differently to move from a position of helplessness, self-sacrifice, or control to one of responsibility, choice, and accountability?

1 **Where is the drama in your life?** Give an example of a time you found yourself in each role of the trauma triangle. (Refer to the diagram and chart for reference). Can you identify the mode you were in?

   a Victim: _____

   _____

   b Rescuer: _____

   _____

   c Persecutor: _____

   _____

2 How were these patterns helpful in the past? _____

   _____

3 How are they unhelpful today? _____

   _____

4 What can you do differently to move out of the roles of the trauma triangle into healthy adult relationships?_____

   _____

   _____

   _____

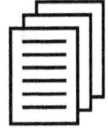

Strengthening the Healthy Adult Mode: Supporting Your Vulnerable Child Mode

1 Label your emotions in the current situation:

   a *Describe your feeling* (e.g., "I am feeling anxious and scared").

   _____

   _____

   _____

2 Validate your emotions:

   a *How can you validate your current emotions?* (e.g., "These emotions are understandable and normal. Relationships are very important to me. It is part of my value system that those relationships reflect respect, love, and appreciation. I want those qualities to be part of my relationships, and it is ok to feel nervous when I sense their absence").

   _____

   _____

   _____

   b *How can you understand your feelings in the context of your personal history?* (e.g., "These emotions are understandable and normal because of my personal history. When I was younger, I often felt that others did not respect or appreciate who I was or what I needed. These needs were often rebuffed, and I felt something was wrong with me").

   _____

   _____

   _____

3 Care for yourself:

   a *What skills can you use to care for yourself?* (e.g., "As a healthy adult, I can manage my emotions. As I reflect upon my feelings and consider my needs, I can calm myself, be mindful of my feelings, and visualize myself asking for what I need. I can also remember that I cannot control how another person receives what I say").

   _____

   _____

   _____

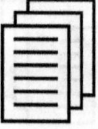

b *What skills can you use to take care of yourself in your relationships?* (e.g., " As a Healthy Adult, I can prepare to speak up for myself and assert my needs. I can write out what I need in my relationships in a way that is more likely to get those needs met and not react in the moment. I can practice what I want to express before I speak with my partner").

_____

_____

_____

Adapted from: van der Wijnhaart (2015). Healthy Adult Mode: Ways to Strengthen the Healthy Adult of Our Patients. ISST Bulletin. Germany: International Society of Schema Therapy.

EXERCISE 12.1

Role Awareness Meditation

This exercise helps group members become more aware of their roles in their relationships and how those roles may relate to the trauma triangle (victim, rescuer, and persecutor).

1 Ask group members to sit comfortably facing a partner.
2 Invite them to close their eyes and take several deep breaths to synchronize their breathing.
3 Suggest that they silently reflect on the following questions:

   - What role do they tend to play in relationships?
   - Does their role change depending on the relationship?
   - When might they act as a victim, rescuer, or persecutor?
   - How does each role affect their interactions?

4 After a few minutes, ask the group to open their eyes. Have them take turns sharing their insights.
5 Discuss ways group members can support each other in breaking free from unhealthy roles and fostering more balanced relationships.

EXERCISE 12.2

Strengthening the Healthy Adult Mode

(Hayes & Brockman 2022)

1 Find a comfortable position and close your eyes. Take a few deep breaths to relax your body and mind.
2 Imagine yourself in a peaceful setting, perhaps a serene garden or a quiet mountaintop. As you look around, you notice a figure approaching—this is your Healthy Adult self. As your Healthy Adult approaches, notice their confident posture, straight shoulders, and heads held high. Listen to their reassuring voice and see the calmness in their eyes and the strength in their stance. Feel the warmth and strength of their presence, the confidence, wisdom, and compassion emanating from them.
3 Now, imagine stepping into your Healthy Adult self. Feel your posture straightening and your breathing becoming steady. Experience a sense of inner calm spreading through your body as you notice a feeling of strength and resilience growing within you.
4 Visualize yourself facing a challenging situation. As your Healthy Adult self, practice these three steps: 1. Acknowledge and validate your emotions. 2. Assess the situation rationally. 3. See yourself taking appropriate action with confidence.
5 As you continue to embody your Healthy Adult, say to yourself. "I am calm, confident, and capable." Feel the sense of accomplishment and inner peace as you visualize yourself successfully navigating various life situations.
6 Slowly bring your awareness back to your surroundings. Open your eyes, carrying the essence of your Healthy Adult with you.
7 Practice this visualization regularly to strengthen your connection to your Healthy Adult Mode.

References

Edwards, D. J. A. (2012). *Overcoming Obstacles to Reparenting the Inner Child*. Workshop presented at the International Society of Schema Therapy Conference, World Trade Center, New York.

Edwards, D. J. A. (2015). Self-pity/victim: a surrender schema mode. *Schema Therapy Bulletin*, 1, 3–6.

Hayes, C., & Brockman, R. (2022). Strengthening the healthy adult mode. *schematherapytrainingonline.com*. https://schematherapysociety.org/techniques

Karpman, S. (1968). Fairy tales and script drama analysis. *Transactional Analysis Bulletin*, 7(26), 39–43.

Lac, A., & Donaldson, C. D., (2022). Development and validation of the drama triangle scale: are you a victim, rescuer, or persecutor? *Journal of Interpersonal Violence*, 37(7–8): NP4057–NP4081. https://doi.org/10.1177/0886260520957696

Liotti, G. (2004). Trauma, dissociation, and disorganized attachment: three strands of a single braid. *Psychotherapy Theory: Research, Practice, and Training*, 41, 472–486.

van der Wijnhaart, R. (2015). *Healthy Adult Mode: Ways to Strengthen the Healthy Adult of Our Patients*. ISST Bulletin. Germany: International Society of Schema Therapy.

Shame and the Inner Critic

Shame and the Inner Critic

> *Rachel never realized what was happening in her home was unusual or different from her friends' homes. "We were told not to talk about what was happening at home. One day, however, when visiting a friend, I saw his mother tousling his hair and affectionately kissing him. That never happened in my home. I suddenly understood that the beatings I got were not the norm elsewhere. How could I know what was 'normal' or 'not normal,' inappropriate or abusive? That was all I knew. I didn't understand why I was being beaten. I thought I deserved it. I felt so defeated".*

The experience of early childhood trauma is characterized by silence, isolation, disconnection, loss, and lack of control. As survivors came forward to disclose their experiences and the veil of secrecy began to lift, we began to learn more about the profound effect of these early experiences and the impact of shrouding them in secrecy. Trauma results in the loss of safety, trust, innocence, family, a normal childhood, identity, and self-worth that perpetuates secrecy, isolation, and disconnection. The inability to speak about the trauma feeds internalized messages of difference and defectiveness that lead to a profound sense of shame and guilt (Brown, 2010; Collin-Vézina. 2015; Alaggia, et al., 2019). Shame, guilt, and the internalized messages of the inner critic are closely related. Group therapy becomes a powerful tool to help mitigate the impact of secrecy, isolation, disconnection, and loss that makes one want to hide away. Breaking the silence within a "cocoon" of others who share similar experiences diminishes feelings of isolation, alienation, shame, and guilt.

Goals

1 Understand the relationship between shame and the inner critic.
2 Identify the functions of the inner critic.

DOI: 10.4324/9781003462958-24

3 Understand why self-compassion is an antidote to shame and the inner critic.
4 Learn ways to quiet the inner critic voice.

Procedure

1 Mindfulness Exercise: Ask the group to practice combining breathing with self-compassion: "Focus on your breath, noticing the physical sensation of breathing in and out. On each inhale, acknowledge your current experience in body, emotions, and thoughts. On each exhale, offer yourself relief or kindness, as you would to a close friend. Continue this pattern, breathing in awareness and breathing out self-compassion."
2 Check-In.
3 Ask the group "How do you relate to yourself when the going gets tough? Ally or enemy?"

> *Consider this situation: There may be two types of parents: one, a critical parent who judges your efforts and criticizes your mistakes. A second parent supports your efforts even when imperfect and works with you to correct errors. Where would you learn best? Who would motivate you more? Why? What happens when that 'critical parent' is the voice in your head? What function does this voice serve? Why do we readily accept the voice of the 'inner critic'? How might you respond if a child told you they were a failure because of a small mistake? How can you convey the same message to yourself?*

4 What is the relationship between shame and the common messages of the Inner Critic? Discuss the cognitive distortions.
5 Discuss the functions of the Inner Critic. Explore how group members identify and challenge their inner critic. What are the messages of their Inner Critic? Refer to the NICABM Idiographic "**Shame vs. Guilt: Understanding the Difference**" https://www.nicabm.com/shame-guilt-client-handout/. Review **Handout 13.1 Talking About Shame and Guilt.**
6 Choose a group exercise to practice challenging the Inner Critic mode. Identify and challenge the myths about self-compassion. **Exercise 13.1 Challenging the Inner Critic's Messages or Exercise 13.2 Compassionate Chair Work With the Critic Mode.**
7 Debrief and discuss the members' reactions and observations to the exercise.
8 Review strategies for practicing self-compassion and quieting the inner critic. Emphasize that developing self-compassion in the face of the inner critic takes patience and practice. "It is a journey, not a destination,

and your commitment to this process will significantly change how you relate to yourself."

9 Summarize the main takeaways from the group discussion.
10 Check-out.
11 Grounding: Suggested practice: **The Self-Compassion Break Meditation** (Neff & Germer, 2018; Germer and Neff, 2019). https://self-compassion.org/self-compassion-practices/).

Main Themes

Shame and guilt are ordinary, universal, and human emotions that confront the threat of disconnection and rejection. Experiencing them does not make someone inherently flawed or weak. "Healthy shame" teaches us how to behave acceptably and fit in with our community. It motivates us to change unhealthy behaviors and mend missteps to avoid disconnection. Guilt motivates repair for a behavior that is wrong or harmful to others. It is an adaptive emotion when it encourages the repair of mistakes. When justified, it does not challenge a person's overall sense of worthiness—"What I *did* was bad," not "I am bad." (Figure 13.1)

Shame becomes toxic when it becomes part of a person's identity, leading them to believe they are inherently defective, inadequate, and unworthy. It often originates in childhood experiences, mainly through repeated exposure to shaming or traumatic events. Its constant presence becomes embedded in a person's self-concept, defining how they view themselves and their place in the world, believing "I am bad (shameful, unworthy)" rather than "I did something terrible (shameful, unworthy)". While it may have been initially a mechanism for self-protection and social regulation, it loses its adaptive value when shame becomes toxic. It can lead to dysfunctional relationships and social isolation (Nathanson, 1992).

Persistent self-judgment and self-punishment reinforce the chronic feelings of unworthiness, inadequacy, and self-hatred. Shame is the pain felt when one believes one is flawed and unworthy of love and belonging (Brown, 2021 Chen et al., 2024). Guilt is often intertwined with shame in the context of complex Post Traumatic Stress Disorder (PTSD), further exacerbating beliefs about self and relationship difficulties. Guilt becomes pernicious when *unjustified* and self-punishing. Unjustified guilt may include guilt for surviving or not suffering as much as another or believing they deserved or caused what happened. "If I had acted differently, I could have prevented it."

Shame and guilt form the core of complex Post Traumatic Stress Disorder (CPTSD). These interpersonal, unpleasant, self-conscious, and self-critical emotions stemming from early emotional neglect, abuse, or betrayal become internalized as feelings of being flawed, unworthy, or unacceptable.

SHAME vs. GUILT

Understanding the difference

SHAME

Shame is feeling bad about yourself as a person.

I am worthless.
Unlovable..
Broken..

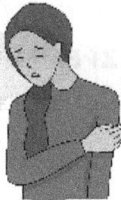

I AM BAD.

GUILT

Guilt is feeling bad about what you did.

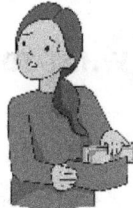

I DID SOMETHING BAD.

WHY DO WE EXPERIENCE SHAME?

Shame is a defense mechanism. It is a way we learned to keep ourselves safe from harm in the past.

It served an important purpose in the past – it kept us safe. But now it may cause problems in our lives and relationships when we no longer need that shame to keep us safe.

Shame can be a way we blame ourselves for something that happened to us that wasn't our fault.

When we feel ashamed, we may feel we can control our safety by controlling our actions and beliefs.

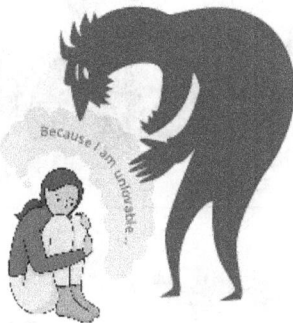

Because I am unlovable..

nicabm
www.nicabm.com

P. 1

Figure 13.1 Shame vs. Guilt

SHAME vs. GUILT
Understanding the difference

WHY IT MATTERS

When we understand the differences between these powerful feelings, we begin to understand and eliminate negative self-judgments and self-talk.

WHAT TO DO WHEN YOU EXPERIENCE ...

SHAME

• Exercise self-compassion.
• Recognize shame as a survival tactic.
• Seek healthy connections with others.
• Talk to your therapist.

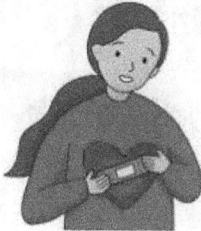

GUILT

• Admit you are wrong.
• Take responsibility.
• Seek forgiveness.
• Change your behavior.

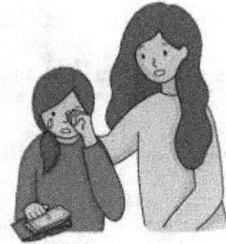

nicabm
www.nicabm.com

P. 2

Figure 13.1 (Continued)

"The abusive and/or neglectful relational misattunement disrupts ongoing developmental growth and binds attachments to abusive caregivers. This shame based relational frame becomes a template for subsequent relationships and self-definitions" (Hohfeler, 2025, p.1).

It is not uncommon to hear statements such as *"I feel damaged, dirty, infected; I deserved it"* or *"I just wanted to forget about it. It was not that big a deal. I dealt with it myself"*, *"I feel unwanted,"* *"I feel like it was it was my fault,"* or even *"How do I explain what happened when I do not understand and am so confused about it? Others will blame and abandon me if they know"*. Efforts to hide from the feelings linked to the trauma lead to coping strategies such as dissociation, substance use, avoidance, or hypervigilance.

Shame and dissociation combine as a protective way to self-regulate, which limits emotional awareness. Individuals can hide from life and themselves to avoid further rejection, humiliation, and criticism. This contributes to the development of a negative self-image and hinders one's ability to form healthy intimate connections, cope with trauma-related symptoms, and maintain emotional well-being.

The Inner Critic modes are the critical, shaming, or demanding voices heard in childhood that become internalized as a challenging and perfectionistic inner critic in adulthood. The inner critic keeps us small and "safe" from perceived threats, potential failures, humiliation, embarrassment, and demanding standards by attacking perceived flaws and shortcomings that might lead to social rejection, failure, or harm. This self-critical voice berates as it echoes the harsh, shaming messages of criticism, failure, rejection, high expectations, or abuse received from others. The critic maintains attachments, contains unexpressed rage, prevents rejection, attacks the self before anyone else can, avoids failure, and provides motivation and control. Perfectionism and refusal to accept mistakes is an attempt to fight the inner critic's voice. Common messages might include, "My parents loved me. I was the problem"; "It is my fault, not my (abusive) father's"; "I attack myself since I cannot get angry at others"; "I won't be attacked or rejected if I keep my head down"; "I'll punish myself first before others can hurt me"; "I won't risk failing if I put myself down"; "I won't do anything if I don't drive myself", "I can't control others, but I can control myself" (Brockman & Behary, 2023; Startup & Breidis, 2024). Common shame and guilt-based beliefs might include "I am bad, unlovable, unworthy, or not good enough"; "There must be something wrong with me." "I cannot seem to do anything right" and "I should have... (done something different)". Internal shaming and self-criticism breed more shame and guilt, creating a vicious cycle that fuels critical self-evaluation, self-doubt, and insecurity. (Paradoxically, the inner critic may be activated after positive experiences or achievements. It can undermine feelings of joy, satisfaction, or self-worth. Good feelings are seen as risky or undeserved).

The Inner Critic can be expressed as Introjected Parent messages and a self-attacking coping mode (the Flagellating Overcontroller (Simpson, 2020). When people believe they are defective or worthless, the inner critic protects them from doing anything that would further hurt and shame them. The self-attacking coping mode redirects anger that might be directed at parents and invites further abuse that may help keep the family stable. This protective instinct helps navigate social situations more effectively and avoid unnecessary risks when balanced. The harmful effects of the inner critic can be mitigated by reframing its purpose as an ally (perhaps misguided) rather than an enemy. Challenging the inner critic, "This was the best way of coping then, but it is not helpful, even harmful now," allows it to morph into a friend with a new job description (Edwards, personal communication, 2025).

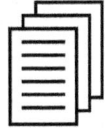

Talking about Shame and Guilt

Shame and guilt thrive in secrecy and isolation. The less we talk about these emotions, the more powerful they become and the more control they have over our lives. They are about the fear of disconnection (Brown et al., 2011; Brown, 2012). The person hides their feelings of defectiveness and fears that something about them or something they did would prevent them from connecting with others. Am I good enough? Am I worthy of connection? Change occurs when we develop a more compassionate relationship with our feelings of shame and guilt. We are seen when we talk about these feelings, name them, own them, and share them. Shame needs light and air; it loses power when spoken.

(DeYoung, 2015, p. 116)

1 **What thoughts, feelings, and physical sensations do you experience when you experience shame and guilt?**

_____

_____

- **Shame and guilt often result in intolerable feelings in the body.** *Physical sensations such as a dry mouth, a pounding heart, and a sinking feeling of doing something wrong may arise. Thoughts like "I am not good enough" or "I'm a bad person"? may arise, as well as urges to run and hide from situations and relationships that trigger these feelings.*

2 **What triggers your feelings of shame and guilt?**

_____

_____

- *Is it a feeling of failure to meet certain expectations? For instance, does looking different from the accepted "norm" trigger body shame? Are these expectations valid or unhealthy and unrealistic? Is this something to be ashamed of? Perfectionism and high expectations for oneself are often evident in statements such as "I should not make mistakes" or "I should be strong."*

3 **What are some of your unhealthy reactions when you feel shame or guilt?**

_____

_____

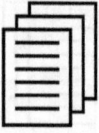

- *In traumatized individuals, it is not the effect of shame itself that impacts relationship difficulties but responses to managing the feeling. Responses such as distancing from others, working to please, or shaming others do not help develop self-empathy or foster feelings of worthiness and self-acceptance.*

4 **How does talking about your feelings of shame and guilt help or hurt you?**

_____

_____

- *Avoiding talking about these feelings may cause them to fester and go unchecked. Their power diminishes when you shed light on them and address them openly. Consider the costs of hiding parts of yourself from others. "What would it feel like if you could be yourself, sharing all these aspects of who you are, and still feel accepted by others?" "Could people accept you even knowing this about you? And what would that be like?" (Padesky, 2021). Sharing these feelings answers the lonely question, "Am I the only one?" with a resounding, "No, you are not alone." (Hartling et al., 2000).*

EXERCISE 13.1

Challenging the Inner Critic's Messages

While challenging the inner critic mode can be difficult, group support allows members to confront their internalized critical messages while strengthening their "Good Parent" (Healthy Adult) mode.

This exercise asks group members to write negative messages about their inner critics on a cloth or paper parent effigy. Once they have written down the messages, the effigy is removed, emphasizing its powerlessness to harm. The members then write "good parent" messages on a similar figure. The group then explores how it felt to challenge and remove the inner critic's negative messages, replacing them with "good parent" messages (Farrell & Shaw, 2012).

EXERCISE 13.2

Compassionate Chair Work with the Critic Mode

(Startup & Breidis, 2024)

1 Ask a volunteer to participate in an experiential chair work exercise with the inner critic mode. Ask the other group members to observe their reactions during the exercise and note similarities to their experiences.

2 Ask the volunteer to describe a situation in which they experienced shame or blame.

3 Identify the modes involved: Critic and the Healthy Adult

4 Set up chairs with the critic in one chair, the patient in the Healthy Adult chair (their usual chair), and the group sitting around them in a circle.

5 Ask the group member to sit in the critic mode chair and guide her to speak from this side: "Be this side for a moment; what is this side of you saying?" Ask the client what it is like to sit in the critic chair; what emotions and physical sensations are they feeling? (If this becomes too dysregulating, have the client remain in their original chair).

6 Explain that the purpose of the exercise is to get to know the critic better, but not to get rid of it. Compassionately enquire about the purpose of the Critic, its origins, and the experience of fulfilling that role. The following questions can guide the conversation:

a Tell me about your role, purpose, and goals.

b What makes it essential to do what you do?

c What do you fear might happen if you stopped?

d Do you model yourself on anyone in X's life? Are you the voice of someone familiar?

e How old was X when you came to be? What was happening then?

f Is there more you would like us to know?

g What is it like for you to carry all that responsibility for X's success/ safety, etc. (whatever the critic's purpose is)?

h How old do you feel X is now? What if you found out that he was x years old? How would that change how you think about/treat him?

i What would it be like if there was someone else helping you with this important task? What if I told you other parts/modes might have some ideas, too? (Introduce the Critic to the Healthy Adult Mode).

7 Remember, the purpose of the exercise is relationship building with the Critic and you/other parts of the client, rather than "winning" or outarguing the Critic. Keep your tone neutral, nonjudgmental, open-minded, and filled with genuine interest and curiosity.

8 If the Critic agrees, arrange a meeting between the Critic and the client's Healthy Adult (HA) mode. Have the client move into the Healthy Adult Chair. What would the HA like the Critic to know? How can the HA mode help the critic in their task? Notice what happens and facilitate a dialogue. See if the Critic and HA can negotiate to share the responsibility of caring for the Vulnerable Child's needs. (If the Critic mode resists meeting the HA, acknowledge this mode's willingness to share up to this point and suggest meeting the HA another time). At the end of the exercise, ask the Critic and the HA to continue their conversation at home to get to know one another better (e.g., imagining conversation for 5–10 minutes/day).

9 Debrief the experience with the volunteer and the other group members. What did they notice in their reactions? What did it feel like from the Critic's Perspective? From the HA perspective? How might the Critic and HA continue the conversation? What might be a challenge?

References

Alaggia, R., Collin-Vézina, D., & Lateef, R. (2019). Facilitators and barriers to child sexual abuse (csa) disclosures: a research update (2000-2016). *Trauma Violence Abuse*, 20(2), 260–283. https://doi.org/10.1177/1524838017697312

Brockman, R., & Behary, W. (2023). Taming the inner critic modes: a contextual schema therapy approach. *Schema Therapy Bulletin*, Summer.

Brown, B. (2010). Shame hates it when we reach out and tell... https://atomicquote. com/author/brene-brown/quote/shame-hates-it-when-we-reach-out-and-tell-our-story-it-hates-having-words-wrapped-around-it-it-cant-survive-being-shared-shame-loves-secrecy-the-most-dangerous-thing-to-do-after-a-shaming-exp

Brown, B. (2012) https://brenebrown.com/videos/ted-talk-listening-to-shame/

Brown, Brené, (2021). *Atlas of the Heart: Mapping Meaningful Connection and the Language of Human Experience*. New York: Random House.

Brown, B., Hernandez, V. R., & Villarreal, Y. (2011). Connections: A 12-session psychoeducational shame resilience curriculum. In R. L. Dearing & J. P. Tangney (Eds.), *Shame in the Therapy Hour*. Washington, DC: American Psychological Association, 355–371. https://doi.org/10.1037/12326-015

Chen, X., Dai, B., Li, S., & Liu, L. (2024). Childhood maltreatment, shame, and self-esteem: an exploratory analysis of influencing factors on criminal behavior in juvenile female offenders. *BMC Psychology* 12, 257. https://doi.org/10.1186/s40359-024-01758-x

Collin-Vézina﹐ D., De La Sablonnière-Griffin, M., Palmer, A. M., & Milne, L. (2015). A preliminary mapping of individual, relational, and social factors that impede disclosure of childhood sexual abuse. *Child Abuse & Neglect*, 43,123–134. https://doi.org/10.1016/j.chiabu.2015.03.010

DeYoung, P. A. (2015). *Understanding and Treating Chronic Shame: A Relational/Neurobiological Approach*. New York: Routledge/Taylor & Francis Group.

Edwards, D. A. (2025). Personal communication.

Farrell, J.M & Shaw, I.A. (2012). *Group Schema Therapy for Borderline Personality Disorder: A Step-By-Step Treatment Manual with Patient Workbook*. New York: John Wiley and Sons.

Germer, C. & Neff, K. (2019). *Teaching the Mindful Self-Compassion Program: A Guide for Professionals*. New York: Guilford Press.

Hartling, L., Rosen, W., Walker, M., & Jordan, J. (2000). Shame and humiliation: from isolation to relational transformation. *Wellesley Centers for Women*, 88, 1–4.

Hohfeler, R. A. III. (2025). Shame as affect regulation in dissociative identity disorder. *Journal of Trauma & Dissociation*, 26(2), 218–238. https://doi.org/10.1080/15299732.2024.2448419

Nathanson, D. L. (1992). *Shame and Pride: Affect, Sex, and the Birth of the Self*, First Edition. New York: W.W. Norton.

Neff, K. & Germer, C. (2018). *The Mindful Self-Compassion Workbook*. New York: Guilford Press.

NICABM (2021). *Shame vs. Guilt: Understanding the Difference Idiographic*. Storrs, CT: NICABM, National Institute for the Clinical Application of Behavioral Medicine. https://www.nicabm.com

Padesky, C. (2021). *Questions That Can Help Your Clients Talk About Shame*. Storrs, CT: NICABM, National Institute for the Clinical Application of Behavioral Medicine. https://www.nicabm.com/questions-that-can-help-your-clients-talk-about-shame.

Simpson, S. (2020). Manual of Group Schema Therapy for Eating Disorders. In S. Simpson & E. Smith (Eds.), *Schema Therapy for Eating Disorders: Theory and Practice for Individual and Group Settings*. London: Routledge, 136–184.

Startup, H., & Breidis, J. (2024). Schema therapy for complex trauma: an experiential skills masterclass. *Schema Therapy School*. Workshop presented May 16-17, 2024.

Session 14

Self-Compassion

Trauma disrupts a person's ability to develop self-compassion, with shame and self-criticism turning up as frequent visitors. The Inner Critic's voice can be excessively critical, demanding, and judgmental. Continually "beating oneself up" makes regulating emotions and managing stress difficult. Compassion provides a buffer against the harmful effects of trauma. It is a powerful antidote to the inner critic as it challenges the toxic self-talk with kindness, acceptance, understanding, and caring. Instead of being controlled by the inner critic, self-compassion empowers us to recognize and validate emotional needs, develop a nurturing inner dialog, and respond to ourselves with kindness when distressed.

Practicing self-kindness, common humanity, and mindfulness directly contradicts the core beliefs and emotional experiences underlying harsh judgments and criticisms. Self-kindness diffuses the power of the cycle of toxic self-attack (shame feeds the inner critic that then perpetuates more shame through relentless self-criticism) and counters the core belief of "I am bad" or "I am not good enough." Mindfulness creates space to observe the inner critic's thoughts and feelings of shame with acceptance and non-judgment. We can become aware of the inner critic without being overtaken by it. Recognizing our common humanity reminds us that everyone struggles and makes mistakes. It does not mean we are fundamentally flawed or unworthy if we do. Meeting the thoughts of the Inner Critic from a kinder, more compassionate, Healthy Adult mode helps heal the relationship one has with oneself and with others.

Goals

1 Highlight the role of self-compassion in healing trauma.
2 Understand how self-compassion challenges the role of shame and the inner critic.
3 Identify Neff's three components of self-compassion.
4 Challenge the five myths commonly believed about self-compassion.

DOI: 10.4324/9781003462958-25

5 Understand the interrelationship of self-compassion and the Affect Regulation Model.
6 Understand the importance of cultivating the soothing system for reassurance and comfort.
7 Identify ways to practice self-compassion.

Procedure

1 Mindfulness: Suggested practice: **Finding Loving-Kindness Phrases** (Germer, 2019, https://www.mindful.org/find-loving-kindness-phrases/). This is a pen-and-paper exercise rather than an informal practice for use in daily life. It is designed to help discover personally meaningful loving-kindness and compassion phrases. If one already has phrases and wishes to continue using them, they don't need to find new words.
2 Check-In: Review the critical points of Neff's Self-Compassion (Kindness, Common Humanity, and Mindfulness) and Gilbert's Affect Regulation Model (The threat, drive, and soothing/caregiving systems) (*Figure 14. 1*). Compare and contrast each approach.
3 Explore how self-compassion supports healing from trauma. Discuss how both models of self-compassion reduce the disruption caused by emotional dysregulation and the activation of survival defenses. How does this affect the brain, body, relationships, and sense of self?
4 Introduce the practice of self-compassion as an antidote to shame and the inner critic. How can the Healthy Adult mode counteract these messages? Refer to **Handout 14.1 Quieting The Voice Of The Inner Critic.**
5 Summarize the main takeaways from the group discussion.
6 Check-out.
7 Grounding: Suggested practice: **Building the Compassionate Self** (The Compassionate Mind Foundation) (https://soundcloud.com/compassionatemind/building-the-compassionate-self?in=compassionatemind/sets/compassionate-minds&utm_source=clipboard&utm_medium=text&utm_campaign=social_sharing). This exercise cultivates self-compassion by developing a compassionate inner voice or self. It activates the soothing system in the brain, creates a more supportive inner dialog, cultivates self-compassion to counter self-criticism, and enhances emotional regulation and resilience.

Main Themes

Self-compassion is rooted in the evolution of caring motives and behavior, seen initially as evolving from the challenges of reproduction and caring for offspring. Caring evolved to provide a source of protection, a secure base to offer support, encouragement, and guidance, and a safe haven that provides ways of regulating threats (and sometimes drives) and emotions that have become destabilizing or overwhelming (i.e., attachment) (Gilbert, 2020). General components of compassion have been identified as the recognition of the universality of suffering, feeling sympathy, empathy, or concern for those who are suffering (emotional resonance), tolerating the distress associated with witnessing suffering, and being motivated to alleviate the suffering (Strauss et al., 2016). Self-compassion helps regulate the complex emotions associated with pain and suffering. Recognizing and accepting that pain and suffering are normal parts of the human experience allow us to approach the pain and reduce the suffering, buffering against the harsh messages and fear-based protection of the inner critic.

Models of Self-Compassion

Mindful Self-Compassion

Mindful Self-Compassion (Germer & Neff, 2019) conceptualizes self-compassion as turning compassion inward in a kind and understanding way rather than being harshly self-critical when we fail, make mistakes, or feel inadequate. This involves three key components: **Self-kindness vs. Self-judgment** (being caring and supportive toward oneself when experiencing difficulties rather than harshly critical), **Common Humanity vs. Isolation** (suffering and imperfection are part of the shared human experience, something we all go through, not something that happens to "me" alone) and **Mindfulness vs. Over-identification** (being present, balanced, non-judgmental, and receptive with one's thoughts and emotions without over-identifying or being swept away by negativity). Neff (2015) describes the five myths often associated with self-compassion (Neff, 2015):

Self-compassion is a form of self-pity. In reality, self-compassion makes us more willing to accept, experience, and acknowledge complicated feelings with kindness and is an antidote to feeling sorry for ourselves. *Self-compassion means weakness*. Rather than being a weakness, self-compassion is one of the most potent sources of coping and resilience. "It's not just what you face in life, but how you relate to yourself when the going gets tough—as an inner ally or enemy—that determines your ability to cope successfully." *Self-compassion will make me complacent*. Self-compassion does not undermine our motivation to push ourselves to do better but motivates us more effectively than self-punishment. *Self-compassion is narcissistic*. Self-compassion is not self-esteem (an evaluation of self-worth that requires feeling better than others). It is kindly accepting our imperfections, especially when we fail or feel inadequate. *Self-compassion is selfish*. Being good to yourself helps you be good to others. When we give ourselves compassion, we create a protective buffer, allowing us to understand and feel for the suffering person without being drained by their suffering. Neff emphasizes the shared human experience and self-kindness.

Drive, excite, vitality

Content, safe, connected.

Incentive/resource-
focused

Non-wanting/
Affiliative focused

Threat-focused
Protection and
Safety-seeking

Threat-based

Sadness

⇕

Shutdown

Anger, Anxiety, Disgust

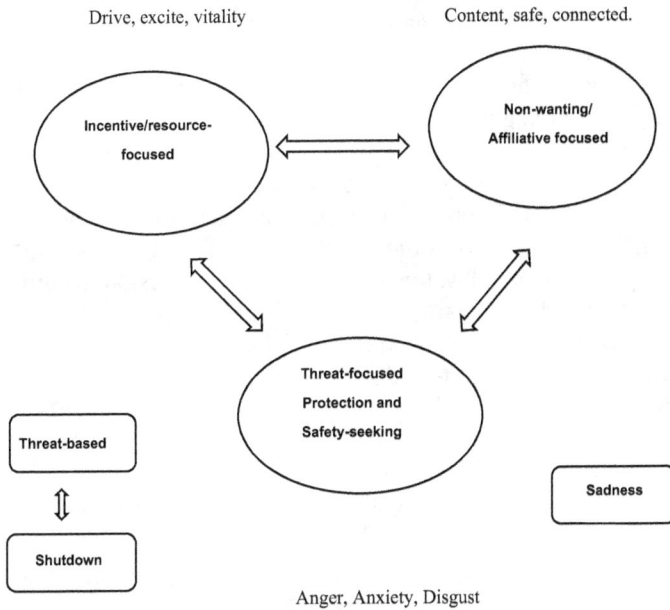

Figure 14.1 The Three Functions of Emotion: Drive, Protection, and Soothing Gilbert, P., & Simos, G. (2022). Compassion-focused therapy: Clinical practice and applications with permission from Routledge. Adapted from Gilbert, P. (2010) The Compassionate Mind (Constable). © P. Gilbert

Compassion-Focused Therapy

Gilbert (2010) has proposed that humans move between three major emotion regulation systems (the threat, drive, and soothing/caregiving systems) to help manage their emotions. The **Drive System** motivates and energizes us to acquire resources, pursue goals, and achieve. It gives us feelings of excitement, anticipation, and joy. The **Threat System** plays a role in detecting perceived threats. It is designed to overreact and respond aggressively to potentially ambiguous threats, prioritizing survival over pleasurable pursuits. It can become easily dysregulated, causing distress in situations that are not currently threatening. The **Soothing System** regulates emotions and restores balance. It provides a respite by downregulating the physiological arousal of the threat system's fight-or-flight response and the drive system's frustration when goals are blocked, or resources cannot be acquired. The threat and drive systems are often overactive, and distress results from an imbalance between these overactive systems and the underactive soothing caring system. Individuals may rely on the drive system to "fix" perceived threats through excessive striving, perfectionism, or unhealthy coping mechanisms like substance use when the soothing system is underdeveloped. Self-compassion activates the soothing system and counterbalances the overactive drive and threat systems. A balanced state occurs when the three systems interact smoothly—the threat system alerts us to real dangers, the drive system motivates goal pursuit, and the soothing system regulates the threat response and allows for rest/contentment between tasks. Gilbert emphasizes proactive motivation to alleviate suffering through self-kindness and compassionate actions.

Mindful Self-Compassion and Compassion-Focused Therapy (CFT) share several similarities and have some key differences. Both approaches emphasize the importance of cultivating kindness and compassion toward oneself, especially during times of suffering or difficulty. Germer and Neff (2019) emphasize Buddhist psychology and mindfulness traditions, highlighting the three core components: self-kindness vs. self-judgment, common humanity vs. isolation, and mindfulness vs. over-identification. Gilbert's focus on developing the soothing system to balance out the threat and drive systems is grounded in evolutionary psychology and neuroscience. This approach was specifically developed for those with high levels of shame and self-criticism.

Self-Compassion and Early Childhood Trauma

Early Childhood Trauma is associated with lower levels of self-compassion. Clients with histories of trauma present with fears and resistance that hinder self-compassion. Gilbert (2020) considered these the 'intuitive wisdom of protection' (in the activated threat system) that is perhaps embodied in the inner critic's voice. In contrast, higher self-compassion is related to lower posttraumatic stress disorder (PTSD) symptom severity, greater resilience, and better emotion regulation.

Both Neff and Germer's Mindful Self-Compassion (MSC) approach and Gilbert's CFT address the intense feelings of shame and self-criticism that often accompany traumatic experiences. Cultivating self-kindness, common humanity, and mindfulness reduces self-judgment, isolation, and emotional dysregulation. Self-compassion activates the soothing system that counterbalances the overactive drive and threat systems. Both approaches focus on reducing the harsh self-criticism, replacing it with a kinder, more understanding inner dialog, and incorporating body-based interventions to address the physical signs of trauma.

Self-compassion involves being aware of your pain, understanding it is a normal human experience, and directing kindness toward yourself. It helps healing by offering yourself the support and love you deserve. It silences the inner critic and reduces the self-blame and shame often associated with trauma. It fosters self-acceptance and promotes emotional regulation. Self-compassion reduces trauma-related emotional reactivity and promotes a balanced emotional state, resilience, growth, inner strength, self-care, and connections with others (Quirke, 2024).

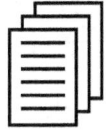

Quieting the Voice of the Inner Critic

Increasing awareness of the inner critic's patterns and messages makes it easier to manage the negative influence. The goal is to reduce the inner critic's power while increasing self-compassion and self-care. Quieting the inner critic is an ongoing practice of questioning the validity of the inner critic mode's unreasonable messages and reframing them in a more balanced, nurturing way grounded in facts. Remember that confronting the critic can be challenging because of the myths about self-compassion and the overactive threat and drive systems. As you strengthen your Healthy Adult mode, you will develop a more compassionate relationship with yourself. Self-compassion is a fundamental shift in how you relate to yourself, particularly in times of difficulty or when facing personal shortcomings.

> *A moment of self-compassion can change your entire day. A string of such moments can change the course of your life.*
>
> Chris Germer (https://chrisgermer.com/about)

1 **Tune into the harsh and judgmental self-talk** when your inner voice is unreasonably self-critical.
2 **Notice what you feel** when you are in a critical or demanding mode (shame, anxiety, hopelessness, frustration). Which situations tend to trigger your inner critic? What emotions are present, and how do they feel in your body?
3 **Label or name the inner critic** to create more distance and separation ("There is that critical voice again," "Judgy Joseph"). Imagine it as an animal or other figure external to yourself.
4 **Identify the need or fear** underlying the critic's harsh words and diffuse its hold by acknowledging its good intentions. Is it trying to protect you from perceived threats like failure or rejection? Where did this voice come from? Is it a familiar message? What is it trying to accomplish?

   a Exercise: Pay attention to that self-critical voice within you. Ask that part, "How are you trying to keep me safe?"; "Thank you. I know you are trying to protect me, but it is not helpful when you judge and criticize me." Can you address those needs rather than attacking?*.

5 **Activate the soothing system**, affiliation, and connection to reduce isolation. **Use soothing self-talk and reassuring affirmations** like "I am not

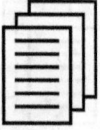

alone in my limitations" or "I am worthy of love and belonging." Diaphragmatic breathing, body scans, or muscle relaxation help calm the body and mind and interrupt negative thought patterns. Remember that everyone sometimes experiences shame, insecurity, and self-criticism (you are part of common humanity).

a Exercise: As you breathe in and out, see if you can allow yourself to enjoy the sensations of breathing. Notice unpleasant emotions, allow them to be momentarily, and then watch them go. Allow in a pleasant sensation and enjoy it as deeply as you can. Repeat for five breaths.*

b Exercise: What would you offer a friend at the end of a hard day that you can offer yourself now?* Treat yourself with the same warmth, understanding, and care you would show a good friend who is struggling. Exercise: Placing a hand over your heart or hugging yourself activates the caregiving compassionate, soothing system. Self-Hug: Wrap your arms around yourself and give yourself a hug for three breaths. Try saying, "I love you just as you are." Notice how these words feel.*

6 **Practice shifting into the Healthy Adult mode** to offer self-compassion when maladaptive modes are activated.

a Dialog with the critical, demanding, shaming part of yourself (threat and drive systems) and the compassionate self (soothing system). Give each "part" a chance to speak from different chairs to better understand their motivations. Give "voice" to the soothing system's perspective of compassion from another chair. Appreciate your successes and positive experiences. The inner critic discounts the positive by dismissing compliments, downplaying successes, or focusing disproportionately on mistakes or flaws.

b Nurture the Happy Child mode by reconnecting with joy and spontaneity, encouraging fun and playfulness, and fostering a sense of fulfillment and zest for life.

i Exercise: Acknowledge progress, not perfection. When did you last do a less-than-perfect job and feel ok about it?

ii Think of a successful experience from your life. How do you deserve credit?*

7 **Schema flashcards:** Encourage yourself with self-kindness when you struggle with self-criticism. ("Others have felt this way before me," "It is ok to be kind to myself," "I can accept that I will make mistakes at times," "This is hard."). Develop personalized, compassionate phrases to

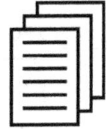

counter negative self-talk. Practice using these phrases regularly, especially when facing challenges or setbacks

8 **Practice compassionate imagery and self-talk** to trigger feelings of safety. Visualize receiving warmth, acceptance, and understanding from a compassionate, wiser, Healthy Adult self. Imagine their words and feelings of care surrounding you with warmth and wisdom, providing them with the compassion they needed but did not receive.

a Exercise: Think of someone who has abundant compassion. Imagine them sending you love right now. Are they saying anything? What is the expression on their face? How does it make you feel? *

*Adapted from Willard et al., 2016.

References

Germer, C. (2019). *Find Your Loving Kindness Phrases*. https://www.mindful.org/find-loving-kindness-phrases/.

Germer, C. & Neff, K. (2019). *Teaching the Mindful Self-Compassion Program: A Guide for Professionals*. New York: Guilford Press.

Gilbert, P. (2010). *The Compassionate Mind: A New Approach to Life's Challenges*. United Kingdom: New Harbinger Publications.

Gilbert, P. (2020). Compassion: from its evolution to a psychotherapy. *Frontiers in Psychology*, 11, 586161. https://doi.org/10.3389/fpsyg.2020.586161

Gilbert, P., & Simos, G. (2022). Compassion-focused therapy: Clinical practice and applications with permission from Routledge. Adapted from Gilbert, P. (2010) *The Compassionate Mind*. Constable. © P. Gilbert https://www.actwithcompassion.com/lovingkindness_for_everyone_in_the_room

Neff, K. D. (2015). The five myths of self-compassion. *Psychotherapy Networker*, 39(5), 30–35.

Neff, K. & Germer, C. (2018). *The Mindful Self-Compassion Workbook: A Proven Way to Accept Yourself, Build Inner Strength, and Thrive*. New York: Guilford Press.

Quirke, M. G. (2024). The synergy between stress and self-compassion in building resilience. *Social and Personality Psychology Compass*, 18(7), e12978. https://doi.org/10.1111/spc3.12978

Strauss, C., Taylor, B. L., Gu, J., Kuyken, W., Baer, R., Jones, F., & Cavanagh, K. (2016). What is compassion, and how can we measure it? A review of definitions and measures. *Clinical Psychology Review*. 47, 15–27. https://doi.org/10.1016/j.cpr.2016.05.004

The Compassionate Mind Foundation. https://soundcloud.com/compassionatemind/building-the-compassionate-self?in=compassionatemind/sets/compassionate-minds&utm_source=clipboard&utm_medium=text&utm_campaign=social_sharing

Willard, C., Abblett, M., & Desmond, T. (2016). *The Self Compassion Deck*. Eau Claire, WI: Pesi Publishing & Media.

Developing Healthy Relationships

Childhood trauma can challenge the ability to form and maintain healthy relationships in adulthood, leaving one feeling insecure and distrustful of others and one's instincts, creating difficulties in emotion regulation, emotional and sexual intimacy, attachment, assertiveness, setting boundaries, and effective communication. Betrayal by those meant to care for and protect shapes expectations for relationships and affects interactions with partners, family, friends, and coworkers. Survivors may find that they are easily triggered in certain situations, misinterpret meanings and intentions, feel misunderstood or that they don't matter, fall into particular roles, push people away, or anxiously cling to them. They may struggle to communicate their needs or be authentic in their interactions. Recognizing the maladaptive patterns characterized by overcontrol, excessive power differential, dependency, subjugation, jealousy, distrust, hypervigilance, contempt, avoidance, or excessive conflict is pivotal in taking control and developing healthy relationships.

Goals

1 Identify the qualities of healthy relationships.
2 Understand how boundaries, roles, trust, authenticity, intimacy, communication, and conflict resolution in current relationships are colored by the "trauma lens."
3 Identify ways to offset the impact of trauma on relational patterns.

Procedure

1 Mindfulness Suggested Practices: **Lovingkindness Meditation** or **Exercise 15.1 Establishing Connections Exercise. Lovingkindness Meditation** has been shown to reduce self-criticism, quiet the inner critic (Shahar et al., 2015), and enhance vagal tone and well-being (Kok et al., 2013). Engaging in compassion and self-love meditations reduces trauma symptoms

DOI: 10.4324/9781003462958-26

and flashbacks (Kearney et al., 2013) and results in improved social relationships (Hutcherson et al., 2008; Don et al., 2022). These can be powerful connecting experiences that help activate peoples' social engagement systems. **Establishing Connections** is a structured group activity that builds the capacity for safe emotional connection, strengthens boundary awareness, develops present-moment awareness during interactions, and reduces relationship anxiety through co-regulation.

2 Check-In.
3 Discuss the characteristics of a healthy relationship.
4 Explore the ways early relational trauma can lead to dysregulation and disconnection in relationships.
5 Review **Handout 15.1 Trauma and Relationships**. Discuss how past beliefs about relationships help or hinder current relationships.
6 Discuss ways to change behaviors that interfere with the development of healthy relationships.
7 Summarize the main takeaways from the group discussion.
8 Check-out.
9 Grounding exercise: **Exercise 15.2 Passing Claps**

Main Themes

A relationship is a state of emotional connection between people. We grow and develop through and toward relationships throughout our lives. There are many different types of relationships with varying levels of intimacy and closeness, as well as different hierarchies and power balances. Our self-worth and sense of self are often grounded in our ability to make and maintain relationships. It takes skill and effort to maintain mutually respectful, trustworthy, and empathetic relationships that share power and influence, manage conflict constructively, encourage independence and self-reliance, set clear boundaries, and encourage direct communication that expresses emotions and vulnerability (Gottman & Silver, 2015).. The Healthy Adult mode (HA) plays a central role in developing and sustaining healthy relationships. It serves as an internal "good parent," promoting empathy in relationships and meeting the unmet emotional needs of the Vulnerable Child mode. The HA helps manage dysfunctional modes and emotional responses by balancing the expression and inhibition of adult and child-mode emotions, which hinder intimacy and connection.

Characteristics of a Healthy Relationship

- **Mutual respect, trust, and empathy** are the cornerstones of healthy relationships. Openness and responsiveness to another's individuality, opinions, and boundaries create a space where partners can feel safe and vulnerable with each other. Consistency, honesty, and reliability build trust. Trauma survivors may struggle to trust others, fearing betrayal or harm. This can make it challenging to form close bonds or maintain existing relationships. Miscommunications and misunderstandings can activate defensive modes and create heightened tension, distancing, and disconnection (Campbell & Renshaw, 2018; Wang, et al, 2017). Understanding these dynamics can help foster healthy relationships.

- **Empowerment** is power with, not over another, where all involved contribute, grow, and benefit. Trauma often results in beliefs that one is powerless and that it is safer to surrender to the other person's demands.

- **Authenticity** is honesty, genuineness, and trust that allows expression of the true self. Trauma may make it feel unsafe to be vulnerable and "unmask" the true self. When the other person fails to respond empathically, we turn away. To maintain some semblance of a relationship, we learn to keep parts of ourselves to ourselves and not risk showing our true selves.

- **Intimacy** is a strong emotional connection and physical affection (as appropriate for the relationship type) that allows vulnerability and openness to private thoughts and feelings. Trauma can lead to difficulty managing emotions that affect not only the individual but also their loved ones (Beck, et al, 2009). Mood swings, irritability, or emotional numbness can make it challenging for partners to connect emotionally. Coping with a roller coaster of emotions (emotional breakdowns, intense anger, irritability, sadness, or numbness) can make others feel like they must walk on eggshells to avoid potential landmines.

  Survivors of sexual trauma may experience difficulties with physical intimacy, potentially dissociating or having extreme emotional reactions during intimate moments. Sex can be experienced as shameful or frightening or as currency to appease others or get needs met.

  Interest in social or sexual activities diminishes. To cope with trauma-related symptoms, individuals may engage in avoidance behaviors that can push partners away or create distance in relationships. The people in your life may feel hurt, frustrated, or angry themselves. They may also detach to avoid conflict or engage in hostile interactions that have the potential to escalate reenactments of past abusive dynamics.

  The HA mode contributes to deeper emotional connections in relationships by addressing unmet emotional needs and fostering self-awareness. Its ability to nurture fondness and admiration facilitates a turning toward each other instead of turning away. It helps build an "emotional bank account" to be drawn upon during conflict.

- **Independence and autonomy**: The two-legged model of relationships describes how we need the leg of assertiveness and autonomy (the "me") and the leg of attachment (the "we") to be balanced in a healthy relationship (Roediger, 2024, personal communication). Trauma may cause relationship boundaries to become too porous, allowing over-dependence or repetition of unhealthy relationship patterns from the past, or too rigid, preventing the connection by pushing others away. Both styles can strain the relationship.

- **Establishing clear boundaries and limits and asserting needs** is asking for what you need and want in the relationship straightforwardly ("I" statements) and being specific about your boundaries and expectations. Trauma can impact a person's sense of self-worth, making it difficult to set healthy boundaries or advocate for their needs in relationships. When past needs are unmet, asking for what you need may be challenging. You may sacrifice your needs to please others and avoid negative consequences. You may feel unworthy of love or healthy relationships.

- **Open communication** is crucial in establishing boundaries. Partners can express themselves freely and listen actively to each other. There is a willingness to engage and turn toward the other person with full attention and presence. Trauma survivors may struggle to express their needs and desires, often because they've internalized negative messages or learned that their needs don't matter.

- **Conflict resolution**—The central paradox is that ruptures (misunderstandings, hurts, disappointments, letting one another down) occur in every relationship. It is not so much that a conflict arises, but more importantly, how it is repaired. **Trauma** can cause a person to be constantly on high alert, which may manifest as overprotectiveness or perceiving threats where none exist. This can create tension and misunderstandings in relationships. Conflict is inevitable in close relationships, and disagreements can be handled constructively without blame, abuse, or manipulation. Empathic, caring responses allow honest, open communication that helps repair any ruptures. Once we turn toward the other person, the connection is re-established, and the relationship is strengthened. The goal is not to eliminate conflict but to deal with it effectively. Psychologist John Gottman states that only about 30% of problems in a relationship will be resolved. The HA helps manage conflicts more effectively by providing a balanced perspective and promoting healthier coping strategies to solve problems that can be solved while recognizing that it is not necessary to solve all problems. Making and receiving repair attempts quickly and compromising overcome the gridlock that represents chronic perpetual relationship problems (Powling, et al., 2024).

- **Honesty, transparency, accountability, ethical actions, and cooperation** are central to healthy relationships. Ask yourself: Is the other person trustworthy? Do they keep promises? Do they consider your needs? Do they have similar values? When another person's presence and vibe communicate calm and comfort, you intuitively feel safe as the relationship provides a sense of reassurance and security.

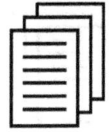

Trauma and Relationships

Early childhood trauma shapes fundamental beliefs about relationships and other people. When people are supposed to care for and protect you and instead hurt and betray you, knowing whom you can trust and what is safe and acceptable in relationships becomes confusing. Many of your early beliefs helped you survive when growing up but may interfere with the development of healthy relationships today.

1 Check which of the following beliefs you identify with.

--- It is not safe to rely on other people.
--- I can't trust anyone.
--- I can't trust myself to know what is safe and acceptable in relationships.
--- I have lost interest in social or sexual activities.
--- Sex is shameful, aversive, and frightening.
--- I feel numb and shut down and tend to avoid painful feelings.
--- It is hard to feel connected when I feel numb or hypervigilant.
--- I use sex to connect to people.
--- It isn't easy to relax, experience pleasure, and connect to others.
--- I feel tense and detached when I engage with others.
--- I am always alert to being hurt by other people.
--- I often misunderstand other people's intentions.
--- Other people often misunderstand me.
--- People tell me they walk on eggshells around me.
--- I avoid conflict in my relationships.
--- I don't know what being in a healthy relationship means.
--- I don't have the right to ask for what I need.
--- I often find myself involved in hurtful and destructive relationships.
--- I depend too much on other people.
--- I frequently get angry and lash out at people I care about.
--- I'm afraid people will not be there for me when I need them.
--- I enjoy being around many people but don't feel close to any of them.
--- It is important to please others.
--- I prefer to be on my own.
--- I worry that people won't be there for me.
--- It makes me uncomfortable if people get too close.

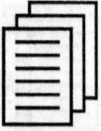

--- It is important that I am in a relationship with someone with the same values.
--- I feel like I wear a mask when interacting with others.
--- No one knows the true me.

2 Which beliefs helped you in the past? Are they still helpful? If so, why? If not, why not?

_____

_____

_____

_____

_____

_____

3 How skills can you use to help change unhelpful patterns?

_____

_____

_____

_____

_____

EXERCISE 15.1

Establishing Connections

This structured group activity builds the capacity for safe emotional connection while staying grounded in the present moment. It helps strengthen
boundary awareness, develop present-moment awareness during interactions, and reduce relationship anxiety through co-regulation, essential skills
for healthy attachment. Ask participants to sit in pairs facing each other,
about arm's length apart. Each person should have enough personal space.
Emphasize that participants can modify or stop the exercise at any time.

1 Synchronized Breathing: Partners observe each other's natural breathing
   rhythm and gradually align breathing patterns without forcing anything.
   Ask them to follow the shared rhythm while maintaining their personal
   boundaries.
2 Have partners describe what they mindfully and non-judgmentally
   observe about the present moment, focusing on environmental details
   like sounds, temperature, or lighting.
3 Partners then place their feet firmly on the floor, grounding their connection. Ask them to share one word describing their current emotional
   state while maintaining their presence.
4 Debrief: Participants briefly share their experience and identify helpful
   grounding elements. Normalize the different comfort levels experienced
   by the group. How can they connect this exercise to their daily relationship interactions?

EXERCISE 15.2

Passing Claps

A great way to get participants back in the present moment is to have them do a simple action together. At the end of the group session, invite participants to form a circle and participate in a clapping exercise. Some examples of short exercises:

1 Everyone claps four times and then pauses. Repeat.
2 The leader counts to four repeatedly, while the participants clap when at numbers one and three.
3 One person claps in any sequence. The person next to them repeats the clapping sequence and then passes a new sequence to the next member. This moves on through the group. Go around the circle a couple of times.
4 Have everyone clap ten times, then say a grounding word such as "calm" or "focus."

References

Beck, J. G., Grant, D. M., Clapp, J. D., & Palyo, S. A. (2009). Understanding the interpersonal impact of trauma: contributions of PTSD and depression. *Journal of Anxiety Disorders*, 23(4):443–450. https://doi.org/10.1016/j.janxdis.2008.09.001

Campbell, S. B., & Renshaw, K. D. (2018). Posttraumatic stress disorder and relationship functioning: a comprehensive review and organizational framework. *Clinical Psychology Review*, 65:152–162. https://doi.org/10.1016/j.cpr.2018.08.003

Don, B. P., Van Cappellen, P., & Fredrickson, B. L. (2022). Training in mindfulness or loving-kindness meditation is associated with lower variability in social connectedness across time. *Mindfulness*, 13, 1173–1184. https://doi.org/10.1007/s12671-022-01856-0

Gottman, J. & Silver, N. (2015). *The Seven Principles for Making Marriage Work: A Practical Guide (Revised Edition)*. Chatsworth, CA: Harmony Publishing.

Hutcherson, C. A., Seppala, E. M., & Gross, J. J. (2008). Loving-kindness meditation increases social connectedness. *Emotion*, 8(5), 720–724. https://doi.org/10.1037/a0013237

Kearney, D. J., Malte, C. A., McManus, C., Martinez, M. E., Felleman, B., & Simpson, T. L. (2013). Loving-kindness meditation for posttraumatic stress disorder: a pilot study. *Journal of Traumatic Stress*, 26(4), 426–434. https://doi.org/10.1002/jts.21832

Kok, B. E., Coffey, K. A., Cohn, M. A., Catalino, L. I., Vacharkulksemsuk, T., Algoe, S. B., Brantley, M., & Fredrickson, B. L. (2013). How positive emotions build physical health: perceived positive social connections account for the upward spiral between positive emotions and vagal tone. *Psychological Science*, 24(7), 1123–1132. https://doi.org/10.1177/0956797612470827

Nortje, A. (2020). 10+ Mindful Grounding techniques. https://positivepsychology.com/grounding-techniques/

Powling, R., Brown, D., Tekin, S., & Billings, J. (2024). Partners' experiences of their loved ones' trauma and PTSD: an ongoing journey of loss and gain. *PloS One*, 19(2), E0292315. https://doi.org/10.1371/journal.pone.0292315

Schwartz, A. (2018). Grounding. Https://Drarielleschwartz.Com/Grounding-Dr-Arielle-Schwartz/

Shahar, B., Szsepsenwol, O., Zilcha-Mano, S., Haim, N., Zamir, O., Levi-Yeshuvi, S., & Levit-Binnun, N. (2015). A wait-list randomized controlled trial of loving-kindness meditation program for self-criticism. *Clinical Psychology and Psychotherapy*, 22(4), 346–356. https://doi.org/10.1002/cpp.1893

The Real Recreational Therapist (2018). Group Therapy Grounding Exercises. Https://Kevingctrs.Com/Group-Therapy-Grounding-Exercises/

Wang, F., Edwards, K., & Hill, P. (2017). Humility as a relational virtue: establishing trust, empowering repair, and building marital well-being. *Journal of Psychology and Christianity*, 36(2), 168–179.

Making Sense of It All
Recovery, Reconnection, and Integration

There is a wholeness about me. I feel like I am no longer floating but am steady and real. A feeling of belonging, not just being. For 52 years, I have lived so fragmented and distant from the world, afraid that some-thing terrible would happen, needing to run away and let other parts take over. This led to more chaos, irritation, frustration, rage, and sad-ness. I am learning that all feelings, good and bad, are part of being human – of being alive and a real person.

(George, 2022)

The impact of early childhood trauma is not all negative, and there is hope for post-traumatic healing, reconnection, integration, recovery, and growth. It does not have to be a life sentence; it can lead to the discovery of inner strength, resilience, and growth (Herman, 1992; Levine, 1997; Courtois, 2014).

Central to a healing process that helps survivors make sense of their experiences is the construction of an organized, coherent narrative from the often fragmented, disjointed, and chaotic memories of the early trauma. As group members move from passive victims to active participants, they begin to understand how their early trauma has shaped their current lives, beliefs, and behaviors. As they recognize recurrent trauma responses, they start to realize that their early experiences no longer need to dictate how they live their lives. The past happened to them, but it is not happening now. They can begin to feel increased control and power over their lives as they are no longer pulled back into the past and begin to live in the present and look toward the future. It is important to remember that, while painful, trauma can also be a powerful force for positive change and a catalyst for continued growth and self-discovery. As the group nears its end, participants appreciate that trauma does define their entire life. Together, they can celebrate their achievements and recognize their strength in surviving and coping with trauma.

DOI: 10.4324/9781003462958-27

*Note that many group members may not be in phase three of treatment at the end of the group. This session highlights the potential for positive change and growth following traumatic experiences to help clients develop a more optimistic outlook on their recovery journey.

Goals

1 Understand the importance of the reconnection and integration phase of recovery. Identify the tasks of this third phase of healing.
2 Understand how each member has made sense of their experiences, how trauma has shaped their lives, and how it can be integrated into their life story.
3 Review the growth and progress throughout the group, highlighting the achievements and growth of each member.
4 Explore participants' visions for their future and identify ways to continue healing.
5 Identify different responses to the pending termination.

Procedure

1 Mindfulness Exercise (group choice).
2 Check-In.
3 Explore critical points about recovery, reconnection, and integration through the quotes about recovering from trauma.
4 Discuss what post-traumatic growth (PTG) means for each group member.
5 Explore how post-traumatic recovery and growth result from increased integration of functioning and reduce the disruptive and dysregulating effects of trauma. Discuss the reiterative spiral from trauma recovery.
6 Discuss what each member has learned about themselves and the impact of their early traumatic experiences. Identify each member's growth and progress throughout the group.
7 Review **Handout 16.1 Your Healing Journey: Recovery, Reconnection And Integration.**
8 Discuss ways to continue healing and identify personal goals as each group member moves forward in their recovery.
9 Practice **Exercise 16.1. Future-Oriented Imagery.** (Mentally visualizing optimistic future scenarios can counter the adverse effects of traumatic experiences. Some may find it difficult to imagine a positive future when they believe their lives have been significantly limited by their trauma. This exercise introduces a strength-based future scenario that imagines the HA self as a powerful resource. Exercises of this type can help instill hope and agency as they reduce fear and anxiety associated

with trauma, motivate recovery efforts, and enhance skills to manage triggers and challenging situations).

10   Identify personal goals as each group member moves forward in their recovery.

11   Explore feelings about pending termination.

12   Final exercise: **Exercise 16.2 The Stone Ceremony.**

13   Check-out

Main Themes

Reconnection and Integration

The third stage of trauma recovery is typically called the reconnection and integration phase, where the individual moves from helplessness and isolation to empowerment and reconnection. This stage focuses on helping the individual reintegrate into their life and society after recognizing and understanding the effects of their trauma. "The survivor no longer feels possessed by her traumatic past; she is in possession of herself" (Herman, 1992, p. 202). During this third phase, with a sturdier Healthy Adult mode, the individual develops greater self-acceptance and self-compassion, appreciating things that might have been taken for granted. Personal needs and values are recognized as the sense of self stabilizes. Increased trust leads to healthier relationships that reflect choice, transparent but permeable boundaries, and personal responsibility. Challenging old trauma-based beliefs, maladaptive schema, and dysfunctional coping modes lead to new ways of being. Fine-tuning self-regulatory skills helps manage stress more effectively with increased personal strength, confidence, emotional balance, and self-control (Tedeschi & Calhoun, 2004, Collier, 2016).

Post-traumatic Growth

PTG describes the positive psychological changes that occur after a struggle with traumatic and highly challenging life circumstances. It is not resilience or "bouncing back." It refers to what can happen when someone experiences a traumatic event that challenges his or her core beliefs, endures psychological struggle, and then ultimately finds a sense of personal growth. PTG focuses on five key domains: personal strength, new possibilities, stronger relationships, appreciation of life, and spiritual change and growth (Tedeschi & Calhoun, 2004). It is about the person evolving into a stronger, more resilient version of themself, and not just returning to their pre-trauma state. New learning and skill development (emotional awareness, expression, and modulation) lead to higher levels of functioning in different life spheres (Doherty & Scannell-Desch, 2023).

With increased stability, a better grasp of the impact of their past and a toolbox of resources to help modulate their emotions, participants can address the traumatic material with less post-traumatic impairment. They can shift their focus to present-day life issues (developing relationships that allow vulnerability and increased intimacy, mourning the losses endured because of the trauma, and forming a new system of meaning and beliefs that allows them to live in the present) and develop a life that is less affected by the trauma and its consequences.

Healing is not linear and usually proceeds in starts and stops as a recursive back-and-forth spiral. Clients will advance and relapse as they heal. Resolution of complex trauma does not have a defined endpoint, but as they heal, the effects of trauma no longer dominate their daily life. Even as they move forward, some may struggle with the extent of the dysfunction and pathology of their past, recognizing that they may never have had the opportunity for a "normal" life. Healing may involve revisiting earlier stages as issues are revisited repeatedly along the spiral. Growth occurs alongside the ongoing challenges with the understanding that although setbacks still occur and old ways of coping may help get through the day, new skills lessen trauma's hold.

Developing a Vision for the Future

Introducing the concept of PTG early in treatment can provide hope and motivation for individuals struggling with complex trauma. Helping clients envision a future beyond their current struggles increases optimism, direction, and purpose for the future. Trauma recovery can be seen as more than symptom reduction; it is also about personal development and finding new meaning in life. Participants can look back on their goals for participating in the group and look forward to what they next want to achieve. They can think about how to apply their new skills and insights. As the group works together to explore feelings of abandonment, grief, fear, and loss that might arise near its end, members can also work on developing a new vision for the future. They can identify ways they have grown or become stronger and find ways to continue building upon those strengths (Wagner et al., 2016).

Termination

As members transition out of the supportive group environment, group leaders can ensure the group's impact continues beyond its end by summarizing trauma-related themes discussed in the group and reinforcing the skills and insights gained during their time together. Reviewing progress is a vital part of the group's closure. Encourage each member to evaluate their progress: Have they achieved their goals? What can they take away from the group? Has it been useful? If so, how? If not, why not? This self-reflection reinforces the value of the group experience.

Provide sufficient time for processing termination. Group leaders may choose to allow two sessions for processing termination and exploring feelings and potential losses that some members may experience with the group ending. As the group ends, remind group members that the healing journey continues. How might they continue moving forward? What does healing mean to them? Provide members with additional resources, ongoing sources of support, and coping strategies they can use after the group ends.

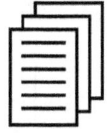

Your Healing Journey: Recovery, Reconnection and Integration

The recovery and reconnection phase is about integrating your past experiences and moving forward. At this point in your journey, you can acknowledge that the past happened; it happened to you, but it is not happening now. Your past experiences no longer drive your behaviors; instead, you can focus on the present and look toward your future. (If you have not yet reached this point in your journey, imagine how you would like it to look).

1 What does "the past happened, it happened to me, but it is not happening now" mean to you?

2 How have you changed or grown since beginning your healing journey? How has your perspective on your trauma changed over time?

3 What have been some of the most challenging aspects of your recovery journey?

4 How have your beliefs about yourself and others changed as you have grown to understand the impact of your early experiences?

5 How have your ideas about relationships evolved?

6 In what ways do you feel more empowered or in control of your life now?

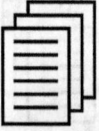

7 How do you handle triggers or difficult emotions when they arise now?

_____

_____

8 What self-care practices have become essential parts of your routine?

_____

_____

9 What do you imagine life beyond trauma looks like? What goals do you have for yourself moving forward?

_____

_____

10 What is your image of your Healthy Adult self? Draw it or write about it.

EXERCISE 16.1

Future-Oriented Imagery

Future-oriented imagery rescripting is used to reinforce the ability of each participant's HA side to meet their needs directly. In imagery, the group members can practice new behaviors to bypass coping mode responses to typical triggering situations (adapted from Simpson & Smith, 2020).

1 "Please close your eyes and identify when you felt connected to your HA side.
2 Anchor the felt sense of this side in the body (e.g., confident, standing tall, and calm).
3 Now imagine a triggering situation. Use all your senses (sight, smell, hearing, touch, and body sensations) to identify the cues that typically trigger your old coping behaviors.
4 Reconnect with your HA side—how would this part of you manage the situation differently (to bypass self-destructive patterns and meet the needs of your vulnerable child)?
5 Invite your HA side to speak to the person (or coping mode) in the image calmly and assertively, expressing the needs of the vulnerable child mode.
6 Let this unfold like a movie, and notice what arises. How does it feel? How does the other person or coping mode respond? How does the vulnerable child react? What does it feel like to act from your HA mode?
7 Open your eyes when you are ready. What did you notice about this experience?"

EXERCISE 16.2

The Stone Ceremony

The Stone Ceremony is a powerful ritual that works well as the final act to close the group. It provides a meaningful way for members to acknowledge their shared journey, celebrate their victories, and say goodbye. Each group member chooses a stone with a word inscribed on it that best captures the meaning of this experience (e.g., strength, resilience, hope, and trust—these inscribed stones are available online). One at a time, each member passes their stone around and receives feedback from the other members and group leaders. The group members share their thoughts and feelings about that member and the progress they have noticed; this ritual allows the group to provide feedback about their shared experience and note the changes in each other. Seeing others positively makes them feel less shame about their experiences and more hope for their future.

References

Collier, L. (2016). Growth after trauma: why are some people more resilient than others—and can it be taught? In *Monitor on Psychology*. Washington, DC: American Psychological Association.

Courtois, C. A. (2014). It's not you, it's what happened to you: complex trauma and treatment. In *Elements Behavioral Health*. Dublin, OH: Telemachus Press.

Doherty, M. E., & Scannell-Desch, E. (2023). *A Conceptual Framework and Model for Posttraumatic Growth. Women's Journeys to Posttraumatic Growth: A Guide for the Helping Professions and Women Who Have Experienced Trauma*. New York: Routledge, 4–8.

Herman, J. (1992). *Trauma and Recovery: The Aftermath of Violence – From Domestic Abuse to Political Terror*. New York: Basic Books.

Levine, P. A. (1997). *Waking the Tiger: Healing Trauma the Innate Capacity to Transform Overwhelming Experiences*. Berkley, California: North Atlantic Books.

Simpson, S., & Smith, E. (Eds.) (2020). *Schema Therapy for Eating Disorders: Theory and Practice for Individual and Group Settings*. New York: Routledge.

Tedeschi, R. G. & Calhoun, L. G. (2004). Posttraumatic growth: conceptual foundations and empirical evidence. *Psychological Inquiry*, 15(1), 1–18.

Wagner, A. C., Torbit, L., Jenzer, T., Landy, M. S., Pukay-Martin, N. D., Macdonald, A., Fredman, S. J., & Monson, C. M. (2016). The role of posttraumatic growth in a randomized controlled trial of cognitive-behavioral conjoint therapy for PTSD. *Journal of Traumatic Stress*, 29(4), 379–83. https://doi.org/10.1002/Jts.22122

Part 3

A Roadmap for Recovery from Complex Trauma

Chapter 10

Recovering from Complex Trauma

Group Therapy for Complex Trauma: A Schema-Informed Approach serves as a vital resource for understanding and treating complex trauma, particularly as it relates to early childhood experiences. Through an integration of Schema Therapy principles and trauma-informed group therapy approaches, it provides a comprehensive framework for clinicians seeking to support individuals grappling with the profound impact of these adverse experiences.

The journey through this group therapy program for Complex Post-Traumatic Stress Disorder (CPTSD) represents a structured, compassionate roadmap for reclaiming agency and rebuilding a life fractured by trauma. It contextualizes the problem within a clinical framework, emphasizing why group therapy is uniquely suited to address the isolation and relational difficulties stemming from CPTSD. Over 20 weeks, participants engage in a transformative process that bridges psychoeducation, experiential learning, and schema-informed interventions, fostering resilience and self-compassion. The program's strength lies in an approach that balances safety, skill-building, and deep therapeutic work while honoring the unique needs of trauma survivors. By combining Schema Therapy principles with trauma-informed care in a group setting, therapists can create an environment that fosters safety, connection, and healing for participants navigating the complex aftermath of their early traumatic experiences.

Several core themes unfold throughout this program that collectively contribute distinct yet interconnected pieces to the overarching framework for understanding and addressing early childhood trauma in a group therapy setting. Each piece provides theoretical depth and practical applications for fostering healing and resilience within a cohesive narrative.

Safety and Connection

Safety and connection are cultivated from the initial sessions, prioritizing a secure and cohesive environment where participants can fully engage in

DOI: 10.4324/9781003462958-29

the group processes without fear of retraumatization. The focus on safety underscores its importance as the cornerstone of practical trauma work. Participants must feel emotionally secure before they can engage in deeper therapeutic work. The groundwork for trust, stability, and collective healing is laid through a predictable structure, clear group guidelines and boundaries, and normalizing shared experiences of trauma.

Impact of Trauma

The exploration of prolonged and repeated trauma in early childhood reveals its profound and enduring consequences, the wide range of symptoms, and complicated presentation. The effects on self-regulation, self-identity, and relational dynamics are addressed throughout the entire book, beginning with discussions about how CPTSD disrupts core aspects of functioning. The concept of the six "D's" (dysregulation, disruption, distortion, disorientation, disconnection, and defensiveness) encapsulates the way trauma fundamentally alters how individuals perceive themselves and the world, disrupting emotions, distorting beliefs and cognitions, disconnecting relationships, disorienting somatic and sensory responses and defending against the pain of the experience. We better understand how attachment and autonomy needs become disrupted when basic needs are unmet, leading to a worldview characterized by mistrust, deprivation, and shame. We can see how these deeply ingrained dysregulation, disconnection, and defensiveness patterns shape an individual's sense of self and interactions with the world. We can understand the wide range of strategies individuals use to protect themselves from the pain of these experiences.

Schema Therapy

Schema Therapy is offered as the theoretical backbone and practical foundation for healing trauma. Its focus on the therapeutic relationship, maladaptive schemas (deeply ingrained beliefs and patterns of behavior that are detrimental to one's well-being), and dysfunctional coping aligns with the relational and identity-based challenges inherent in CPTSD; ST is introduced as a lens through which to understand and treat the maladaptive schemas formed by childhood trauma. Group therapy provides a corrective interpersonal environment for healing. The Group Schema Therapy approach is uniquely structured to resolve CPTSD's core issues. Dysregulation is reduced through psychoeducation and resource development (emotion management, mindfulness, and grounding) as the group's coregulation helps stabilize arousal.

Relationships, Roles, and the Group

The relational aspect of group therapy is a central theme throughout the program. Many of the principles of Schema Therapy have been integrated into this model of group treatment for Complex Trauma to enhance the influence of the group and the strength of its common therapeutic factors (support, belonging, universality, vicarious and observational learning, and instillation of hope). Group settings provide unique opportunities for individuals to experience connection, reduce isolation, and practice healthier interpersonal dynamics. Healing from trauma often requires relational repair, which group therapy facilitates through mutual support and modeled trust. The group acts as a "corrective emotional experience," challenging isolation and shame through shared vulnerability. Members reshape relational templates and internalize healthier attachment dynamics as limited reparenting and empathic confrontation are practiced by the whole group within a supportive cohort. The collective journey from chaos to coherence mirrors the broader trauma recovery arc, reinforcing that healing is not solitary but communal.

The therapist's role within the group is identified as a "good parent," a "healthy adult" model, and a stabilizing anchor, managing intense emotions, fostering cohesion, and maintaining boundaries. The therapist's role is highlighted as both authoritative and empathetic. Balancing leadership with flexibility allows therapists to manage group dynamics while considering both individual and the group's collective needs. Therapists play a pivotal role in modeling trust, authenticity, and emotional stability for participants, providing a reassuring and secure environment for healing.

Therapists and group members alike provide corrective emotional experiences, nurturing unmet childhood needs within therapeutic boundaries. The group mirrors relational dynamics, offering opportunities to practice trust, vulnerability, and assertiveness in a safe space. It reduces isolation through shared experiences that combat shame and stigma and reinforces universality and hope. Peer modeling and co-regulation help members stay within their Window of Tolerance, enhancing emotional regulation during triggering discussions. As emotional triggers are reduced, traumatic narratives can be rescripted through the multiple exercises practiced in the group. Self-defeating behaviors are empathically confronted while understanding and validating their origins. Group feedback challenges maladaptive behaviors (e.g., avoidance or overcompensation) more effectively than individual therapy alone. Moreover, the emphasis on building safety within the group context allows participants to confront their past traumas while developing healthier coping mechanisms supported by their peers and therapists.

This program emphasizes the therapeutic power of shared experiences and mutual support by addressing these issues within an environment where healing can occur. The group provides the container to practice healthier interactions, countering relational distortions and maladaptive schemas perpetuating lifelong issues. Group members learn to identify the self-defeating patterns rooted in unmet childhood needs by learning about ST concepts such as Early Maladaptive Schemes and Schema modes. Specific therapeutic tools like limited reparenting, empathic confrontation, imagery rescripting, and mode dialogues are central interventions in the group. Empathic confrontation softens defensiveness and maladaptive coping without shaming. Mode dialogues and imagery rescripting integrate fragmented self-states into a coherent narrative, reducing identity fragmentation. Exercises throughout the sessions encourage dialogues between dysfunctional modes and the emerging Healthy Adult that foster self-compassion and adaptive responses. Incorporating experiential techniques (mindfulness, grounding exercises, imagery, and the Stone Ceremony) throughout the sessions promotes somatic awareness, enhances participants' ability to navigate their emotional landscapes, and celebrates their progress.

Emotion Regulation

The ability to regulate emotions is repeatedly emphasized as both a challenge for trauma survivors and a key goal of therapy. Emotion regulation resources offered throughout the book equip participants to navigate triggers without resorting to maladaptive coping. The Window of Tolerance and the River of Integration metaphors help members visualize dysregulation (hyper/hypoarousal) and the path to emotional equilibrium as they learn to recognize triggers and practice techniques to help regulate their affect. The focus on widening the Window of Tolerance ensures gradual exposure to distressing emotions within a manageable framework.

Teaching emotional regulation skills enables participants to process trauma safely and effectively. Mindfulness techniques, grounding exercises, and psychoeducation about the Window of Tolerance are critical tools for helping participants manage distress and counteract dysfunctional modes, which are central to developing a Healthy Adult. They foster flexibility and resilience and help clients develop present-moment awareness, expand their Window of Tolerance, and reconnect with their bodies. The concept of the Healthy Adult mode represents a hopeful theme focused on resilience and growth. A strong Healthy Adult mode enables members to adaptively meet their emotional needs, quiet their Inner Critic, and care for their Vulnerable Child mode. Empowering the Healthy Adult mode fosters self-compassion, autonomy, and long-term recovery. Mindfulness expands participants' capacity to process trauma safely by cultivating self-awareness and emotional regulation. The focus on strengthening the Healthy Adult mode provides a hopeful counterpoint to earlier discussions of dysfunction.

The Range of Coping Responses

The complex interplay between trauma and maladaptive coping behaviors like substance abuse or eating disorders is also examined. These behaviors are framed not as failures but as coping mechanisms developed to manage overwhelming emotions caused by trauma. While not designed as a separate protocol, it is essential to integrate psychoeducation about these patterns into group therapy together with promoting healthier coping strategies. It broadens the narrative to include secondary effects of trauma, ensuring that therapy addresses not just core wounds but also their behavioral manifestations. Framing these behaviors as coping modes encourages a compassionate approach within therapy that helps members replace maladaptive coping strategies with healthier alternatives. It shifts the narrative toward recovery and empowerment, highlighting participants' capacity for healing and self-compassion.

Psychoeducation

The structured session protocols outlined in Part Two guide practitioners in facilitating meaningful discussions and interventions that promote emotional awareness, regulation, and recovery. A primary therapeutic goal is cultivating the Healthy Adult mode, which moderates dysfunctional modes, sets boundaries, and fosters self-compassion. The progressive nature of these sessions is designed to meet the client's needs in such a way that strengthens their ability to manage life's stressors and challenges. Psychoeducation on complex trauma, the neurobiology of trauma, the body, memory, attachment, relationships, shame and self-criticism, self-compassion, and post-traumatic growth helps clients increase their understanding of the impact of trauma. It increases their capacity to overcome debilitating emotions such as shame, fear, and mistrust, to increase self-compassion and self-acceptance, to empower a sense of autonomy and agency, and to increase the capacity to set limits and be assertive within healthy and satisfying relationships. An intense, healthy adult mode helps survivors regulate emotions, reframe negative self-concepts, and build healthier relationships. While CBT-based therapies target symptoms, this approach addresses identity fragmentation and relational patterns through schema work.

Recovery and Growth

As the program progresses, the emphasis shifts to recovery and sustaining gains. New knowledge, resources, skills, and a deepened understanding of triggers and strengths help the members recover. They are encouraged to continue practicing the new skills acquired during the group session. Regular use of mindfulness and grounding resources helps to maintain emotional equilibrium while applying relational skills in personal and professional contexts reinforces trust and boundaries.

Trauma recovery is not about erasing the past but integrating it into a narrative of resilience. The themes running throughout the book collectively underscore the complexity of early childhood trauma while offering a roadmap for healing through structured group therapy grounded in Schema Therapy principles. As we move forward in our understanding of trauma treatment, it is essential to recognize that recovery is not linear; it is a complex journey that requires patience, compassion, and a tailored approach to each individual's needs. This book equips therapists with the knowledge and tools necessary for effective intervention and instills hope for those on the path to healing from complex trauma. This book advances trauma care by merging Schema Therapy's depth and complexity with group therapy's relational power. It offers a structured yet flexible framework that prioritizes safety, skill-building, and identity coherence—addressing gaps in traditional models. Focusing on the interplay between schemas and trauma responses delivers the roadmap for sustainable recovery from CPTSD.

The overarching theme presented here is one of hope—despite the deep scars left by early childhood trauma, recovery is possible through compassionate care, relational repair, and skill-building. Safety, connection, emotional regulation, empowerment, and resilience are essential for recovery. While trauma narrows the Window of Tolerance, it cultivates profound strengths—sensitivity, adaptability, and survival. Emphasizing empowerment through schema healing and strengthening the Healthy Adult reinforces this optimistic outlook. Group members transform survival into a testament of courage as they reclaim their stories by nurturing the Healthy Adult and honoring their Vulnerable Child.

We can collectively contribute to a more compassionate and informed approach to trauma recovery by fostering resilience and empowering individuals to reclaim their narratives. With the proper support, they can move from surviving to thriving by regaining their sense of agency and connection. While their work may not be done, they have more tools to light the way. Trauma is about dysregulation, disruption, distortion, disorientation, defensiveness, and disconnection. Healing involves regulation, integration, flexibility, clarity, coherence, and reconnection. Herein lies the power to thrive.

Index

Note: *Italic* page numbers refer to figures.

action tendencies 19, 31, 225, 226, 231, 236–237; *see also* survival defenses
addiction (Substance Use Disorder and Behavioral Addictions) 5, 43, 82–87, 240; and emotion regulation deficits 83–84; in group schema therapy 85–87; comorbidity with trauma/eating disorders 82–87; *see also* eating disorders
amygdala 180—182, *183*
attachment: core needs and schema 28–29, 127, 144; relationship to emotion regulation 245–246; attachment styles/disruption 246–250; effects of early trauma on attachment 4, 227–228, 244–253; attachment repair and trauma 244–253; corrective attachment experiences in group 46, 73, 83, 85–87, 91, 93, 96, 245, 246, 257
autonomic nervous system: trauma impact 179, 185; Polyvagal theory & diagrams *184*; *see also* parasympathetic nervous system; sympathetic nervous system; Polyvagal theory; window of tolerance

Behary, W. 54, 106, 273
body memories 83, 192–193, 204, 214; 'the body keeps score' 191–192; hijacking 178, 179, 182, 185
body scan 76, 78, 159, 187, 191, 195, 288

bottom-up approaches 180, 193; interventions 47–50; and embodiment 194; and schema therapy 193–194
boundaries 19, 28, 31; and safety in the group 43–45, 48, 50, 51, 53, 55, 57, 63, 68, 73, 77, 104, 117; and structural dissociation 240–241; and attachment 249–250; and roles in relationships 256, 257, 260, 292, 294, 303, 314, 315

centering 106, 194–195
chair work 35, 55, 61, 94, 133, 216; Compassionate Chair Work 278–279; *see also* mode dialogues
cohesion 6, 17, 19, 39, 46, 56, 57, 66, 110, 315
Complex Post-Traumatic Stress Disorder (CPTSD) 8–19, 103, 141–150, 270; symptoms instead of memories 9
comorbidity 82–87
compassion focused therapy 285–286; *see also* self-compassion
Connecting Web exercise 46, 110, 114–115
containment 48–49, 150, 160
conflict/conflict resolution 39, 54, 56, 59, 62, 64–66, 69, 96, 117–119, 130, 258, 291, 294, 295
coping modes *see* schema modes
core needs 6, 85, 109, 123; *see also* identifying needs
coregulation 4, 46, 47, 257, 314

corrective emotional experience 35, 37, 45–46, 55, 86, 87, 91, 125, 126, 133, 315
countertransference 67–69
Courtois, C. 8, 9, 12–14, 17, 18, 36, 62, 116, 119, 143

defensiveness: impact of trauma 3, 5, 44, 65, 66, 92, 103, 104, 228, 314, 316, 318
disconnection 3–5, 28, 29, 52, 92, 93, 103, 127–129, 153, 155, 167, 183, 185, 198, 227, 231, 268, 270, 275, 293, 314, 318
dissociation 3, 9, 11, 12, 17, 18, 59, 63–64, 76, 83–84, 120, 131, 144, 155, 167, 184, 185, 215, 224–241, 258, 273
distortion 3, 5, 38, 92, 93, 103, 227, 314, 316, 318
diversity 57–58, 96, 143, 145
dysregulation 3, 5; emotional 6, 13, 16–18, 62–63, 83, 93, 96, 316; in group 53–59, 62; and lack of integration 144–145; and the nervous system 182; and the body 192; and diagnoses 227

Early Childhood Trauma 3–6, 8–9, 27, 31, 34, 43, 47, 82, 103–104, 112, 141–145, 165, 178, 224, 244, 257, 268, 286, 295, 300, 318
early maladaptive schemas (EMS) 9, 27, 29–31, 66–68, 93, 95, 112–114, 125–129, 246
eating disorders 82–83; and schema therapy 85–86; see also addictions
Edwards, D.J.A. 28, 31–34, 129, 132, 217, 231, 258, 260, 274
Ella and the Thunderstorm 6, 110, 111, 114, 122; see also Identifying Needs
emotional contagion 56–57
emotional deprivation (early maladaptive schema) 28–29, 31, 94, 95, 127, 128, 155
emotion dysregulation 6, 13, 18, 53, 62–63, 69, 93, 94, 96, 142, 145, 205, 215, 227, 245, 283, 286
emotions: and groups 14, 18, 36, 38, 53, 56, 65, 76, 92, 117; and schema 28–29, 128, 130;

resources 47, 48, 174–176; and the healthy adult mode 55–56, 73, 172, 263; challenges 75, 77; and window of tolerance 152–156; and survival tendencies 240–241; and relationships 292–293, 316; see also emotion regulation
emotion regulation 11, 13, 37, 63, 83, 165–176, 316–317; core emotions 167; understanding emotion 165–166; and the healthy adult mode 168; and trauma 167–168; in group 43, 46, 153, 165–176; regulation strategies 174–176; DBT 168; see also self-regulation, co regulation
empathy/empathic attunement 54, 55, 58, 59, 284, 292–293
empathic failure 54–55
empathic confrontation 27, 34, 36–38, 45, 60–61, 92, 93, 125, 315, 316
embodiment 75, 191, 194

facilitation, group: art and science 52; role of leadership 52–53, 58–59, 66, 96
failure of integration (six D's) xii, 3, 7, 103, 142; impact of trauma 314
Farrell, J. 36–38, 45, 46, 86, 92, 93, 114–115, 122, 126, 135–137, 150, 277
feedback 38, 46, 53, 55, 57–59, 76, 91, 104, 117, 120, 308, 315
felt sense 46, 114, 307
felt sense focusing 197
Fisher, J. 9, 10, 63, 84, 143, 190, 193, 224, 227, 228, 236, 241, 247
flashbacks 63, 75, 83, 96, 143, 179, 204, 207, 212–217, 227, 231
future vision and future imagery 303, 307

Gilbert, P. 11, 283–286; see also compassion focused therapy; self-compassion
good parent: and the healthy adult mode 33–35, 73, 114, 131, 132, 134, 136–138, 149, 277, 292; in the group 37, 39, 45, 52, 55; role of therapist 52, 55, 69, 315; see also limited reparenting

grounding 6, 49; and emotion dysregulation 62, 63, 76, 77; in the group 76, 114; as somatic intervention 78, 94, 96, 106, 110, 114, 121, 160, 163, 194, 196, 210, 215, 217, 220, 232, 233
Group Schema Therapy 36–37, 91–92, 112–115; and trauma 36–39, 92–93; challenges 96; interventions 133–136, 314
group therapy 5, 13, 103–107, 313–315; dynamics 43–44, 52–62; goals 112; group formation 109–116; structure & format 103–107; sample format 120–121; guidelines 57, 61, 111; sample guidelines 116–119; cohesion 46; safety 43–44; models 16–17, 92, 103, 109–115; norms 57, 111–113; limitations 18, 47, 59–62, 113; effectiveness 15–18, 37, 112; for complex trauma 5, 14–16; individual vs. group treatment 15–16; contraindications 18; and risk management 47; termination 303–304; therapist role 44–46, 52–53, 315; see also phased based approach
guilt 10, 53, 144, 270–277, 271; see also shame

healthy adult (HA) mode 27, 31, 33–35, 55–56, 114, 131–133, 155, 167–168, 172–174, 231, 235–238; and mindfulness 72–74, 79; strengthening 55–56, 92, 93, 96, 260, 263–264, 266, 277, 302, 313, 318; and self-compassion 278–279, 288; see also the good parent
healthy relationships 10, 14, 36, 39, 73, 92, 104, 291–296; characteristics 292–294; and the group 315; and trauma 295–296
Herman, J.L. 8, 9, 11–12, 16, 94, 143, 302
hippocampus 179, 181, 182, 183, 185, 203, 204
hypothalamus 181, 182, 183
hyperarousal 49, 96, 145, 153–155, 157, 215, 316; and downregulating 49, 83, 159; and the body 185, 192

hypoarousal 49, 96, 145, 153–155; and upregulating 49, 83, 161, 192, 215, 316

ice cream shoppe imagery 135
identifying needs 113–114; see also Ella and the Thunderstorm and The Orchid and the Dandelion
imagery/imagery rescripting 34–35, 38, 64, 86, 93–96, 133, 135, 149, 161, 193, 216, 220–221, 289, 301, 307, 316
information processing 154, 178, 181–182; sensory processing (brainstem): 181–182; emotional processing (limbic system) 182; cognitive processing (neocortex) 181
inner critic 32, 33, 35, 39, 73, 80, 130, 132, 136, 228, 236, 260, 268–274, 277, 278–279, 282–289
integration 3, 11, 39, 80, 103, 106, 144; and the window of tolerance 154–155; and emotions 167; and the nervous system 180–181; and memory 207–208; and recovery 300–307
interventions: general concepts 10–14; schema-informed 34–35, 45, 85, 91, 93, 96, 193; resourcing 48–50; mindfulness and embodiment 194–196, 317
intrusive memories 206, 212–213, 215
intrusive symptoms 10, 39, 48, 212–222; imagery rehearsal therapy 216–217; triggers 218–219; managing intrusive symptoms 219–221; see also flashbacks, nightmares, intrusive memory

leadership: role 52–69, 315
limbic system 180, 181, 193
limited reparenting 27, 34, 37; in the group 45–46; and attachment repair 93, 96, 125; as a bottom-up approach 193, 315, 316; see also good parent

memory: in trauma 185, 202–208; memory processing 11, 12, 16, 62, 141; and emotion dysregulation 62–63; and dissociation 227;

body memory 192; memory
reconsolidation 205–206; symptoms
instead of memories 9; explicit
179, 180, 185, 203–204; implicit
192, 203–204; and group therapy
206; see also intrusive symptoms/
memories
meta-awareness 33, 131
Mindful Self-Compassion 46,
72–80, 284; see also Neff; self
compassion
mindfulness 46, 62, 64, 72–80, 133,
160, 175, 176, 194–195; and
the healthy adult 72–74, 79; and
intrusive symptoms 217, 220; and
dissociation 232; challenges 75–76;
and groups 76–78; exercises 78–80,
160, 209; and self-compassion 282,
284, 286
Modes on the Bus 136–137
mode dialogues 34–35, 40, 96, 316
mode flipping 132–133
mode interventions (mode tracking;
schema diary, flashcards) 133–134
MUPS (Multiple Unexplained Physical
Symptoms) 145, 182, 192; see also
somatic symptoms
mountain meditation 78, 163

Neff, K. 11, 270, 284, 286; see also
Mindful Self-Compassion
neocortex 180
nervous system response to threat 180
neurobiology of trauma 178–186
neuroplasticity 96, 185–186
neuroception 179, 183 ; see also
autonomic nervous system;
Polyvagal theory
nightmares 212–222; and Schema
Therapy 215–216; and imagery
rehearsal 216–217; rescripting 221

Orchid and the Dandelion 111, 114,
123; see also identifying needs

pacing 48, 62, 63, 65, 196
pain paradox 74–75
parasympathetic nervous system
182–183; see also autonomic
nervous system
pendulation 49, 94, 196
phase/stage based treatment 9–13, 94

Polyvagal Theory/ladder 183–184;
and schema modes 184–185; and
impact of trauma 184, 185; see
also autonomic nervous system;
parasympathetic nervous system;
sympathetic nervous system; vagus
nerve
post-traumatic growth 14, 303–304
Post-Traumatic Stress Disorder (PTSD)
74, 143

risk management 47
recovery 50, 75, 80, 86–87, 187,
212–213, 300–304, 315, 317–318;
see also future vision and future
imagery; post traumatic growth
recovery spiral 7, 10, 303
resilience 13, 15, 74, 91, 93, 208, 302,
313, 318
resource development 47–50,
114–115; see also containment;
grounding; mindfulness
pendulation; orienting; pacing;
titration
Roediger, E. 27, 28, 30, 35, 293
roles in relationships 231, 255–261,
291, 315; see also Trauma Triangle

safety: and treatment 9–11; building in
groups 43–50, 111–113, 121,
313–314; and conflict 64–66;
and the healthy adult 73; and
the Polyvagal Theory 183; and
intrusive symptoms 220–221; safe
place imagery 149; safety bubble
150, 160; and therapist role 43–44;
and therapy relationship 44–46,
315–316
Sample Group Format 120–121
Sample Group Guidelines 111, 116–119
schema healing 34–35, 126, 318
schema modes 31–34, 129–132; and
mode imagery 38; and chair work
61; and modes on the bus exercise
136–137; coping modes 47, 228,
231, 258; and the healthy adult 55,
73, 93; and dissociation 228–231;
and arousal 155, 167, 193, 217;
addiction 86, 193; and needs 112,
113, 129; and Polyvagal Theory
184–185; and intrusive symptoms
215–216

Schema Therapy 27–40; goals 35, 132; in groups 91, 133, 313–315; interventions 27–40, 125–139, 282–287; *see also* early maladaptive schema; empathic confrontation; group schema therapy; imagery rescripting; limited reparenting; mode dialogues; schema modes

self-compassion 46, 282–289; and trauma 283, 286; mindful self-compassion 284; myths of self-compassion 284; compassion focused therapy 285–286

self-criticism 33, 282, 286–287

self-regulation 44–49, 114, 152, 165–174

shame: and schema 30, 125; and addiction 84; and the inner critic 268–279, 316; as consequence of trauma 9, 10, 12, 14–15; and the body 192–193, 270, *271*; *see also* guilt

Shaw, I. 36–38, 45, 46, 86, 92, 93, 114–115, 122, 126, 135, 136, 138, 150, 277

Siegel, D.J. 47; and the window of tolerance 153–154

stabilization 11–12, 19, 93, 94, 106, 303

stress hormones 145, 182, 192

survival defenses 3, 33, 103, 142, 184, 226, 228, 283

Stone Ceremony 7, 14, 308

structural dissociation 227–231; and action tendencies/survival defenses *229–230*, 236–241

somatic dysregulation: definition 145; somatic symptoms 190–199

somatic therapies (somatic experiencing; somatosensory psychotherapy; somatic awareness; somatic resourcing) 10, 11, 48, 49, 63, 78, 94, 145, 190, 193, 196, 316

sympathetic nervous system 75, 178, 183, 184

sympathetic reassurance 54, 59

symptom management 85, 95, 157–161, 231

termination 106, 303–304

therapeutic challenges 52–69

therapy-interfering/destroying behaviors 59–60, 62–69

threat detection system 181–182, *183*, 194

titration 49; monitoring arousal 196

transference 66–67

trauma triangle 255–264; and attachment 257–258; roles and coping modes 258–259, 262; changing roles 260–264

Triune brain 180, *181*; *see also* information processing

vagus nerve, ventral vagal state 178, 195

van der Kolk, B. 9, 94, 144; threat detection system 181; the body keeps score 191, 206

Window of Tolerance 39, 44, 47, 152–162, 315, 316; zones of arousal *154*; bottom up approaches 47–49, 193; management 159–162; *see also* hyperarousal; hypoarousal; integration; river of integration

For Product Safety Concerns and Information please contact our EU
representative GPSR@taylorandfrancis.com
Taylor & Francis Verlag GmbH, Kaufingerstraße 24, 80331 München, Germany